B A T E S' *Pocket Guide to*
Physical Examination
AND History Taking

Bates' Pocket Guide to Physical Examination AND History Taking

EIGHTH EDITION

Lynn S. Bickley, MD, FACP
Clinical Professor of Internal Medicine
School of Medicine
University of New Mexico
Albuquerque, New Mexico

Peter G. Szilagyi, MD, MPH
Professor of Pediatrics and Executive Vice-Chair
Department of Pediatrics
University of California at Los Angeles (UCLA)
Los Angeles, California

Guest Editor

Richard M. Hoffman, MD, MPH, FACP
Professor of Internal Medicine and Epidemiology
Director, Division of General Internal Medicine
University of Iowa Carver College of Medicine
Iowa City, Iowa

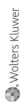

Wolters Kluwer

Philadelphia • Baltimore • New York • London
Buenos Aires • Hong Kong • Sydney • Tokyo

Acquisitions Editor: Crystal Taylor
Product Development Editor: Greg Nicholl
Marketing Manager: Michael McMahon
Production Project Manager: Cynthia Rudy
Design Coordinator: Holly McLaughlin
Art Director: Jennifer Clements
Illustrator: Body Scientific International
Manufacturing Coordinator: Margie Orzech
Prepress Vendor: Aptara, Inc.

Eighth Edition

Copyright © 2017 Wolters Kluwer.

Library of Congress Cataloging-in-Publication Data
Names: Bickley, Lynn S., author. | Szilagyi, Peter G., author. | Hoffman, Richard M., editor. | Abridgement of (expression): Bickley, Lynn S. Bates' guide to physical examination and history-taking / Lynn S. Bickley, Peter G. Szilagyi ; guest editor, Richard M. Hoffman.
Title: Bates' pocket guide to physical examination and history taking / Lynn S. Bickley, Peter G. Szilagyi.
Other titles: Pocket guide to physical examination and history taking
Description: Eighth edition. | Philadelphia : Wolters Kluwer, [2017] | Abridgement of: Bates' guide to physical examination and history-taking / Lynn S. Bickley, Peter G. Szilagyi. Twelfth edition. [2017] | Includes bibliographical references and index.
Identifiers: LCCN 2016030575 | ISBN 9781496338488 (alk. paper)
Subjects: | MESH: Physical Examination—methods | Medical History Taking—methods | Handbooks
Classification: LCC RC76 | NLM WB 39 | DDC 616.07/54—dc23
LC record available at https://lccn.loc.gov/2016030575

We would like to dedicate this book to all our students, trainees, and mentees who have taught us the true value of both the science and the art of medicine.

Faculty Reviewers

J. D. Bartleson Jr., MD
Associate Professor of Neurology
Mayo Clinic
Rochester, Minnesota

John D. Bartlett, MD
Assistant Clinical Professor of
    Ophthalmology
Jules Stein Eye Institute
David Geffen School of Medicine
Los Angeles, California

Amy E. Blatt, MD
Assistant Professor
Department of Medicine
School of Medicine and Dentistry
University of Rochester Medical Center
Rochester, New York

Adam Brodsky, MD
Associate Professor
Medical Director
Geriatric Psychiatry Services
Department of Psychiatry and
    Behavioral Sciences
School of Medicine
University of New Mexico Psychiatric
    Center & Sandoval Regional
    Medical Center
Albuquerque, New Mexico

Thomas M. Carroll, MD, PhD
Assistant Professor
Department of Medicine
School of Medicine and Dentistry
University of Rochester Medical Center
Rochester, New York

Adam J. Doyle, MD
Assistant Professor
Department of Surgery
School of Medicine and Dentistry
University of Rochester Medical Center
Rochester, New York

Amit Garg, MD
Dermatologist
Northwell Health Physician Partners
Manhasset, New York

Catherine F. Gracey, MD
Associate Professor
Department of Medicine
School of Medicine and Dentistry
University of Rochester Medical
    Center
Rochester, New York

Carla Herman, MD, MPH
Chief
Division of Geriatrics and Palliative
    Medicine
Professor
Department of Internal Medicine
School of Medicine
University of New Mexico
Albuquerque, New Mexico

William C. Hulbert, MD
Professor
Department of Urology
School of Medicine and Dentistry
University of Rochester Medical Center
Rochester, New York

Mark Landig, OD
Department of Ophthalmology
Jules Stein Eye Institute
David Geffen School of Medicine
Los Angeles, California

Helen R. Levey, DO, MPH
PGY5 Resident
School of Medicine and Dentistry
University of Rochester Medical
    Center
Rochester, New York

Patrick McCleskey, MD
Dermatologist
Oakland Medical Center
Oakland, California

Jeanne H. S. O'Brien, MD
Associate Professor
Department of Urology
School of Medicine and Dentistry
University of Rochester Medical Center
Rochester, New York

Alec B. O'Connor, MD, MPH
Director, Internal Medicine
Associate Professor
Department of Medicine
School of Medicine and Dentistry
University of Rochester Medical Center
Rochester, New York

A. Andrew Rudmann, MD
Associate Professor
Department of Medicine
University of Rochester Medical Center
School of Medicine and Dentistry
Rochester, New York

Moira A. Szilagyi, MD, PhD
Professor of Pediatrics
University of California at Los Angeles
(UCLA)
Los Angeles, California

Loralei Lacina Thornburg, MD
Associate Professor
Department of Obstetrics and
Gynecology
School of Medicine and Dentistry
University of Rochester Medical Center
Rochester, New York

Scott A. Vogelgesang, MD
Director
Division of Immunology
Clinical Professor
Department of Internal Medicine–
Immunology
University of Iowa Carver College
of Medicine
Iowa City, Iowa

Brian P. Watkins, MD
Surgeon
Genesee Surgical Associates
Rochester, New York

Paula Zozzaro-Smith, DO
Fellow of Maternal-Fetal Medicine
Department of Obstetrics and
Gynecology
The University of Rochester
Rochester, New York

STUDENT REVIEWERS

Ayala Danzig
University of Rochester School of
Medicine and Dentistry

Benjamin Edmonds
University of Central Florida College
of Medicine

Nicholas P. N. Goldstein
University of Rochester School of
Medicine and Dentistry

Preface

Bates' Pocket Guide to Physical Examination and History Taking, eighth edition, is a concise, portable text, with new chapters on assessing clinical evidence and examination of the skin, hair, and nails, that:

- Recommends how to sequence the physical examination and document an accurate written record.
- Clarifies assessment of clinical evidence.
- Describes how to interview the patient and take the health history.
- Details and illustrates the steps of each of the regional physical examinations.
- Reminds students of common, normal, and abnormal physical findings.
- Provides visual aids and comparative tables to guide recognition of common and selected findings.

There are several ways to use the *Pocket Guide:*

- To review and remember the content of a health history.
- To review and rehearse the techniques of examination. This can be done while learning a single section and again while combining the approaches to several body systems or regions into an integrated examination (see Chapter 1).
- To review common variations of normal and selected abnormalities. Observations are keener and more precise when the examiner knows what to look, listen, and feel for.
- To look up special techniques as the need arises. Maneuvers such as The Timed Get Up and Go test are included in the Special Techniques section in each chapter.
- To look up additional information about possible findings, including abnormalities and standards of normal.

The *Pocket Guide* is not intended to serve as a primary text for learning the skills of history taking or physical examination. Its detail is too brief. It is intended instead as an aid for student recall of the regional examinations and examinations for special populations and as a convenient, brief, and portable reference.

Contents

Foundations for Clinical Proficiency

This chapter provides a road map to clinical proficiency in two critical areas: the health history and the physical examination.

For adults, the comprehensive history includes Identifying Data and Source of the History, Chief Complaint(s), Present Illness, Past History, Family History, Personal and Social History, and Review of Systems. New patients in the office or hospital merit a comprehensive health history; however, in many situations, a more flexible focused, or problem-oriented, interview is appropriate. The components of the comprehensive health history structure the patient's story and the format of your written record, but the order shown below should not dictate the sequence of the interview. The interview is more fluid and should follow the patient's leads and cues, as described in Chapter 3.

Overview: Components of the Adult Health History

Identifying Data	• Identifying data—such as age, gender, occupation, marital status
	• Source of the history—usually the patient, but can be a family member or friend, letter of referral, or the clinical record
	• If appropriate, establish source of referral because a written report may be needed
Reliability	• Varies according to the patient's memory, trust, and mood
Chief Complaint(s)	• The one or more symptoms or concerns causing the patient to seek care
Present Illness	• Amplifies the Chief Complaint; describes how each symptom developed
	• Includes patient's thoughts and feelings about the illness
	• Pulls in relevant portions of the Review of Systems, called "pertinent positives and negatives" (see p. 3)
	• May include medications, allergies, habits of smoking and alcohol, which frequently are pertinent to the present illness

(continued)

Overview: Components of the Adult Health History (Continued)

Past History	• Lists childhood illnesses
	• Lists adult illnesses with dates for at least four categories: medical, surgical, obstetric/gynecologic, and psychiatric
	• Includes health maintenance practices such as immunizations, screening tests, lifestyle issues, and home safety
Family History	• Outlines or diagrams age and health, or age and cause of death, of siblings, parents, and grandparents
	• Documents presence or absence of specific illnesses in family, such as hypertension, coronary artery disease, etc.
Personal and Social History	• Describes educational level, family of origin, current household, personal interests, and lifestyle
Review of Systems	• Documents presence or absence of common symptoms related to each major body system

Decide if your assessment will be *comprehensive* or *focused.* Be sure to distinguish *subjective* from *objective* data.

Subjective Data	**Objective Data**
What the patient tells you	What you detect during the examination, laboratory information, and test data
The symptoms and history, from Chief Complaint through Review of Systems	All physical examination findings, or signs

The Comprehensive Adult Health History

As you elicit the adult health history, be sure to include the following: date and time of history; identifying data, which include age, gender, marital status, and occupation; and reliability, which reflects the quality of information the patient provides.

Chief Complaint(s)

Quote the patient's own words. "My stomach hurts and I feel awful"; or "I have come for my regular check-up."

Present Illness

This section is a complete, clear, and chronologic account of the problems prompting the patient to seek care. It should include the problem's onset, the setting in which it has developed, its manifestations, and any treatments.

Every principal symptom should be well characterized, with descriptions of the seven features listed below and *pertinent positives* and *negatives* from relevant areas of the Review of Systems that help clarify the *differential diagnosis*.

The Seven Attributes of Every Symptom

- Location
- Quality
- Quantity or severity
- Timing, including onset, duration, and frequency
- Setting in which it occurs
- Aggravating and relieving factors
- Associated manifestations

In addition, list **medications**, including name, dose, route, and frequency of use; **allergies**, including *specific reactions* to each medication; **tobacco** use; and **alcohol** and **drug** use.

Past History

List **childhood illnesses**, then list **adult illnesses** in each of four areas:

- *Medical* (e.g., diabetes, hypertension, hepatitis, asthma, HIV), with dates of onset; also information about hospitalizations with dates; number and gender of sexual partners; risky sexual practices

- *Surgical* (dates, indications, and types of operations)

- *Obstetric/gynecologic* (obstetric history, menstrual history, birth control, and sexual function)

- *Psychiatric* (illness and time frame, diagnoses, hospitalizations, and treatments)

Also discuss **Health Maintenance**, including *immunizations,* such as tetanus, pertussis, diphtheria, polio, measles, rubella, mumps, influenza, varicella, hepatitis B virus (HBV), human papillomavirus (HPV), *Haemophilus influenzae* type B, pneumococcal vaccine, and herpes zoster vaccine; and *screening tests,* such as tuberculin tests, Pap smears, mammograms, stool tests for occult blood, colonoscopy, and cholesterol tests, together with the results and the dates they were last performed.

Family History

Outline or diagram the age and health, or age and cause of death, of each immediate relative, including grandparents, parents, siblings, children, and grandchildren. Record the following conditions as either *present or absent* in the family: hypertension, coronary artery disease, elevated cholesterol levels, stroke, diabetes, thyroid or renal disease, cancer (specify type), arthritis, tuberculosis, asthma or lung disease, headache, seizure disorder, mental illness, suicide, alcohol or drug addiction, and allergies, as well as conditions that the patient reports.

Personal and Social History

Include occupation and the last year of schooling; home situation and significant others; sources of stress, both recent and long term; important life experiences, such as military service; leisure activities; religious affiliation and spiritual beliefs; and activities of daily living (ADLs). Also include lifestyle habits such as *exercise* and *diet, safety measures,* and *alternative health care* practices.

Review of Systems (ROS)

These "yes/no" questions go from "head to toe" and conclude the interview. Selected sections can also clarify the Chief Complaint; for example, the respiratory ROS helps characterize the symptom of cough. Start with a fairly general question. This allows you to shift to more specific questions about systems that may be of concern. For example, "How are your ears and hearing?" "How about your lungs and breathing?" "Any trouble with your heart?" "How is your digestion?" The *Review of Systems* questions may uncover problems that the patient overlooked. *Remember to move major health events to the Present Illness or Past History in your write-up.*

Some clinicians do the *Review of Systems* during the physical examination. If the patient has only a few symptoms, this combination can be efficient but may disrupt the flow of both the history and the examination.

General. Usual weight, recent weight change, clothing that fits more tightly or loosely than before; weakness, fatigue, fever.

Skin. Rashes, lumps, sores, itching, dryness, color change; changes in hair or nails; changes in size or color of moles.

Head, Eyes, Ears, Nose, Throat (HEENT). *Head:* Headache, head injury, dizziness, lightheadedness. *Eyes:* Vision, glasses or contact lenses, last examination, pain, redness, excessive tearing, double or blurred vision, spots, specks, flashing lights, glaucoma, cataracts. *Ears:* Hearing, tinnitus, vertigo, earache, infection, discharge. If hearing is decreased, use or nonuse of hearing aid. *Nose and sinuses:* Frequent colds, nasal stuffiness, discharge or itching, hay fever, nosebleeds, sinus trouble. **Throat (or mouth and pharynx):** Condition of teeth and gums; bleeding gums; dentures, if any, and how they fit; last dental examination; sore tongue; dry mouth; frequent sore throats; hoarseness.

Neck. Lumps, "swollen glands," goiter, pain, stiffness.

Breasts. Lumps, pain or discomfort, nipple discharge, self-examination practices.

Respiratory. Cough, sputum (color, quantity), hemoptysis, dyspnea, wheezing, pleurisy, last chest x-ray. You may wish to include asthma, bronchitis, emphysema, pneumonia, and tuberculosis.

Cardiovascular. "Heart trouble," hypertension, rheumatic fever, heart murmurs, chest pain or discomfort, palpitations, dyspnea, orthopnea, paroxysmal nocturnal dyspnea, edema, past electrocardiographic or other cardiovascular tests.

Gastrointestinal. Trouble swallowing, heartburn, appetite, nausea. Bowel movements, color and size of stools, change in bowel habits, rectal bleeding or black or tarry stools, hemorrhoids, constipation, diarrhea. Abdominal pain, food intolerance, excessive belching or passing of gas. Jaundice, liver or gallbladder trouble, hepatitis.

Peripheral Vascular. Intermittent claudication; leg cramps; varicose veins; past clots in veins; swelling in calves, legs, or feet; color change in fingertips or toes during cold weather; swelling with redness or tenderness.

Urinary. Frequency of urination, polyuria, nocturia, urgency, burning or pain on urination, hematuria, urinary infections, kidney stones, incontinence; in males, reduced caliber or force of urinary stream, hesitancy, dribbling.

Genital. *Male:* Hernias, discharge from or sores on penis, testicular pain or masses, history of sexually transmitted infections (STIs) and treatments, testicular self-examination practices. Sexual habits, interest, function, satisfaction, birth control methods, condom use, problems. Concerns about HIV infection. *Female:* Age at menarche; regularity, frequency, and duration of periods; amount of bleeding, bleeding between periods or after intercourse, last menstrual period; dysmenorrhea, premenstrual tension. Age at menopause, menopausal symptoms, postmenopausal bleeding. In patients born before 1971, exposure to diethylstilbestrol (DES) from maternal use during pregnancy. Vaginal discharge, itching, sores, lumps, STIs and treatments. Number of pregnancies, number and type of deliveries, number of abortions (spontaneous and induced), complications of pregnancy, birth control methods. Sexual preference, interest, function, satisfaction, problems (including dyspareunia). Concerns about HIV infection.

Musculoskeletal. Muscle or joint pain, stiffness, arthritis, gout, backache. If present, describe location of affected joints or muscles, any swelling, redness, pain, tenderness, stiffness, weakness, or limitation of motion or activity; include timing of symptoms (e.g., morning or evening), duration, and any history of trauma. Neck or low back pain. Joint pain with systemic features such as fever, chills, rash, anorexia, weight loss, or weakness.

Psychiatric. Nervousness; tension; mood, including depression, memory change, suicide attempts, if relevant.

Neurologic. Changes in mood, attention, or speech; changes in orientation, memory, insight, or judgment; headache, dizziness, vertigo; fainting, blackouts, seizures, weakness, paralysis, numbness or loss of sensation, tingling or "pins and needles," tremors or other involuntary movements, seizures.

Hematologic. Anemia, easy bruising or bleeding, past transfusions, transfusion reactions.

Endocrine. "Thyroid trouble," heat or cold intolerance, excessive sweating, excessive thirst or hunger, polyuria, change in glove or shoe size.

The Comprehensive Physical Examination

Conduct a *comprehensive physical examination* on most new patients or patients being admitted to the hospital. For more *problem-oriented,* or *focused, assessments,* the presenting complaints will dictate which segments you elect to perform.

■ *The key to a thorough and accurate physical examination is a systematic sequence of examination.* With effort and practice, you will acquire your own routine sequence. This book recommends examining from the patient's *right side.*

■ Apply the techniques of inspection, palpation, auscultation, and percussion to each body region, but be sensitive to the whole patient.

■ *Minimize the number of times you ask the patient to change position* from supine to sitting, or standing to lying supine.

■ For an overview of the physical examination, study the sequence that follows. *Note that clinicians vary in where they place different segments, especially for the musculoskeletal and nervous systems.*

Beginning the Examination: Setting the Stage

Take the following steps to prepare for the physical examination.

Steps in Preparing for the Physical Examination

1. Reflect on your approach to the patient.
2. Adjust the lighting and the environment.
3. Check your equipment.
4. Make the patient comfortable.
5. Observe standard and universal precautions.
6. Choose the sequence, scope, and positioning of examination.

Think through your approach, your professional demeanor, and how to make the patient comfortable and relaxed. *Always wash your hands in the patient's presence before beginning the examination.*

Reflect on Your Approach to the Patient. Identify yourself as a student. Try to appear calm, organized, and competent, even if you feel differently. If you forget to do part of the examination, this is not uncommon, especially at first! Simply examine that area out of sequence, but smoothly.

Adjust Lighting and the Environment. Adjust the bed to a convenient height (be sure to lower it when finished!). Ask the patient to move toward you if this makes it easier to do your physical examination. Good lighting and a quiet environment are important. *Tangential lighting* is optimal for structures such as the jugular venous pulse, the thyroid gland, and the apical impulse of the heart. It throws contours, elevations, and depressions, whether moving or stationary, into sharper relief.

Check Your Equipment. Be sure your stethoscope, reflex hammer, and other equipment are readily at hand.

Make the Patient Comfortable. Show concern for privacy and modesty.

- Close nearby doors and draw curtains before beginning.

- Acquire the art of *draping the patient* with the gown or draw sheet as you learn each examination segment in future chapters. *Your goal is to visualize one body area at a time.*

- As you proceed, keep the patient informed, especially when you anticipate embarrassment or discomfort, as when checking for the femoral pulse. Also try to gauge how much the patient wants to know.

- Make sure your instructions to the patient at each step are courteous and clear.

- Watch the patient's facial expression and even ask "Is it okay?" as you move through the examination.

When you have finished, tell the patient your general impressions and what to expect next. Lower the bed to avoid risk of falls and raise the bedrails if needed. As you leave, clean your equipment, dispose of waste materials, and wash your hands.

Standard and MRSA Precautions. Observe standard and universal precautions. Use rigorous handwashing before and after all patient contact and, whenever indicated, personal protective equipment (gloves; gowns; and mouth, nose, and eye protection); safe injection practices; safe handling of contaminated equipment or surfaces; respiratory hygiene and cough etiquette; patient isolation criteria; and precautions relating to equipment, toys, solid surfaces, and laundry handling.

Universal Precautions. Universal precautions are a set of precautions designed to prevent transmission of HIV, HBV, and other bloodborne pathogens when providing first aid or health care. The following fluids are considered potentially infectious: all blood and other body fluids containing visible blood, semen, and vaginal secretions; and cerebrospinal, synovial, pleural, peritoneal, pericardial, and amniotic fluids. Protective barriers include gloves, gowns, aprons, masks, and protective eyewear. All health care workers should observe the important precautions for safe injections and prevention of injury from needlesticks, scalpels, and other sharp instruments and devices. Report to your health service immediately if such injury occurs.

Choose the Sequence, Scope, and Positioning of the Examination. The sequence of the examination should

- maximize the patient's comfort

- avoid unnecessary changes in position, and

- enhance the clinician's efficiency.

The Physical Examination: Suggested Sequence and Positioning

- General survey
- Vital signs
- Skin: upper torso, anterior and posterior
- Head and neck, including thyroid and lymph nodes
- *Optional:* Nervous system (mental status, cranial nerves, upper extremity motor strength, bulk, tone, cerebellar function)
- Thorax and lungs
- Breasts
- Musculoskeletal as indicated: upper extremities
- Cardiovascular, including jugular venous pressure (JVP), carotid upstrokes and bruits, point of maximal impulse (PMI), S_1, S_2, murmurs, extra sounds
- Cardiovascular, for S_3 and murmur of mitral stenosis
- Cardiovascular, for murmur of aortic insufficiency

- *Optional:* thorax and lungs—anterior
- Breasts and axillae
- Abdomen
- Peripheral vascular
- *Optional:* skin—lower torso and extremities
- Nervous system: lower extremity motor strength, bulk, tone, sensation; reflexes; Babinski reflex
- Musculoskeletal, as indicated
- *Optional:* skin, anterior and posterior
- *Optional:* nervous system, including gait
- *Optional:* musculoskeletal, comprehensive
- *Women:* pelvic and rectal examination
- *Men:* prostate and rectal examination

Key to the Symbols for the Patient's Position

Sitting		Lying supine	
Lying supine, with head of bed raised 30 degrees		Standing	
Same, turned partly to left side		Lying supine, with hips flexed, abducted, and externally rotated, and knees flexed (lithotomy position)	
Sitting, leaning forward			
		Lying on the left side (left lateral decubitus)	

Each symbol pertains until a new one appears. Two symbols separated by a slash indicate either or both positions.

Choose whether to do a *comprehensive* or *focused examination.* In general, move from "head to toe." An important goal as a student is to develop your own sequence with these principles in mind.

Examine the patient from the patient's *right side*. Note that the right side is more reliable to estimate jugular venous pressure from the right, the palpating hand rests more comfortably on the apical impulse, the right kidney is more frequently palpable than the left, and examining tables are frequently positioned to accommodate a right-handed approach.

To examine the *supine patient,* you can examine the head, neck, and anterior chest. Then roll the patient onto each side to listen to the lungs, examine the back, and inspect the skin. Roll the patient back and finish the rest of the examination with the patient again supine.

The Physical Examination: Head to Toe
General Survey. Continue this survey throughout the patient visit. Observe general state of health, height, build, and sexual development. Note posture, motor activity, and gait; dress, grooming, and personal hygiene; and any odors of the body or breath. Watch facial expressions and note manner, affect, and reactions to persons and things in the environment. Listen to the patient's manner of speaking and note the state of awareness or level of consciousness.

ⓘ Vital Signs. *Ask the patient to sit on the edge of the bed or examining table,* unless this position is contraindicated. Stand in front of the patient, moving to either side as needed. Measure the blood pressure. Count pulse and respiratory rate. If indicated, measure body temperature.

Skin. Observe the face. Identify any lesions, noting their location, distribution, arrangement, type, and color. Inspect and palpate the hair and nails. Study the patient's hands. Continue to assess the skin as you examine the other body regions.

HEENT. *Head:* Examine the hair, scalp, skull, and face. *Eyes:* Check visual acuity and screen the visual fields. Note position and alignment of the eyes. Observe the eyelids. Inspect the sclera and conjunctiva of each eye. With oblique lighting, inspect each cornea, iris, and lens. Assess extraocular movements. Darken the room to promote pupillary dilation and visibility of the fundi. Compare the pupils, and test their reactions to light. With an ophthalmoscope, inspect the ocular fundi. *Ears:* Inspect the auricles, canals, and drums. Check auditory acuity. If acuity is diminished, check lateralization (Weber test) and compare air and bone conduction (Rinne test). *Nose and sinuses:* Examine the external nose; using a light and nasal speculum, inspect nasal mucosa, septum, and turbinates. Palpate for tenderness of the frontal and maxillary sinuses. *Throat (or mouth and pharynx):* Inspect the lips, oral mucosa, gums, teeth, tongue, palate, tonsils, and pharynx. You may wish to assess the cranial nerves at this point in the examination.

Neck. *Move behind the sitting patient* to feel the thyroid gland and to examine the back, posterior thorax, and lungs. Inspect and palpate the cervical lymph nodes. Note any masses or unusual pulsations in the neck. Feel for any deviation of the trachea. Observe sound and effort of the patient's breathing. Inspect and palpate the thyroid gland.

Back. Inspect and palpate the spine and muscles.

Posterior Thorax and Lungs. Inspect and palpate the spine and muscles of the *upper* back. Inspect, palpate, and percuss the chest. Identify the level of diaphragmatic dullness on each side. Listen to the breath sounds; identify any adventitious (or added) sounds; and, if indicated, listen to transmitted voice sounds (see p. 151).

Breasts, Axillae, and Epitrochlear Nodes. *The patient is still sitting.* Move to the front again. In a woman, inspect the breasts with patient's arms relaxed, then elevated, and then with her hands pressed on her hips. In either sex, inspect the axillae and feel for the axillary nodes; feel for the epitrochlear nodes.

A Note on the Musculoskeletal System. By now, you have made preliminary observations of the musculoskeletal system, including the hands, the upper back, and, in women, the shoulders' range of motion (ROM). Use these observations to decide whether a full musculoskeletal examination is warranted: *With the patient still sitting,* examine the hands, arms, shoulders, neck, and temporomandibular joints. Inspect and palpate the joints and check their ROM. (You may choose to examine upper extremity muscle bulk, tone, strength, and reflexes at this time, or you may decide to wait until later.)

Palpate the breasts, while continuing your inspection.

Anterior Thorax and Lungs. *The patient position is supine.* Ask the patient to lie down. Stand at the *right side* of the patient's bed. Inspect, palpate, and percuss the chest. Listen to the breath sounds, any adventitious sounds, and, if indicated, transmitted voice sounds.

Cardiovascular System. *Elevate head of bed to about 30 degrees,* adjusting as necessary to see the jugular venous pulsations. Observe the jugular venous pulsations, and measure the jugular venous pressure in relation to the sternal angle. Inspect and palpate the carotid pulsations. Listen for carotid bruits.

Ask the patient to roll partly onto the left side while you listen at the apex. Then have the patient roll back to supine while you listen to the rest of the heart. Ask the patient to sit, lean forward, and exhale while you listen for the murmur of aortic regurgitation. Inspect and palpate the precordium.

Note the location, diameter, amplitude, and duration of the apical impulse. Listen at the apex and the lower sternal border with the bell of a stethoscope. Listen at each auscultatory area with the diaphragm. Listen for S_1 and S_2 and for physiologic splitting of S_2. Listen for any abnormal heart sounds or murmurs.

o— Abdomen. Lower the head of the bed to the flat position. *The patient should be supine.* Inspect, auscultate, and percuss. Palpate lightly, then deeply. Assess the liver and spleen by percussion and then palpation. Try to feel the kidneys; palpate the aorta and its pulsations. If you suspect kidney infection, percuss posteriorly over the costovertebral angles.

o—/ Peripheral Vascular System. *With the patient supine,* palpate the femoral pulses and, if indicated, popliteal pulses. Palpate the inguinal lymph nodes. Inspect for edema, discoloration, or ulcers in the lower extremities. Palpate for pitting edema. *With the patient standing,* inspect for varicose veins.

o—/ Lower Extremities. Examine the legs, assessing the peripheral vascular, musculoskeletal, and nervous systems *while the patient is still supine.* Each of these systems can be further assessed when the patient stands.

/o— Nervous System. *The patient is sitting or supine.* The examination of the nervous system can also be divided into the upper extremity examination (when the patient is still sitting) and the lower extremity examination (when the patient is supine) after examination of the peripheral nervous system.

Mental Status. If indicated and not done during the interview, assess orientation, mood, thought process, thought content, abnormal perceptions, insight and judgment, memory and attention, information and vocabulary, calculating abilities, abstract thinking, and constructional ability.

Cranial Nerves. If not already examined, check sense of smell, funduscopic examination, strength of the temporal and masseter muscles, corneal reflexes, facial movements, gag reflex, strength of the trapezia and sternocleidomastoid muscles, and protrusion of tongue.

Motor System. Muscle bulk, tone, and strength of major muscle groups. *Cerebellar function:* rapid alternating movements (RAMs), point-to-point movements such as finger to nose ($F \rightarrow N$) and heel to shin ($H \rightarrow S$); gait. Observe patient's gait and ability to walk heel to toe, on toes, and on heels; to hop in place; and to do shallow knee bends. Do a Romberg test; check for pronator drift.

Sensory System. Pain, temperature, light touch, vibrations, and discrimination. Compare right and left sides and distal with proximal areas on the limbs.

Reflexes. Include biceps, triceps, brachioradialis, patellar, Achilles deep tendon reflexes; also plantar reflexes or Babinski reflex (see pp. 327–328).

Additional Examinations. The *rectal* and *genital* examinations are often performed at the end of the physical examination.

⚬⃥/Ⅱ Male Genitalia and Hernias. Examine the penis and scrotal contents. Check for hernias.

⚬⃥ Rectal Examination in Men. *The patient is lying on his left side* for the rectal examination. Inspect the sacrococcygeal and perianal areas. Palpate the anal canal, rectum, and prostate. (If the patient cannot stand, examine the genitalia before doing the rectal examination.)

⋏⋏ Genital and Rectal Examination in Women. *The patient is supine in the lithotomy position.* Sit during the examination with the speculum, then stand during bimanual examination of uterus, adnexa, and rectum. Examine the external genitalia, vagina, and cervix. Obtain a Pap smear. Palpate the uterus and adnexa. Do a bimanual and rectal examination.

Clinical Reasoning, Assessment, and Plan

Using sound clinical reasoning, you must now analyze your findings and identify the patient's problems. You must share your impressions with the patient and document your findings in the patient's record in a succinct legible format that communicates the patient's story and physical findings, and the rationale for your assessment and plan, to other members of the health care team. As you make clinical decisions, you will turn to clinical evidence, calling on your knowledge of sensitivity, specificity, predictive value, and the analytical tools detailed in Chapter 2, Evaluating Clinical Evidence.

The comprehensive health history and physical examination form the foundation of your clinical *Assessment*. The *Plan* is often wide-ranging and incorporates patient education, changes in medications, needed tests, referrals to other clinicians, and return visits for counseling and support. A successful *Plan* includes the patient's responses to the problems identified and to the interventions that you recommend. It requires good interpersonal skills and sensitivity to the patient's goals, economic means, competing responsibilities, and family structure and dynamics.

Clinical Reasoning and Assessment

Because assessment takes place in the clinician's mind, the process of clinical reasoning may seem opaque and even mysterious to beginning students. Study the steps described below. Focus on determining "What explains this patient's concerns?" and "What are the findings, problems, and diagnoses?"

Steps for Identifying Problems and Making Diagnoses

1. Identify abnormal findings.
2. Localize findings anatomically.
3. Cluster the clinical findings.
4. Search for the probable cause of the findings.
5. Cluster the clinical data.
6. Generate hypotheses about the causes of the patient's problems.
7. Test the hypotheses and establish a working diagnosis.

Identify Abnormal Findings.   Make a list of the patient's *symptoms,* the *signs* you observed during the physical examination, and any laboratory reports available to you.

Localize These Findings Anatomically.   Often this step is straightforward. The symptom of scratchy throat and the sign of an erythematous inflamed posterior pharynx, for example, clearly localize the problem to the pharynx. A complaint of headache leads you quickly to the structures of the skull and brain. Other symptoms, however, may present greater difficulty. Chest pain, for example, can originate in the coronary arteries, the stomach and esophagus, or the muscles and bones of the thorax. If the pain is exertional and relieved by rest, either the heart or the musculoskeletal components of the chest wall may be involved. If the patient notes pain only when carrying groceries with the left arm, the musculoskeletal system becomes the likely culprit.

When localizing findings, be as specific as your data allow; however, you may have to settle for a body region, such as the chest, or a body system, such as the musculoskeletal system. On the other hand, you may be able to define the exact structure involved, such as the left pectoral muscle. Some symptoms and signs are constitutional and cannot be localized, such as fatigue or fever, but are useful in the next set of steps.

Cluster the Clinical Findings.   Several clinical characteristics may help.

■ *Patient age:* The patient's *age* may help; younger adults are more likely to have a single disease, whereas older adults tend to have multiple diseases.

■ *Timing of symptoms:* The *timing* of symptoms is often useful. For example, an episode of pharyngitis 6 weeks ago is probably unrelated to the fever, chills, pleuritic chest pain, and cough that prompted an office visit today. To use timing effectively, you need to know the natural history of various diseases and conditions. A yellow penile discharge followed 3 weeks later by a painless penile ulcer suggests two problems: gonorrhea and primary syphilis.

■ *Involvement of different body systems:* If symptoms and signs occur in a single system, one disease may explain them. Problems in different, apparently unrelated, systems often require more than one explanation. For example, you might decide to group a patient's high blood pressure and sustained apical impulse together with flame-shaped retinal hemorrhages, place them in the cardiovascular system, and label the constellation "hypertensive cardiovascular disease with hypertensive retinopathy."

■ *Multisystem conditions:* With experience, you will become increasingly adept at recognizing *multisystem conditions* and building plausible explanations that link manifestations that are seemingly unrelated. To explain cough, hemoptysis, and weight loss in a 60-year-old plumber who has smoked cigarettes for 40 years, you would rank lung cancer high in your differential diagnosis. You might support your diagnosis with your observation of the patient's cyanotic nailbeds.

■ *Key questions:* You can also *ask a series of key questions* that may steer your thinking in one direction and allow you to temporarily ignore the others. For example, you may ask what produces and relieves the patient's chest pain. If the answer is exercise and rest, you can focus on the cardiovascular and musculoskeletal systems and set the gastrointestinal (GI) system aside. If the pain is epigastric, you can logically focus on the GI tract. A series of discriminating questions helps you analyze the clinical data and reach logical explanations.

Search for the Probable Cause of the Findings. Patient complaints often stem from a *pathologic process* involving diseases of a body system or structure. These processes are commonly classified as congenital, inflammatory or infectious, immunologic, neoplastic, metabolic, nutritional, degenerative, vascular, traumatic, and toxic.

Other problems are *pathophysiologic,* reflecting derangements of biologic functions, such as heart failure or migraine headache. Still other problems are *psychopathologic,* such as disorders of mood like depression or headache as an expression of a somatic symptom disorder.

Generate Hypotheses About the Causes of the Patient's Problem. Draw on the full range of your knowledge and experience, and read widely. By consulting the clinical literature, you embark on the lifelong goal of *evidence-based decision making and clinical practice.* The following steps may help.

Steps for Generating Clinical Hypotheses

1. Select the most specific and critical findings to support your hypothesis.
2. Match your findings against all the conditions that can produce them.
3. Eliminate the diagnostic possibilities that fail to explain the findings.
4. Weigh the competing possibilities and select the most likely diagnosis.
5. Give special attention to potentially life-threatening conditions.

Test Your Hypotheses. You are likely to need further history, additional maneuvers on physical examination, or laboratory studies or x-rays to confirm or rule out your tentative diagnosis or to clarify which diagnosis is most likely.

Establish a Working Diagnosis. Establish a working definition of the problem at the highest level of explicitness and certainty that the data allow. You may be limited to a symptom, such as "tension headache, cause unknown." At other times, you can define a problem more specifically based on its anatomy, disease process, or cause. Routinely listing *Health Maintenance* helps you track several important health concerns more effectively: immunizations, screening tests such as mammograms or colonoscopies, instructions regarding nutrition and breast or testicular self-examinations, recommendations about exercise or use of seat belts, and responses to important life events.

Use Shared Decision-Making to Develop a Plan

Identify and record a *Plan* for each patient problem. Specify the next steps for each problem, ranging from tests and procedures to subspecialty consultations to new or changed medications to arranging a family meeting. It is critical to not only obtain patient agreement but to have the patient participate in the decision making whenever possible.

The Quality Clinical Record: The Case of Mrs. N.

The *clinical record* serves a dual purpose—it reflects your analysis of the patient's health status, and it documents the unique features of the patient's history, examination, laboratory and test results, assessment, and plan in a formal written format. In a well-constructed record, each problem in the *Assessment* is listed in order of priority with an explanation of supporting findings and a differential diagnosis, followed by a *Plan* for addressing that problem.

Compose the clinical record as soon after seeing the patient as possible, before your findings fade from memory, and follow the tips below for a quality patient record.

Tips for Ensuring Quality Patient Data

- Ask open-ended questions and listen carefully to the patient's story.
- Craft a thorough and systematic sequence to history taking and physical examination.
- Keep an open mind toward both the patient and the clinical data.
- Always include "the worst-case scenario" in your list of possible explanations of the patient's problem, and make sure it can be safely eliminated.
- Analyze any mistakes in data collection or interpretation.
- Confer with colleagues and review the pertinent clinical literature to clarify uncertainties.
- Apply the principles of evaluating clinical evidence to patient information and testing.

Study the case of Mrs. N. and scrutinize the history, physical examination, assessment, and plan. Note the standard format of the clinical record.

The Case of Mrs. N.

HEALTH HISTORY
8/25/16 11:00 AM
Mrs. N. is a pleasant, 54-year-old widowed saleswoman residing in Espanola, New Mexico.
Referral. None
Source and Reliability. Self-referred; seems reliable.

Chief Complaint
"My headaches."

Present Illness
Mrs. N. reports increasing problems with frontal headaches over the past 3 months. These are usually bifrontal, throbbing, and mild to moderately severe. She has missed work on several occasions because of associated nausea and vomiting. Headaches now average once a week, usually related to stress, and last 4 to 6 hours. They are relieved by sleep and putting a damp towel over her forehead. There is little relief from aspirin. There are no associated visual changes, motor-sensory deficits, or paresthesias.

She had headaches with nausea and vomiting beginning at age 15 years. These recurred throughout her mid-20s, then decreased to one every 2 or 3 months and almost disappeared.

(continued)

The Case of Mrs. N. (Continued)

The patient reports increased pressure at work from a demanding supervisor; she is also worried about her daughter (see *Personal and Social History*). She thinks her headaches may be like those in the past, but wants to be sure because her mother had a headache just before she died of a stroke. She is concerned because her headaches interfere with her work and make her irritable with her family. She eats three meals a day and drinks three cups of coffee a day and tea at night.

Medications. Acetaminophen, 1 to 2 tablets every 4 to 6 hours as needed. "Water pill" in the past for ankle swelling, none recently.

Allergies. Ampicillin causes rash.

Tobacco. About 1 pack of cigarettes per day since age 18 (36 pack-years).

Alcohol/drugs. Wine on rare occasions. No illicit drugs.

Past History
Childhood Illnesses: Measles, chickenpox. No scarlet fever or rheumatic fever.
Adult Illnesses: Medical: Pyelonephritis, 1998, with fever and right flank pain; treated with ampicillin; developed generalized rash with itching several days later. Reports x-rays were normal; no recurrence of infection. *Surgical:* Tonsillectomy, age 6; appendectomy, age 13. Sutures for laceration, 2001, after stepping on glass. *Ob/Gyn:* 3–3–0–3, with normal vaginal deliveries. Three living children. Menarche age 12. Last menses 6 months ago. Little interest in sex, and not sexually active. No concerns about HIV infection. *Psychiatric:* None.
Health Maintenance: Immunizations: Oral polio vaccine, year uncertain; tetanus shots × 2, 1982, followed with booster 1 year later; flu vaccine, 2000, no reaction. *Screening tests:* Last Pap smear, 2014, normal. No mammograms to date.

Family History
The family history is depicted below.

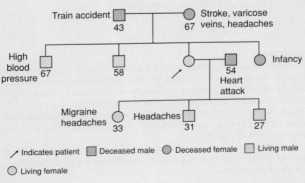

/ Indicates patient ▪ Deceased male ● Deceased female ☐ Living male

○ Living female

(continued)

The Case of Mrs. N. (Continued)

OR, alternatively: Father died at age 43 years in a train accident. Mother died at age 67 years from stroke; had varicose veins, headaches.

One brother, age 61 years, with hypertension, otherwise well; one brother, age 58 years, well except for mild arthritis; one sister, died in infancy of unknown cause.

Husband died at age 54 of heart attack

Daughter, age 33 years, with migraine headaches, otherwise well; son, age 31 years, with headaches; son, age 27 years, well.

No family history of diabetes, tuberculosis, heart or kidney disease, cancer, anemia, epilepsy, or mental illness.

Personal and Social History

Born and raised in Las Cruces, finished high school, married at age 19 years. Worked as sales clerk for 2 years, then moved with husband to Espanola, had three children. Returned to work 15 years ago to improve family finances. Children all married. Four years ago Mr. N. died suddenly of a heart attack, leaving little savings. Mrs. N. has moved to a small apartment to be near daughter, Isabel. Isabel's husband, John, is deployed overseas. Mrs. N.'s apartment is now a haven for Isabel and her two children, Kevin, age 6 years, and Lucia, age 3 years. Mrs. N. feels responsible for helping them; she feels tense and nervous but denies depression. She has friends but rarely discusses family problems: "I'd rather keep them to myself. I don't like gossip." No church or other organizational support. She is typically up at 7:00 AM, works 9:00 AM to 5:30 PM, and eats dinner alone.

Exercise and diet. Gets little exercise. Diet high in carbohydrates.

Safety measures. Uses seat belt regularly. Uses sunblock. Medications kept in an unlocked medicine cabinet. Cleaning solutions in unlocked cabinet below sink. Mr. N's shotgun and box of shells in unlocked closet upstairs.

Review of Systems

General: Has gained 10 lb in the past 4 years.

Skin: No rashes or other changes.

Head, Eyes, Ears, Nose, Throat (HEENT): See *Present Illness.* **Head:** No history of head injury. *Eyes:* Reading glasses for 5 years, last checked 1 year ago. No symptoms. *Ears:* Hearing good. No tinnitus, vertigo, infections. *Nose, sinuses:* Occasional mild cold. No hay fever, sinus trouble. ***Throat (or mouth and pharynx):*** Some bleeding of gums recently. Last dental visit 2 years ago. Occasional canker sore.

Neck: No lumps, goiter, pain. No swollen glands.

Breasts: No lumps, pain, discharge. Does breast self-examination sporadically.

Respiratory: No cough, wheezing, shortness of breath. Last chest x-ray, 1986, St. Mary's Hospital; unremarkable.

Cardiovascular: No known heart disease or high blood pressure; last blood pressure taken in 2007. No dyspnea, orthopnea, chest pain, palpitations. Has never had an electrocardiogram (ECG).

(continued)

The Case of Mrs. N. *(Continued)*

Gastrointestinal: Appetite good; no nausea, vomiting, indigestion. Bowel movement about once daily, though sometimes has hard stools for 2 to 3 days when especially tense; no diarrhea or bleeding. No pain, jaundice, gallbladder or liver problems.

Urinary: No frequency, dysuria, hematuria, or recent flank pain; nocturia × 1, large volume. Occasionally loses urine when coughing.

Genital: No vaginal or pelvic infections. No dyspareunia.

Peripheral vascular: Varicose veins appeared in both legs during first pregnancy. For 10 years, has had swollen ankles after prolonged standing; wears light elastic support hose; tried "water pill" 5 months ago, but it didn't help much; no history of phlebitis or leg pain.

Musculoskeletal: Mild low backaches, often at the end of the workday; no radiation into the legs; used to do back exercises but not now. No other joint pain.

Psychiatric: No history of depression or treatment for psychiatric disorders. (See also *Present Illness* and *Personal and Social History.*)

Neurologic: No fainting, seizures, motor or sensory loss. Memory good.

Hematologic: Except for bleeding gums, no easy bleeding. No anemia.

Endocrine: No known thyroid disorders or heat or cold intolerance. No symptoms or history of diabetes.

PHYSICAL EXAMINATION

Mrs. N. is a short, overweight, middle-aged woman, who is animated and responds quickly to questions. She is somewhat tense, with moist, cold hands. Her hair is well groomed. Her color is good, and she lies flat without discomfort.

Vital signs: Ht (without shoes) 157 cm (5′2″). Wt (dressed) 65 kg (143 lb). BMI 26. BP 164/98 right arm, supine; 160/96 left arm, supine; 152/88 right arm, supine with wide cuff. Heart rate (HR) 88 and regular. Respiratory rate (RR) 18. Temperature (oral) 98.6°F.

Skin: Palms cold and moist, but color good. Scattered cherry angiomas over upper trunk. Nails without clubbing, cyanosis.

Head, Eyes, Ears, Nose, Throat (HEENT): Head: Hair of average texture. Scalp without lesions, normocephalic/atraumatic (NC/AT). *Eyes:* Vision 20/30 in each eye. Visual fields full by confrontation. Conjunctiva pink; sclera white. Pupils 4 mm constricting to 2 mm, round, regular, equally reactive to light. Extraocular movements intact. Disc margins sharp, without hemorrhages, exudates. No arteriolar narrowing or A-V nicking. *Ears:* Wax partially obscures right tympanic membrane (TM); left canal clear, TM with good cone of light. Acuity good to whispered voice. Weber midline. AC > BC. *Nose:* Mucosa pink, septum midline. No sinus tenderness. *Mouth:* Oral mucosa pink. Several interdental papillae red, slightly swollen. Dentition good. Tongue midline, with 3 × 4 mm shallow white ulcer on red base on undersurface near tip; tender but not indurated. Tonsils absent. Pharynx without exudates.

(continued)

The Case of Mrs. N. (Continued)

Neck: Neck supple. Trachea midline. Thyroid isthmus barely palpable, lobes not felt.

Lymph nodes: Small (<1 cm), soft, nontender, and mobile tonsillar and posterior cervical nodes bilaterally. No axillary or epitrochlear nodes. Several small inguinal nodes bilaterally, soft and nontender.

Thorax and lungs: Thorax symmetric with good excursion. Lungs resonant. Breath sounds vesicular with no added sounds. Diaphragms descend 4 cm bilaterally.

Cardiovascular: Jugular venous pressure 1 cm above the sternal angle, with head of examining table raised to 30°. Carotid upstrokes brisk, without bruits. Apical impulse discrete and tapping, barely palpable in the 5th left interspace, 8 cm lateral to the midsternal line. Good S_1, S_2; no S_3 or S_4. A II/VI medium-pitched midsystolic murmur at the lower left sternal border. No diastolic murmurs.

Breasts: Pendulous, symmetric. No masses; nipples without discharge.

Abdomen: Protuberant. Well-healed scar, right lower quadrant. Bowel sounds active. No tenderness or masses. Liver span 7 cm in right midclavicular line; edge smooth, palpable 1 cm below right costal margin (RCM). Spleen and kidneys not felt. No costovertebral angle tenderness (CVAT).

Genitalia: External genitalia without lesions. Mild cystocele at introitus on straining. Vaginal mucosa pink. Cervix pink, parous, and without discharge. Uterus anterior, midline, smooth, not enlarged. Adnexa not palpated due to obesity and poor relaxation. No cervical or adnexal tenderness. Pap smear taken. Rectovaginal wall intact.

Rectal: Rectal vault without masses. Stool brown, negative for fecal blood.

Extremities: Warm and without edema. Calves supple, nontender.

Peripheral vascular: Trace edema at both ankles. Moderate varicosities of saphenous veins both in lower extremities. No stasis pigmentation or ulcers. Pulses (2+ = brisk, or normal):

	Radial	Femoral	Popliteal	Dorsalis Pedis	Posterior Tibial
RT	2+	2+	2+	2+	2+
LT	2+	2+	2+	Absent	2+

Musculoskeletal: No joint deformities. Good range of motion in hands, wrists, elbows, shoulders, spine, hips, knees, ankles.

Neurologic: Mental Status: Tense, but alert and cooperative. Thought coherent. Oriented to person, place, and time. *Cranial nerves:* II to XII intact.

Motor: Good muscle bulk and tone. Strength 5/5 throughout. *Cerebellar:* Rapid alternating movements (RAMs), point-to-point movements intact. Gait stable, fluid. *Sensory:* Pinprick, light touch, position sense, vibration, and stereognosis intact. Romberg negative.

(continued)

The Case of Mrs. N. (Continued)

Reflexes:

	Biceps	Triceps	Brachio-radialis	Patellar	Achilles	Plantar
RT	2+	2+	2+	2+	1+	↓
LT	2+	2+	2+	2+/2+	1+	↓

OR

ASSESSMENT AND PLAN

1. **Migraine headaches.** A 54-year-old woman with migraine headaches since childhood, with a throbbing vascular pattern and frequent nausea and vomiting. Headaches are associated with stress and relieved by sleep and cold compresses. There is no papilledema, and there are no motor or sensory deficits on the neurologic examination. The differential diagnosis includes tension headache, also associated with stress, but there is no relief with massage, and the pain is more throbbing than aching. There are no fever, stiff neck, or focal findings to suggest meningitis, and the lifelong recurrent pattern makes subarachnoid hemorrhage unlikely (usually described as "the worst headache of my life").

   Plan:
   - Discuss features of migraine versus tension headaches.
   - Discuss biofeedback and stress management.
   - Advise patient to avoid caffeine, including coffee, colas, and other carbonated beverages.
   - Start nonsteroidal anti-inflammatory drugs (NSAIDs) for headache, as needed.
   - If needed next visit, begin prophylactic medication if headaches are occurring more than 2 days a week or 8 days a month.

2. **Elevated blood pressure.** Systolic hypertension is present. May be related to anxiety from first visit. No evidence of end-organ damage to retina or heart.

   Plan:
   - Discuss standards for assessing blood pressure; check BP in 1 month.
   - Recheck systolic murmur.
   - Check basic metabolic panel; review urinalysis.
   - Discuss weight reduction and exercise programs (see #4).
   - Reduce salt intake.

3. **Cystocele with occasional stress incontinence.** Cystocele on pelvic examination, probably related to bladder relaxation. Patient is perimenopausal. Incontinence reported with coughing, suggesting alteration in bladder neck anatomy. No dysuria, fever, flank pain. Not taking any contributing medications. Usually involves small amounts of urine, no dribbling, so doubt urge or overflow incontinence.

(continued)

The Case of Mrs. N. (Continued)

Plan:
- Explain cause of stress incontinence.
- Review urinalysis.
- Recommend Kegel exercises.
- Consider topical estrogen cream to vagina during next visit if no improvement.

4. **Overweight.** Patient 5'2", weighs 143 lbs. BMI is ~26.

   Plan:
   - Explore diet history, ask patient to keep food intake diary.
   - Explore motivation to lose weight, set target for weight loss by next visit.
   - Schedule visit with dietitian.
   - Discuss exercise program, specifically, walking 30 minutes most days a week.

5. **Family stress.** Son-in-law deployed, rarely at home; daughter and grandchildren often at patient's home, leading to tensions in these relationships. Patient also has financial constraints. Stress currently situational. No current evidence of major depression.

   Plan:
   - Explore patient's views on strategies to cope with stress.
   - Explore sources of support, including Al-Anon for daughter and financial counseling for patient.
   - Continue to monitor for depression.

6. **Occasional musculoskeletal low back pain.** Usually with prolonged standing. No history of trauma or motor vehicle accident. Pain does not radiate; no tenderness or motor-sensory deficits on examination. Doubt disc or nerve root compression, trochanteric bursitis, sacroiliitis.

   Plan:
   - Review benefits of weight loss and exercises to strengthen low back muscles.

7. **Tobacco abuse.** 1 pack per day for 36 years.

   Plan:
   - Check peak flow or FEV_1/FVC on office spirometry.
   - Give strong warning to stop smoking.
   - Offer referral to tobacco cessation program.
   - Offer patch, current treatment to enhance abstinence.

8. **Varicose veins, lower extremities.** No complaints currently.

9. **History of right pyelonephritis, 1998.**

10. **Ampicillin allergy.** Developed rash but no other allergic reaction.

11. **Health maintenance.** Last Pap smear 2014; has never had a mammogram.

    Plan:
    - Schedule mammogram.
    - Pap smear sent today.
    - Provide three cards to test for fecal blood; next visit, discuss screening colonoscopy.
    - Suggest dental care for mild gingivitis.
    - Advise patient to move medications and caustic cleaning agents to locked cabinet above shoulder height. Urge patient to move gun and cartridges to a locked gun cabinet.

The Importance of the Problem List

After you complete the clinical record, it is good clinical practice to generate a *Problem List* that summarizes the patient's problems that can be placed in the front of the office or hospital chart. *List the most active and serious problems first, and record their date of onset.* Some clinicians make separate lists for active or inactive problems; others make one list in order of priority. A sample *Problem List* for Mrs. N. is provided below.

Problem List: The Case of Mrs. N.

Date Entered	Problem No.	Problem
8/25/16	1	Migraine headaches
	2	Elevated blood pressure
	3	Cystocele with occasional stress incontinence
	4	Overweight
	5	Family stress
	6	Low back pain
	7	Tobacco abuse since age 18 years
	8	Varicose veins
	9	History of right pyelonephritis 1998
	10	Allergy to ampicillin
	11	Health maintenance

Recording Your Findings

A clear, well-organized clinical record is one of the most important adjuncts to patient care. Think especially about the *order and readability* of the record and the *amount of detail* needed. Use the following checklist to make sure your record is informative and easy to follow.

Checklist to Ensure a Quality Clinical Record

Is the Order Clear?
Order is imperative. Make sure that readers can easily find specific points of information. Keep the *subjective* items of the history, for example, in the history; do not let them stray into the physical examination. Did you:

- Make the headings clear?
- Accent your organization with indentations and spacing?
- Arrange the *Present Illness* in chronologic order, starting with the current episode, then filling in relevant background information?

(continued)

Checklist to Ensure a Quality Clinical Record (Continued)

Do the Data Included Contribute Directly to the Assessment?
Spell out the supporting evidence, both positive and negative, for each problem or diagnosis. Make sure there is sufficient detail to support your differential diagnosis and plan.

Are Pertinent Negatives Specifically Described?
Often portions of the history or examination suggest that an abnormality might exist or develop in that area. For example, for the patient with notable bruises, record the "pertinent negatives," such as the absence of injury or violence, familial bleeding disorders, or medications or nutritional deficits that might lead to bruising. For the patient who is depressed but not suicidal, recording both facts is important. In the patient with a transient mood swing, on the other hand, a comment on suicide is unnecessary.

Are There Overgeneralizations or Omissions of Important Data?
Remember that data not recorded are data lost. No matter how vividly you can recall clinical details today, you will probably not remember them in a few months. The phrase "neurologic exam negative," even in your own handwriting, may leave you wondering in a few months' time, "Did I really check the reflexes?"

Is There Too Much Detail?
Is there excess information or redundancy? Is important information buried in a mass of detail, to be discovered by only the most persistent reader? Make your descriptions concise. "Cervix pink and smooth" indicates you saw no redness, ulcers, nodules, masses, cysts, or other suspicious lesions, but this description is shorter and more easily read. You can omit unimportant structures even though you examined them, such as normal eyebrows and eyelashes.

Omit most of your negative findings unless they relate directly to the patient's complaints or specific exclusions in your differential diagnosis. *Instead, concentrate on major negative findings* such as "no heart murmurs."

Is the Written Style Succinct? Are Phrases, Short Words, and Abbreviations Used Appropriately? Is Data Unnecessarily Repeated?
Omit repetitive introductory phrases such as "The patient reports no …" because readers assume the patient is the source of the history unless otherwise specified.

- Using words or brief phrases instead of whole sentences is common, but abbreviations and symbols should be used only if they are readily understood. Use shorter words when possible such as "felt" for "palpated" or "heard" for "auscultated." Omit unnecessary words, such as those in parentheses in the examples below. For example, "Cervix is pink (in color)." "Lungs are resonant (to percussion)."
- Describe what you observed, not what you did. "Optic discs seen" is less informative than "disc margins sharp."

(continued)

Checklist to Ensure a Quality Clinical Record *(Continued)*

Are Diagrams and Precise Measurements Included Where Appropriate?
Diagrams add greatly to the clarity of the record.

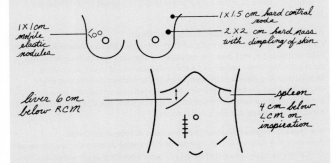

To ensure accurate evaluations and future comparisons, make measurements in centimeters, not in fruits, nuts, or vegetables.

- "1 × 1 cm lymph node" versus a "pea-sized lymph node . . ."
- Or "2 × 2 cm mass on the left lobe of the prostate" versus a "walnut-sized prostate mass."

Is the Tone of the Write-up Neutral and Professional?
It is important to be objective. Hostile or disapproving comments have no place in the patient's record. Never use inflammatory or demeaning words or punctuation.

Comments such as "Patient DRUNK and LATE TO CLINIC AGAIN!!" are unprofessional and set a bad example for other clinicians reading the chart. They also might prove difficult to defend in a legal setting.

Evaluating Clinical Evidence

Excellence in clinical care requires integrating clinical expertise, patient preferences, and the best available clinical evidence. Carefully study the clear descriptions of how the history and physical examination can be viewed as diagnostic tests; how to assess the accuracy of laboratory tests, radiographic imaging, and diagnostic procedures; and how to evaluate clinical research studies and disease prevention guidelines.

Throughout the regional examination chapters, you will find evidence-based recommendations for health promotion interventions, especially screening and prevention. These recommendations are also based on evidence from the clinical literature that can be evaluated according to criteria presented in this chapter.

The History and Physical Examination as Diagnostic Tests

The process of diagnostic reasoning begins with the history. As you learn about your patient, you will start to develop a *differential diagnosis*. You will assign probabilities to the various diagnoses that correspond to how likely you consider them to be explanations for your patient's problem. As you approach clinical problems, your goal is to determine whether you need to perform additional testing (Fig. 2-1).

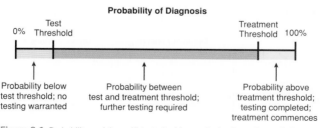

Figure 2-1 Probability revisions. (Adapted with permission from Guyatt G, Rennie D, Meade M, et al. *Users' Guides to the Medical Literature.* 2nd ed. New York, NY: McGraw-Hill Company; 2008; Chapter 14, Figure 14–2.)

If your probability for a disease based on your history and examination is very high (i.e., exceeds the treatment threshold), then you can move ahead and initiate treatment. Conversely, if your probability for a disease is very low (i.e., below the test threshold), then you do not need further testing. The area between the test and treatment thresholds represents clinical uncertainty, and you need further testing to revise probabilities and guide your clinical management.

Evaluating Diagnostic Tests

Two concepts in evaluating diagnostic tests are the validity of the findings and the reproducibility of the test results.

Validity

Does the test provide valid results and accurately identify whether the patient has a disease? This involves comparing the test against a gold standard—the best measure of whether a patient has disease. This could be a biopsy, a structured psychiatric examination, or a colonoscopy.

The *2 × 2 table* is the basic format for evaluating the performance characteristics of a diagnostic test, which means how much the test results revise probabilities for disease.

There are two columns—patients with disease present and patients with disease absent. These categorizations are based on the gold standard test. The two rows correspond to positive and negative test results. The four cells (a, b, c, d) correspond to true positives, false positives, false negatives, and true negatives, respectively.

Setting up the 2 × 2 Table

	Gold Standard: Disease Present	Gold Standard: Disease Absent
Test positive	a True positive	b False positive
Test negative	c False negative	d True negative

Sensitivity and Specificity. The first test statistics to estimate are *sensitivity* and *specificity*.

Sensitivity and Specificity

- **Sensitivity** is the probability that a person with disease has a positive test. This is represented as a/(a + c) in the disease present column of the 2 × 2 table. Sensitivity is also known as the true positive rate.
- **Specificity** is the probability that a nondiseased person has a negative test, represented as d/(b + d) in the disease absent column of the 2 × 2 table. Specificity is also known as the true negative rate.
- *Examples.* An example of these statistics would be the probability that splenomegaly (see Chapter 11, p. 210) is associated with percussion dullness below the left costal margin (sensitivity). Conversely, the probability that a patient without splenomegaly will have percussion dullness is the false-positive rate (1 − specificity) for this physical maneuver.

A negative result from a test with a high sensitivity (i.e., a very low false-negative rate) usually excludes disease. This is represented by the acronym SnNOUT—a **Sen**sitive test with a **N**egative result rules **OUT** disease. Conversely, a positive result in a test with high specificity (e.g., a very low false-positive rate) usually indicates disease. This is represented by the acronym SpPIN—a **Sp**ecific test with a **P**ositive result rules **IN** disease.

Positive and Negative Predictive Values. To determine the probability that a patient actually has disease based on a test result that is either positive or negative, calculate positive and negative predictive values.

Positive and Negative Predictive Values

- The **positive predictive value (PPV)** is the probability that a person with a positive test has disease, represented as a/(a + b) from the test positive row in the 2 × 2 table.
  An example of this statistic is found in prostate cancer screening (see Chapter 15, p. 266), where a man with a PSA value greater than 4.0 ng/mL has only a 30% probability of having prostate cancer found on biopsy.
- The **negative predictive value (NPV)** is the probability that a person with a negative test does not have disease, represented as d/(c + d) in the test negative row in 2 × 2 table.
  An example is: Among men with a PSA level of 4.0 ng/mL or below, 85% are found to be cancer-free on biopsy.

Prevalence of Disease. Predictive value statistics vary substantially according to the prevalence of disease (i.e., the proportion of patients in the disease present column), which is based on the characteristics of the patient population and the clinical setting. The box below shows a 2 × 2 table where both the sensitivity and specificity of the diagnostic test are 90% and the prevalence is 10%. The positive predictive value calculated from the test positive row of the table would be 90/180 = 50%. This means that half of the people with a positive test have disease.

Predictive Values: Prevalence of 10% with Sensitivity and Specificity = 90%

	Disease Present	Disease Absent	Total
Test positive	a 90	b 90	180
Test negative	c 10	d 810	820
Total	100	900	1,000

Sensitivity = a/(a + c) = 90/100 or 90%; specificity = d/(b + d) = 810/900 = 90%

Positive predictive value = a/(a + b) = 90/180 = 50%

However, if the sensitivity and specificity remained the same, but prevalence was only 1%, then the cells would look very different.

Predictive Values: Prevalence of 1% with Sensitivity and Specificity = 90%

	Disease Present	Disease Absent	Total
Test positive	a 9	b 99	108
Test negative	c 1	d 891	892
Total	10	990	1,000

Sensitivity = a/(a + c) = 9/10 or 90%; specificity = d/(b + d) = 891/990 = 90%

Positive predictive value = a/(a + b) = 9/108 = 8.3%

Likelihood Ratios. To evaluate the performance of a diagnostic test that can account for the varying disease prevalence observed in different patient populations, you can use *likelihood ratio* statistics, defined as the probability of obtaining a given test result in a diseased patient divided by the probability of obtaining a given test result in a nondiseased patient. The likelihood ratio tells us how much a test result changes the pre-test disease probability (prevalence) to the post-test disease probability.

The *likelihood ratio for a positive test* is the ratio of getting a positive test result in a diseased person divided by the probability of getting a positive test result in a nondiseased person. The 2 × 2 table shows that this is the same as saying the ratio of the true positive rate (sensitivity) over the false-positive rate (1 − specificity). A higher value (much >1) indicates that a positive test is much more likely to be coming from a diseased person than from a nondiseased person, increasing our confidence that a person with a positive result has disease.

The likelihood ratio for a negative test is the ratio of the probability of getting a negative test result in a diseased person divided by the probability of getting a negative test result in a nondiseased person. The 2 × 2 table shows that this is the same as saying the ratio of the false-negative rate (1 − sensitivity) divided by the true negative rate (specificity). A lower value (much <1) indicates that the negative test is much more likely to be coming from a nondiseased person than from a diseased person, increasing our confidence that a person with a negative result does not have disease.

Interpreting Likelihood Ratios

Likelihood Ratios[a]	Effect on Pre- to Post-test Probability
LRs > 10 or < 0.1	Generate large changes
LRs 5–10 or 0.1–0.2	Generate moderate changes
LRs 2–5 and 0.5–0.2	Generate small (sometimes important) changes
LRs 1–2 and 0.5–1	Alter the probability to a small degree (rarely important)

[a]*Likelihood ratios* >1 are associated with positive results and an increased probability for disease. *Likelihood ratios* <1 are associated with negative results and a decreased probability of disease. A test with a *likelihood ratio of 1* provides no additional information about the probability of disease.

Bayes Theorem. One way to use likelihood ratios to revise probabilities for disease is with the Bayes theorem. This theorem requires converting the estimated prevalence (pre-test probability) to odds using the equation:

$$\text{Pre-test odds} = \text{pre-test probability}/(1 - \text{pre-test probability})$$

The pre-test odds are multiplied by the likelihood ratio to estimate the post-test odds using the following equation:

$$\text{Post-test odds} = \text{Pre-test odds} \times \text{likelihood ratio}$$

The post-test odds are then converted to a probability using the equation:

$$\text{Post-test probability} = \text{post-test odds}/(1 + \text{post-test odds})$$

Fagan Nomogram. If you are more comfortable thinking in terms of probability of having disease, then the Fagan nomogram may be an easier way for you to use likelihood ratios (Fig. 2-2). With this nomogram, you read the pre-test probabilities from the line on the left, then take a straight edge and draw a line from the pre-test probability through the likelihood

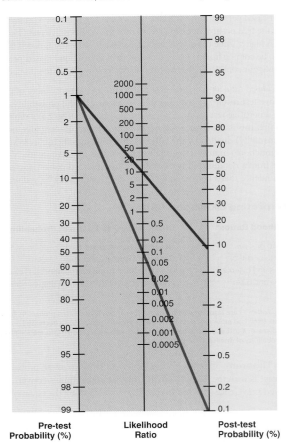

Figure 2-2 Fagan nomogram. (Adapted with permission from Fagan TJ. Letter: nomogram for Bayes theorem. *N Engl J Med*. 1975;293:257.)

ratio in the middle line, and then read the post-test probability on the line on the right.

Figure 2.2 shows how the Fagan nomogram displays probability revisions. In this example, the diagnostic test has a sensitivity of 90% and specificity of 91%. With a pre-test probability (prevalence) of 1%, a positive test result (blue line) leads to a post-test probability of 9%. A negative test result (red line) leads to a post-test probability of 0.1%.

Reproducibility

Kappa Score. Two clinicians examining a patient may not always agree upon the presence of a given finding. Understanding whether there is agreement well beyond chance is important in knowing whether the finding is useful enough to support clinical decision making. The *kappa score* measures the amount of agreement that occurs beyond chance. The box shows how to interpret Kappa values.

Interpreting Kappa Values

Value of Kappa	Strength of Agreement
<0.20	Poor
0.21–0.40	Fair
0.41–0.60	Moderate
0.61–0.80	Good
0.81–1.00	Excellent

For example, although clinicians agree 75% of the time that a patient has an abnormal physical finding, the expected agreement based on chance is 50%. This means that the potential agreement beyond chance is 50% and the actual observer agreement beyond chance is 25%. The kappa level is then 25%/50% = 0.5, which indicates moderate agreement.

Precision. In the context of reproducibility, precision refers to being able to apply the same test to the same unchanged person and obtain the same results. Precision is often used when referring to laboratory tests. A statistical test used to characterize precision is the coefficient of variation, defined as the standard deviation divided by the mean value. Lower values indicate greater precision.

Health Promotion

Throughout the book you will find health promotion sections that make recommendations for *primary prevention* (interventions designed to prevent disease) as well as *secondary prevention* (screening tests designed to find disease or disease processes at an early, asymptomatic stage). The rationale for secondary prevention is that treatment for early-stage disease is often more effective than treatment for later-stage disease. We highlight guidelines from professional organizations that are evidence-based, such as those of the U.S. Preventive Services Task Force (USPSTF) that consider the quality of the evidence and the strength of the recommendation to either provide or withhold the intervention. The strongest health promotion recommendations are based on results from randomized controlled trials (or

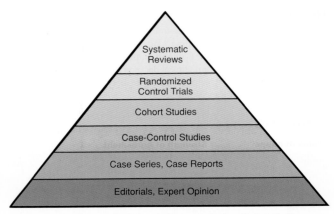

Figure 2-3 Evidence pyramid. (Adapted with permission from Sackett DL, Straus SE, Richardson WS, et al. *Evidence-Based Medicine: How to Practice and Teach EBM.* 2nd ed. Edinburgh: Churchill Livingstone; 2000.)

syntheses of multiple such trials) of therapy or prevention. When searching for evidence-based information, you should select the highest level of available evidence (Fig. 2-3).

Critical Appraisal

Learn the process of critically appraising the clinical literature in order to interpret new studies and guidelines as they appear throughout your professional career. The Evidence-Based Working Group, which consists of experts in epidemiology, has created a rigorous and standardized approach for evaluating studies that has been applied to a wide range of clinical topics, including therapeutic and prevention trials, diagnostic tests, meta-analysis, cost-effectiveness analyses, and practice guidelines. This approach asks three basic questions:

1. Are the results valid (can you believe them)?
2. What are the results (magnitude and precision)?
3. How can you apply the results to patient care?

Understanding Bias

When evaluating study results, it is important to have a thorough understanding of bias. The key sources of bias in clinical research are selection bias, performance bias, detection bias, and attrition bias.

Types of Biases Affecting Evidence

Selection Bias
- Occurs when comparison groups have systematic differences in their baseline characteristics that can affect the outcome of the study
- Creates problems in interpreting observed differences in outcomes because they could result from the interventions or the baseline differences between groups
- Randomly allocating subjects to the intervention is the best approach to minimizing this bias

Performance Bias
- Occurs when there are systematic differences in the care received between comparison groups (other than the intervention)
- Creates problems in interpreting outcome differences
- Blinding subjects and providers to the intervention is the best approach to minimizing this bias

Detection Bias
- Occurs when there are systematic differences in efforts to diagnose or ascertain an outcome
- Blinding outcomes assessors (ensuring that they are unaware of the intervention received by the subject) is the best approach to minimizing this bias

Attrition Bias
- Occurs when there are systematic differences in the comparison groups in the number of subjects who do not complete the study
- Failing to account for these differences can lead to incorrectly estimating the effectiveness of an intervention
- Using an intention-to-treat analysis, where all analyses consider all subjects who were assigned to a comparison group, regardless of whether they received or completed the intervention, can minimize this bias

Results

Assessing Performance of a Treatment or Prevention Intervention. The statistics used to characterize the performance of a treatment or prevention intervention include relative risks, relative risk differences (can be a reduction or increase, reflecting benefit or harm), absolute risk differences (can be a reduction or increase, reflecting benefit or harm), numbers needed to treat, and numbers needed to harm.

2 × 2 Tables for Evaluating Studies of Treatment or Prevention

	Event Occurred	No Event	Total
Experimental group	a	b	a + b
Control group	c	d	c + d

Calculating these performance statistics from the 2×2 table begins with determining probabilities for outcomes.

■ The probability that an intervention subject had the outcome is described by $a/(a + b)$ from row 1 (experimental group); this also called the experimental event rate (EER).

■ The probability that a control subject had the outcome is $c/(c + d)$ from row 2 (control group), or the control event rate (CER).

■ The relative risk, the probability of an outcome in the intervention group compared to the probability of an outcome in the control group, is expressed as the EER/CER.

■ The relative risk difference is defined as |CER − EER|/CER × 100% or 100% − the relative risk, which describes the proportion of baseline risk is reduced/increased by the therapy.

■ The absolute risk difference, the difference in outcome rates between the comparisons groups, is expressed by the |CER − EER|.

■ The reciprocal of the absolute risk difference (reported as a fraction) is the number of subjects who need to be treated over a specific period of time to prevent one outcome. If the intervention actually increases the risk for a bad outcome, then this statistic becomes the number needed to harm.

In many studies these calculations are used to measure treatment effectiveness between control and treatment interventions comparing medications, procedures, or diagnostic tests.

Generalizability

To make this determination, you need to first look at the demographics of the study subjects (e.g., age, gender, race/ethnicity, socioeconomic status, clinical conditions). Then, you need to determine: Are the study demographics applicable to your patient? Is the intervention feasible in your clinical setting? And, most importantly, is the range of potential benefits and harm of the intervention acceptable for your patient?

Guideline Recommendations

There are many approaches for rating the strength of recommendations and we will discuss several grading systems. Review the rating systems in Tables 2-1 to 2-3 (pp. 37–40).

Aids to Interpretation

Table 2-1   U.S. Preventive Services Task Force Ratings: Grade Definitions and Implications for Practice

Grade	Definition	Suggestions for Practice
A	The USPSTF recommends the service. There is high certainty that the net benefit is substantial.	Offer or provide this service.
B	The USPSTF recommends the service. There is high certainty that the net benefit is moderate or there is moderate certainty that the net benefit is moderate to substantial.	Offer or provide this service.
C	The USPSTF recommends selectively offering or providing this service to individual patients based on professional judgment and patient preferences. There is at least moderate certainty that the net benefit is small.	Offer or provide this service for selected patients depending on individual circumstances.
D	The USPSTF recommends against the service. There is moderate or high certainty that the service has no net benefit or that the harms outweigh the benefits.	Discourage the use of this service.
I	The USPSTF concludes that the current evidence is insufficient to assess the balance of benefits and harms of the service. Evidence is lacking, of poor quality, or conflicting, and the balance of benefits and harms cannot be determined.	If the service is offered, patients should understand the uncertainty about the balance of benefits and harms.

The USPSTF defines *certainty* as the "likelihood that the USPSTF assessment of the net benefit of a preventive service is correct." The *net benefit* is defined as benefit minus harm of the preventive service as implemented in a general, primary care population.

Source: Grade Definitions. U.S. Preventive Services Task Force. October 2014. http://www.uspreventiveservicestaskforce.org/Page/Name/grade-definitions.

Table 2-2 U.S. Preventive Services Task Force Levels of Certainty Regarding Benefit

Level of Certainty	Description
High	The available evidence usually includes consistent results from well-designed, well-conducted studies in representative primary care populations. These studies assess the effects of the preventive service on health outcomes. This conclusion is therefore unlikely to be strongly affected by the results of future studies.
Moderate	The available evidence is sufficient to determine the effects of the preventive service on health outcomes, but confidence in the estimate is constrained by such factors as: ■ The number, size, or quality of individual studies. ■ Inconsistency of findings across individual studies. ■ Limited generalizability of findings to routine primary care practice. ■ Lack of coherence in the chain of evidence. As more information becomes available, the magnitude or direction of the observed effect could change, and this change may be large enough to alter the conclusion.
Low	The available evidence is insufficient to assess effects on health outcomes. Evidence is insufficient because of: ■ The limited number or size of studies. ■ Important flaws in study design or methods. ■ Inconsistency of findings across individual studies. ■ Gaps in the chain of evidence. ■ Findings not generalizable to routine primary care practice. ■ Lack of information on important health outcomes. More information may allow estimation of effects on health outcomes.

Source: Update on Methods: Estimating Certainty and Magnitude of Net Benefit. U.S. Preventive Services Task Force. February 2014: http://www.uspreventiveservicestaskforce.org/Page/Name/update-on-methods-estimating-certainty-and-magnitude-of-net-benefit.

Table 2-3   American College of Chest Physicians: Grading Recommendations

Grade of Recommendation/ Description	Benefit vs. Risk and Burdens	Methodologic Quality of Supporting Evidence	Implications
1A/Strong recommendation; high-quality evidence	Benefits clearly outweigh risk and burdens, or vice versa	RCTs without important limitations or overwhelming evidence from observational studies	Strong recommendation; can apply to most patients in most circumstances without reservation
1B/Strong recommendation; moderate-quality evidence	Benefits clearly outweigh risk and burdens, or vice versa	RCTs with important limitations (inconsistent results, methodologic flaws, indirect, or imprecise) or exceptionally strong evidence from observational studies	Strong recommendation; can apply to most patients in most circumstances without reservation
1C/Strong recommendation; low-quality or very low-quality evidence	Benefits clearly outweigh risk and burdens, or vice versa	Observational studies or case series	Strong recommendation but may change when higher-quality evidence becomes available
2A/Weak recommendation; high-quality evidence	Benefits closely balanced with risk and burdens	RCTs without important limitations or overwhelming evidence from observational studies	Weak recommendation; best action may differ depending on circumstances or patients' societal values

(table continues on page 40)

Table 2-3 American College of Chest Physicians: Grading Recommendations (*continued*)

Grade of Recommendation/ Description	Benefit vs. Risk and Burdens	Methodologic Quality of Supporting Evidence	Implications
2B/Weak recommendation; moderate-quality evidence	Benefits closely balanced with risk and burdens	RCTs with important limitations (inconsistent results, methodologic flaws, indirect, or imprecise) or exceptionally strong evidence from observational studies	Weak recommendation; best action may differ depending on circumstances or patients' societal values
2C/Weak recommendation; low-quality or very low-quality evidence	Uncertainty in the estimates of benefits, risks, and burden; benefits, risks, and burdens may be closely balanced	Observational studies or case series	Very weak recommendation; other alternatives may be equally reasonable

Source: Guyatt G, Gutterman D, Baumann MH, et al. Grading strength of recommendations and quality of evidence in clinical guidelines: report from an American college of chest physicians task force. *Chest.* 2006;129(1):174.

Interviewing and the Health History

The health history is a conversation with a purpose. In social conversation, you express your own needs and interests with responsibility only for yourself. The primary goal of the clinician–patient interview is to *listen* and improve the well-being of the patient through a trusting and supportive relationship. The interviewing process differs significantly from the format for the health history presented in Chapter 1. Both are fundamental to your work with patients but serve different purposes.

■ The *interviewing process* that generates the patient's story is fluid and requires empathy, effective communication, and the relational skills to respond to patient cues, feelings, and concerns. It is "open-ended," drawing on a range of techniques that affirm and empower the patient—active listening, guided questioning, nonverbal affirmation, empathic responses, validation, reassurance, summarization, and partnering. These techniques are especially pertinent to eliciting the patient's chief concerns and the History of the Present Illness.

■ The *health history format* is a structured framework for organizing patient information into written or verbal form. This format focuses your attention on the specific kinds of information you need to obtain, facilitates clinical reasoning, and clarifies communication of patient concerns, diagnoses, and plans to other health care providers involved in the patient's care. More "clinician-centered" closed-ended yes/no questions are more pertinent to the Past History, the Family History, the Personal and Social History, and, most closed-ended of all, the Review of Systems.

For new patients in the office, hospital, or long-term care setting, you will do a *comprehensive health history,* described for adults in Chapter 1. For patients who seek care for a specific complaint, such as painful urination, a more limited interview, tailored to that specific problem—sometimes called a *focused* or *problem-oriented history*—may be indicated.

The Fundamentals of Skilled Interviewing

Skilled interviewing requires the use of specific learnable techniques perfected over a lifetime. Practice these techniques and find ways to be observed or recorded so that you can receive feedback on your progress.

Active Listening. This requires listening closely to what the patient is communicating, being aware of the patient's emotional state, and using verbal and nonverbal skills to encourage the patient to continue and expand both concerns and fears.

Empathic Responses. Patients may express—with or without words—feelings they have not consciously acknowledged. Empathic responses are vital to patient rapport and convey that you experience some of the patient's suffering. *To express empathy, you must first recognize the patient's feelings.* Elicit these feelings rather than assume how the patient feels.

Respond with understanding and acceptance. Responses may be as simple as "I understand," "That sounds upsetting," or "You seem sad." Empathy also may be nonverbal—for example, placing your hand on the patient's arm if the patient is crying.

Guided Questioning. It is important to adapt your questioning to the patient's verbal and nonverbal cues.

Techniques of Guided Questioning

- Moving from open-ended to focused questions
- Using questioning that elicits a graded response
- Asking a series of questions, one at a time
- Offering multiple choices for answers
- Clarifying what the patient means
- Encouraging with continuers
- Using echoing

Proceed from the general to the specific. Directed questions should not be leading questions that call for a "yes" or "no" answer: not "Did your stools look like tar?" but "Please describe your stools."

Ask questions that require *a graded response* rather than a single answer. "What physical activity do you do that makes you short of breath?" is better than "Do you get short of breath climbing stairs?" Be sure to *ask one question at a time*. Try "Do you have any of the following problems?" Be sure to pause and establish eye contact as you list each problem.

Sometimes patients seem unable to describe symptoms. *Offer multiple-choice answers.*

For patients using words that are ambiguous, *request clarification,* as in "Tell me exactly what you meant by 'the flu.'"

Posture, actions, or words encourage the patient to say more but do not specify the topic. Nod your head or remain silent. Lean forward, make eye contact, and use *continuers* like "Mm-hmm," "Go on," or "I'm listening."

Repetition and *echoing* of the patient's words encourage the patient to express both factual details and feelings.

Nonverbal Communication. Being sensitive to nonverbal messages allows you to both "read the patient" more effectively and send messages of your own. Pay close attention to eye contact, facial expression, posture, head position and movement such as shaking or nodding, interpersonal distance, and placement of the arms or legs, such as crossed, neutral, or open. Physical contact (like placing your hand on the patient's arm) can convey empathy or help the patient gain control of feelings. You also can mirror the patient's *paralanguage,* or qualities of speech such as pacing, tone, and volume, to increase rapport. Be sensitive to cultural variations in uses and meanings of nonverbal behaviors.

Validation. An important way to make a patient feel accepted is to provide verbal support that legitimizes or validates the patient's emotional experience.

Reassurance. Avoid premature or false reassurance. Such reassurance may block further disclosures, especially if the patient feels that exposing anxiety is a weakness. *The first step to effective reassurance is identifying and accepting the patient's feelings without offering reassurance at that moment.*

Partnering. Express your desire to work with patients in an ongoing way. Reassure patients that regardless of what happens with their disease, as their provider, you are committed to a continuing partnership. Even in your role as a student, such support makes a big difference.

Summarization. Giving a capsule summary lets the patient know that you have been listening carefully. It also clarifies what you know and what you don't know. Summarization allows you to organize your clinical reasoning and to convey your thinking to the patient, which makes the relationship more collaborative.

Transitions. Tell patients when you are changing directions during the interview. This gives patients a greater sense of control.

Empowering the Patient. The clinician–patient relationship is inherently unequal. Patients have many reasons to feel vulnerable: pain, worry, feeling overwhelmed with the health care system, lack of familiarity with the clinical evaluation process. Differences of gender, ethnicity, race, or class may also create power differentials. Ultimately, patients must be empowered to take care of themselves and follow through on your advice. Review the principles below.

Empowering the Patient: Techniques for Sharing Power

- Evoke the patient's perspective.
- Convey interest in the person, not just the problem.
- Follow the patient's lead.
- Elicit and validate emotional content.
- Share information with the patient, especially at transition points during the visit.
- Make your clinical reasoning transparent to the patient.
- Reveal the limits of your knowledge.

The Sequence and Context of the Interview

Preparation, Sequence, and Cultural Context

Interviewing patients to elicit their health history requires planning.

■ **Review the clinical record.** Before seeing the patient, review the clinical record or chart. It often provides valuable information about past diagnoses and treatments; however, data may be incomplete or even disagree with what you learn from the patient, so be open to developing new approaches or ideas.

■ **Set goals for the interview.** Clarify your goals for the interview. A clinician must balance **provider-centered goals** with **patient-centered goals.** The clinician's task is to balance these multiple agendas.

■ **Review your clinical behavior and appearance.** Consciously or not, you send messages through your behavior. Posture, gestures, eye contact, and tone of voice all can express interest, attention, acceptance, and understanding. The skilled interviewer is calm and unhurried, even when time is limited. Reactions that betray disapproval, embarrassment, impatience, or boredom block communication. Patients find cleanliness, neatness, conservative dress, and a name tag reassuring.

■ **Adjust the environment.** Always consider the patient's privacy. Pull shut any bedside curtains. Suggest moving to an empty room rather than having a conversation that can be overheard.

The Sequence of the Interview

In general, an interview moves through several stages. Throughout this sequence, as the clinician, you must always stay attuned to the patient's feelings, help the patient express them, respond to their content, and validate their significance.

■ **Greet the patient and establish rapport.** *Greet the patient* by name and introduce yourself, giving your name. If possible, shake hands. If this is the first contact, explain your role, including your status as a student and how you will be involved in the patient's care. Using a title to address the patient (e.g., Mr. O'Neil, Ms. Wu) is always best. Avoid first names unless you have specific permission from the patient.

Whenever visitors are present, *maintain confidentiality.* Let the **patient** decide if visitors or family members should remain in the room, and ask for the patient's permission before conducting the interview in front of them.

Attend to the patient's comfort. Ask how he or she is feeling and if you are coming at a convenient time. Look for signs of discomfort, such as frequent changes of position or facial expressions that show pain or anxiety. Arranging the bed may make the patient more comfortable.

Consider the best way to *arrange the room.* Choose a distance that facilitates conversation and good eye contact. Try to sit at eye level with the patient. Move any physical barriers between you and the patient, such as desks or bedside tables, out of the way.

Give the patient your undivided attention. Spend enough time on small talk to put the patient at ease. If necessary, jot down short phrases, specific dates, or words rather than trying to put them into a final format. Maintain good eye contact, especially when using the electronic clinical record. Whenever the patient is talking about sensitive or disturbing material, put down your pen.

■ **Establish an agenda.** It is important to identify both your own and the patient's issues at the beginning of the encounter. Often, you may need to focus the interview by asking the patient which problem is most pressing. For example, "Do you have some special concerns today? Which one are you most concerned about?" Some patients may not have a specific complaint or problem. *It is still important to start with the patient's story.*

■ **Invite the patient's story.** Encourage patients to tell their own stories, using their own words. Begin with **open-ended questions** that allow full freedom of response: "Tell me more about…" Avoid questions that restrict the patient to a minimally informative "yes" or "no" answer. *Listen to the patient's answers without interrupting.*

Train yourself to *follow the patient's leads.* Use verbal and nonverbal cues that prompt patients to recount their stories spontaneously. Use *continuers,* especially at the outset, such as nodding your head and using phrases such as "Uh huh," "Go on," and "I see."

■ **Explore the patient's perspective.** The *disease/illness model* helps you understand the difference between your perspective and the patient's perspective. In this model, **disease** is the explanation that the *clinician* uses to organize symptoms that lead to a clinical diagnosis. **Illness** is a construct that explains how the patient experiences the disease, including its effects on relationships, function, and sense of well-being. *The health history interview needs to include both of these views of reality.*

Learning how patients perceive illness means asking patient-centered questions in the four domains listed below, which follow the mnemonic "FIFE"—Feelings, Ideas, effect on Function, and Expectations. This is crucial to patient satisfaction, effective health care, and patient follow-through.

Exploring the Patient's Perspective (F-I-F-E)

- The patient's Feelings, including fears or concerns, about the problem
- The patient's Ideas about the nature and the cause of the problem
- The effect of the problem on the patient's life and Function
- The patient's Expectations of the disease, of the clinician, or of health care, often based on prior personal or family experiences

■ **Identify and respond to the patient's emotional cues.** Patients offer various clues to their concerns that may be direct or indirect, verbal or nonverbal; they may express them as ideas or emotions. Acknowledging and responding to these clues help build rapport, expand the clinician's understanding of the illness, and improve patient satisfaction. Clues to the patient's perspective on illness are provided in the box below.

Clues to the Patient's Perspective on Illness

- Direct statement(s) by the patient of explanations, emotions, expectations, and effects of the illness
- Expression of feelings about the illness without naming the illness
- Attempts to explain or understand symptoms
- Speech clues (e.g., repetition, prolonged reflective pauses)
- Sharing a personal story
- Behavioral clues indicative of unidentified concerns, dissatisfaction, or unmet needs such as reluctance to accept recommendations, seeking a second opinion, or early appointment

Source: Lang F, Floyd MR, Beine KL. Clues to patients' explanations and concerns about their illnesses: a call for active listening. *Arch Fam Med.* 2000;9(3):222–227.

■ **Expand and clarify the patient's story.** Each symptom has attributes that must be clarified, including context, associations, and chronology, especially for pain. It is critical to understand fully every symptom's essential characteristics. *Always elicit the seven features of every symptom.*

To pursue the seven attributes, two mnemonics may help:

■ OLD CARTS, or **O**nset, **L**ocation, **D**uration, **C**haracter, **A**ggravating/**A**lleviating Factors, **R**adiation, and **T**iming; and

■ OPQRST, or **O**nset, **P**alliating/**P**rovoking Factors, **Q**uality, **R**adiation, **S**ite, and **T**iming

The Seven Attributes of a Symptom

1. **Location.** Where is it? Does it radiate?
2. **Quality.** What is it like?
3. **Quantity or severity.** How bad is it? (For pain, ask for a rating on a scale of 1 to 10.)
4. **Timing.** When did (does) it start? How long did (does) it last? How often did (does) it occur?
5. **Onset (setting in which symptom occurs).** Include environmental factors, personal activities, emotional reactions, or other circumstances that may have contributed to the illness.
6. **Remitting or exacerbating factors.** Does anything make it better or worse?
7. **Associated manifestations.** Have you noticed anything else that accompanies it?

Use language that is understandable and appropriate to the patient. Technical language confuses patients and blocks communication. Whenever possible, *repeat back the patient's words and expressions* as the history unfolds, to affirm the patient's experience as you clarify what he or she means.

Facilitate the patient's story by using different types of questions and the techniques of skilled interviewing on pp. 42–44. Often you will need to *use directed questions* (see pp. 42–43) that ask for specific information the patient has not already offered. *In general, an interview moves back and forth from open-ended questions to increasingly focused questions and then on to another open-ended question, returning the lead in the interview to the patient.*

Establishing the sequence and time course of the patient's symptoms is important. Encourage a chronologic account by asking such questions as "What then?" or "What happened next?"

■ **Generate and test diagnostic hypotheses.** As you listen to the patient's concerns, you will *generate and test diagnostic hypotheses* about which disease process might be present. Identifying all the features of each symptom is fundamental to recognizing patterns of disease and to generating the *differential diagnosis.* It is important to fully flesh out the patient's story. This avoids the common trap of *premature closure,* or shutting down the patient's story too quickly, which can lead to errors in diagnosis.

It is helpful to visualize the process of evoking a full description of each symptom(s) as "the cone" (Fig. 3-1). Each symptom has its own "cone," which becomes a paragraph in the History of Present Illness in the written record.

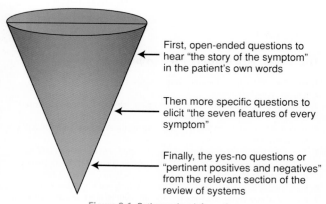

First, open-ended questions to hear "the story of the symptom" in the patient's own words

Then more specific questions to elicit "the seven features of every symptom"

Finally, the yes-no questions or "pertinent positives and negatives" from the relevant section of the review of systems

Figure 3-1 Gather patient information.

■ **Share the treatment plan.** Learning about the disease and conceptualizing the illness give you and the patient the basis for planning further evaluation (physical examination, laboratory tests, consultations, etc.). Shared decision-making involves a three-step process: introducing choices and describing options, using patient decision support tools when available; exploring patient preferences; and moving to a decision, checking that the patient is ready to make a decision and offering more time if needed. *Motivational interviewing* may help the patient achieve desired behavior changes.

The Guiding Style of Motivational Interviewing

- "Ask" open-ended questions—invite the patient to consider how and why they might change
- "Listen" to understand your patient's experience—"capture" their account with brief summaries or reflective listening statements such as "quitting smoking feels beyond you at the moment"; these express empathy, encourage the patient to elaborate, and are often the best way to respond to resistance
- "Inform"—by asking permission to provide information, and then asking what the implications might be for the patient.

Source: Quoted directly from Rollnick S, Butler CC, Kinnersly P, et al. Motivational Interviewing. *BMJ*. 2010;340:1242.

■ **Close the interview and visit.** Make sure the patient fully understands the plans you have developed together. You can say, "We need to stop now. Do you have any questions about what we've covered?" Review future evaluation, treatments, and follow-up. Give the patient a chance to ask any final questions. Ask the patient to "teach back" the plan of care to you in his or her own words.

■ **Take time for self-reflection.** As clinicians, we encounter a wide variety of people, each one unique. Because we bring our own values, assumptions, and biases to every encounter, we must look inward to clarify how our expectations and reactions may affect what we hear and how we behave. *Self-reflection brings a deepening personal awareness to our work with patients and is one of the most rewarding aspects of providing patient care.*

The Cultural Context of the Interview

Cultural Humility—a Changing Paradigm. As you provide care for an ever-expanding and diverse group of patients, it is important to understand how culture shapes not just the patient's beliefs, but your own. *Culture* is a system of shared ideas, rules, and meanings that influences how we view the world, experience it emotionally, and behave in relation to other people. This definition of culture is broader than the term *ethnicity.* The influence of culture is not limited to minority groups—it is relevant to everyone, including the culture of clinicians and their training. *Cultural competence* commonly is viewed as: "a set of attitudes, skills, behaviors, and policies that enable organizations and staff to work effectively in cross-cultural situations. It reflects the ability to acquire and use knowledge of the health-related benefits, attitudes, practices, and communication patterns of clients and their families to improve services, strengthen programs, increase community participation, and close the gaps in health status among diverse population groups."

Clinicians are increasingly challenged to adopt *cultural humility,* a "process that requires humility as individuals continually engage in self-reflection and self-critique as lifelong learners and reflective practitioners." This process includes "the difficult work of examining cultural beliefs and cultural systems of both patients and providers to locate the points of cultural dissonance or synergy that contribute to patients' health outcomes." It calls for clinicians to "bring into check the power imbalances that exist in the dynamics of (clinician)–patient communication" and maintain mutually respectful and dynamic partnerships with patients and communities. The following three-point framework will help you.

The Three Dimensions of Cultural Humility

1. *Self-awareness.* Learn about your own biases; we all have them.
2. *Respectful communication.* Work to eliminate assumptions about what is "normal." Learn directly from your patients; they are the experts on their culture and illness.
3. *Collaborative partnerships.* Build your patient relationships on respect and mutually acceptable plans.

Advanced Interviewing

Interviewing the Challenging Patient

Always remember the importance of listening to the patient and clarifying the patient's agenda.

Silent Patient. Silence has many meanings. Watch closely for nonverbal cues such as difficulty controlling emotions. You may need to shift your inquiry to symptoms of depression or begin an exploratory mental status examination. Silence may be the patient's response to how you are asking questions. Are you asking too many direct questions? Have you offended the patient?

Confusing Patient. Some patients have *multiple symptoms* or a somatization disorder. Focus on the context of the symptoms and guide the interview into a psychosocial assessment. At other times, you may be frustrated or confused. The history is vague and difficult to understand, and patients may describe symptoms in bizarre terms. Try to learn more about the unusual symptoms. Watch for delirium in acutely ill or intoxicated patients and for dementia in the elderly. When you suspect a psychiatric or neurologic disorder, shift to a mental status examination, focusing on level of consciousness, orientation, and memory.

Patient with Altered Cognition. Some patients cannot provide their own histories because of delirium, dementia, or other conditions. Others cannot relate certain parts of the history. In such cases, determine whether the patient has *decision-making capacity,* or the ability to understand information related to health, to make clinical choices based on reason and a consistent set of values, and to declare preferences about treatments. *Capacity* is a clinical designation and can be assessed by clinicians, whereas *competence* is a legal designation and can only be decided by a court. If a patient lacks capacity to make a health care decision, then identify the health care proxy or the agent with power of attorney for health care. If the patient had not identified a surrogate decision maker, then that role may shift to a spouse or family member. *It is critical to remember that decision-making capacity is both "temporal and situational."* It can fluctuate depending on the condition of the patient and the complexity of the decision involved. Many patients with psychiatric or cognitive deficits still retain the ability to make decisions.

Elements of Decision-Making Capacity

Patients must have the ability to:

1. Understand the relevant information about proposed diagnostic tests or treatment,
2. Appreciate their situation (including their underlying values and current clinical situation),
3. Use reason to make a decision, and
4. Communicate their choice.

Source: Sessums LL, Zembrzuska H, Jackson JL. Does this patient have medical decision-making capacity? *JAMA.* 2011;306:420.

For patients with capacity, obtain their consent before talking about their health with others. Consider dividing the interview into two segments—one with the patient and the other with both the patient and a second informant. Also learn the tenets of the *Health Insurance Portability and Accountability Act (HIPAA)* passed by Congress in 1996, which sets strict standards for disclosure for both institutions and providers when sharing patient information.

For patients with impaired capacity, find a *surrogate informant* or *decision maker* to assist with the history. Check whether the patient has a *durable power of attorney for health care* or a *health care proxy*. If not, in many cases, a spouse or family member can represent the patient's wishes.

Talkative Patient. Several techniques are helpful. For the first 5 or 10 minutes, listen closely. Does the patient seem obsessively detailed or unduly anxious? Is there a flight of ideas or disorganized thought process? Try to focus on what seems most important to the patient. "You've described many concerns. Let's focus on the hip pain first. Can you tell me what it feels like?" Or you can ask, "What is your #1 concern today?"

Crying Patient. Usually crying is therapeutic, as is quiet acceptance of the patient's distress. Make a facilitating or supportive remark like "I'm glad that you were able to express your feelings."

Angry or Disruptive Patient. Many patients have reasons to be angry: they are ill, they have suffered a loss, they lack accustomed control over their own lives, and they feel relatively powerless. They may direct this anger toward you. *Accept angry feelings from patients and allow them to express such emotions without getting angry in return.* Validate their feelings without agreeing with their reasons. "I understand that you felt very frustrated by the long wait and answering the same questions over and over." Some angry patients become hostile and disruptive. Before approaching them, alert security. Stay calm, appear accepting, and avoid being challenging. Keep your posture relaxed and nonthreatening. Once you have established rapport, gently suggest moving to a different location.

Patient with a Language Barrier. If the patient speaks a different language, make every effort to find a trained interpreter. The ideal interpreter is a neutral, objective person trained in both languages and cultures. Avoid using family members or friends: confidentiality may be violated. As you work with the interpreter, *make questions clear, short, and simple.* Speak directly to the patient. Bilingual written questionnaires are valuable.

Guidelines for Working with an Interpreter: "INTERPRET"

I   **Introductions:** Make sure to introduce all the individuals in the room. During the introduction, include information as to the roles individuals will play.

N   **Note Goals:** Note the goals of the interview. What is the diagnosis? What will the treatment entail? Will there be any follow-up?

T   **Transparency:** Let the patient know that everything said will be interpreted throughout the session.

(continued)

Guidelines for Working with an Interpreter: "INTERPRET" (Continued)

E   **Ethics:** Use qualified interpreters (not family members or children) when conducting an interview. Qualified interpreters allow the patient to maintain autonomy and make informed decisions about his or her care.

R   **Respect Beliefs:** Limited English Proficient (LEP) patients may have cultural beliefs that need to be taken into account as well. The interpreter may be able to serve as a cultural broker and help explain any cultural beliefs that may exist.

P   **Patient Focus:** The patient should remain the focus of the encounter. Providers should interact with the patient and not the interpreter. Make sure to ask and address any questions the patient may have prior to ending the encounter. If you don't have trained interpreters on staff, the patient may not be able to call in with questions.

R   **Retain Control:** It is important as the provider that you remain in control of the interaction and not let the patient or the interpreter take over the conversation.

E   **Explain:** Use simple language and short sentences when working with an interpreter. This will ensure that comparable words can be found in the second language and that all the information can be conveyed clearly.

T   **Thanks:** Thank the interpreter and the patient for their time. On the chart, note that the patient needs an interpreter and who served as an interpreter this time.

Source: U.S. Department of Health and Human Services. Interpret Tool: working with interpreters in cultural settings. Available at https:www.thinkculturalhealth.hhs.gov/pdfs/InterpretTool.pdf. Accessed May 3, 2016.

Patient with Low Literacy or Low Health Literacy.   Assess the ability to read. Some patients may try to hide their reading problems. Ask the patient to read whatever instructions you have written. Simply handing the patient written material upside down to see if the patient turns it around may settle the question. Assess *health literacy*, or the skills to function effectively in the health care system: interpreting documents, reading labels and medication instructions, and speaking and listening effectively.

Patient with Hearing Loss.   Find out the patient's preferred method of communicating. Patients may use American Sign Language, a unique language with its own syntax, or various other communication forms combining signs and speech. Determine whether the patient identifies with the Deaf or Hearing culture. Handwritten questions and answers may be the best solution. When patients have *partial hearing impairment* or can *read lips,* face them directly, in good light. If the patient has a *unilateral hearing loss,* sit on the hearing side. If the patient has a *hearing aid,* make sure it is working. Eliminate background noise such as television.

Patient with Impaired Vision. Shake hands to establish contact and explain who you are and why you are there. If the room is unfamiliar, orient the patient to the surroundings.

Patient with Limited Intelligence. Patients of moderately limited intelligence usually can give adequate histories. Pay special attention to the patient's schooling and ability to function independently. How far has the patient gone in school? If he or she didn't finish, why not? Assess simple calculations, vocabulary, memory, and abstract thinking. For patients with severe mental retardation, obtain the history from the family or caregivers. Avoid "talking down" or using condescending behavior. The sexual history is equally important and often overlooked.

Patient with Personal Problems. Patients may ask you for advice about personal problems outside the range of health. Letting the patient talk through the problem is usually more valuable and therapeutic than any answer you could give.

Seductive Patient. The emotional and physical intimacy of the clinician–patient relationship may lead to sexual feelings. If you become aware of such feelings, accept them as a normal human response, and bring them to the conscious level so they will not affect your behavior. Denying these feelings makes it more likely that you will act inappropriately. *Any* sexual contact or romantic relationship with patients is *unethical;* keep your relationship with the patient within professional bounds and seek help if you need it.

Sensitive Topics

Guidelines for Broaching Sensitive Topics

- The single most important rule is to be nonjudgmental. Your role is to learn from the patient and help the patient achieve better health. Acceptance is the best way to reach this goal.
- Explain why you need to know certain information. This makes patients less apprehensive. For example, say to patients, "Because sexual practices put people at risk for certain diseases, I ask all of my patients the following questions."
- Find opening questions for sensitive topics and learn the specific kinds of information needed for your shared assessment and plan.
- Consciously acknowledge whatever discomfort you are feeling. Denying your discomfort may lead you to avoid the topic altogether.

The Sexual History. You can introduce questions about sexual function and practices at multiple points in a patient's history. An orienting sentence or two is often helpful. "Now I'd like to ask you some questions about your sexual health and practices" or "I routinely ask all patients about their sexual function."

The Sexual History: Sample Questions

- "When was the last time you had intimate physical contact with someone?" "Did that contact include sexual intercourse?" The term "sexually active" can be ambiguous. Patients have been known to reply, "No, I just lie there."
- "Do you have sex with men, women, or both?" Patients may have same-sex partners yet not consider themselves gay, lesbian, or bisexual. Some gay and lesbian patients have had opposite-sex partners.
- "How many sexual partners have you had in the last 6 months? In the last 5 years? In your lifetime?" These questions make it easy for the patient to acknowledge multiple partners. Ask, "Have you had any new partners in the past 6 months?" If patients question why this information is important, explain that new partners or multiple partners over a lifetime can raise the risk for STIs. Ask about routine use of condoms. "How often do you use condoms?" is an open-ended question that does not presume an answer.
- It is important to ask all patients, "Do you have any concerns about HIV infection or AIDS?" since infection can occur in the absence of risk factors.

Mental Health History. Cultural constructs of mental illness vary widely, causing marked differences in acceptance and attitudes. Ask open-ended questions initially: "Have you ever had any problem with emotional or mental illnesses?" Then move to more specific questions: "Have you ever visited a counselor or psychotherapist?" "Have you taken medication for emotional issues?" "Have you or a family member ever been hospitalized for a mental health problem?"

Be sensitive to reports of mood changes or symptoms such as fatigue, tearfulness, appetite or weight changes, insomnia, and vague somatic complaints. Two validated screening questions are: "Over the past 2 weeks, have you felt down, depressed, or hopeless?" and "Over the past 2 weeks, have you felt little interest or pleasure in doing things?" Ask about thoughts of suicide: "Have you ever thought about hurting yourself or ending your life?" Evaluate severity.

Many patients with schizophrenia or other psychotic disorders can function in the community and tell you about their diagnoses, symptoms, hospitalizations, and medications. Investigate their symptoms and assess any effects on mood or daily activities.

Alcohol and Prescription and Illicit Drugs. Clinicians should routinely ask about current and past use of alcohol or drugs, patterns of use, and family history. Be familiar with the definitions below:

Addiction, Physical Dependence, and Tolerance

Tolerance: A state of adaptation in which exposure to a drug induces changes that result in a diminution of one or more of the drug's effects over time.

Physical Dependence: A state of adaptation that is manifested by a drug class-specific withdrawal syndrome that can be produced by abrupt cessation, rapid dose reduction, decreasing blood level of the drug, and/or administration of an antagonist.

Addiction: A primary, chronic, neurobiologic disease, with genetic, psychosocial, and environmental factors influencing its development and manifestations. It is characterized by behaviors that include one or more of the following: impaired control over drug use, compulsive use, continued use despite harm, and craving.

Source: American Pain Society. Definitions Related to the Use of Opioids for the Treatment of Pain. A consensus statement from the American Academy of Pain Medicine, the American Pain Society, and the American Society of Addiction Medicine, 2001. Available at http://www.asam.org/docs/publicy-policy-statements/1opioid-definitions-consensus-2-011.pdf?sfvrsn=0. Accessed May 3, 2016.

Alcohol. For assessing alcohol intake, "What do you like to drink?" or "Tell me about your use of alcohol" are good opening questions that avoid the easy yes or no response. The most widely used screening questions are the CAGE questions about Cutting down, Annoyance when criticized, Guilty feelings, and Eye-openers. Two or more affirmative answers to the CAGE questions suggest alcoholism. The CAGE Questionnaire is readily available online.

Also ask about blackouts (loss of memory for events during drinking), seizures, accidents or injuries while drinking, job loss, marital conflict, or legal problems. Ask specifically about drinking while driving or operating machinery.

Prescription and Illicit Drugs. Questions about drugs are similar. "How much marijuana do you use? Cocaine? Heroin? Amphetamines?" (Ask about each one by name.) "How about prescription drugs such as sleeping pills?" "Diet pills?" "Painkillers?" Use the CAGE questions but relate them to drug use. With adolescents, it may be helpful to ask about substance use by friends or family members first. "A lot of young people are using drugs these days. How about at your school? Your friends?"

Intimate Partner Violence and Domestic Violence. Many authorities recommend routine screening of all female and older adult patients for domestic violence. Start with general "normalizing" questions: "Because abuse is common in many women's lives, I've begun to ask about it routinely." "Are there times in your relationships that you feel unsafe or afraid?" "Have you ever been hit, kicked, punched, or hurt by someone you know?"

Clues to Physical and Sexual Abuse

- Injuries that are unexplained, seem inconsistent with the patient's story, are concealed by the patient, or cause embarrassment
- Delay in getting treatment for trauma
- History of repeated injuries or "accidents"
- Presence of alcohol or drug abuse in patient or partner
- Partner tries to dominate the visit, will not leave the room, or seems unusually anxious or solicitous
- Pregnancy at a young age; multiple partners
- Repeated vaginal infections and STIs
- Difficulty walking or sitting due to genital/anal pain
- Vaginal lacerations or bruises
- Fear of the pelvic examination or physical contact
- Fear of leaving the examination room

Death and the Dying Patient. Work through your own feelings with the help of reading and discussion. Kübler-Ross has described five stages in our response to loss or the anticipatory grief of impending death: denial and isolation, anger, bargaining, depression or sadness, and acceptance. These stages may occur sequentially or overlap in different combinations. Dying patients rarely want to talk about their illnesses all the time, nor do they wish to confide in everyone they meet. Give them opportunities to talk and then listen receptively, but be supportive if they prefer to stay at a social level.

Understanding the patient's wishes about treatment at the end of life is an important clinician responsibility. Even if discussions of death and dying are difficult, you must learn to ask specific questions. Ask about Do Not Resuscitate (DNR) status. Find out about the patient's frame of reference. "What experiences have you had with the death of a close friend or relative?" "What do you know about cardiopulmonary resuscitation (CPR)?" Assure patients that relieving pain and taking care of their other spiritual and physical needs will be a priority. Encourage any adult, but especially the elderly or chronically ill, to establish a *health care proxy,* an individual who can act for the patient in life-threatening situations.

Ethics and Professionalism

Clinical ethics come into play in almost every patient interaction. Fundamental maxims are as follows:

Building Blocks of Professional Ethics in Patient Care

- *Nonmaleficence* or *primum non nocere*, commonly stated as, "First, do no harm."
- *Beneficence*, or the dictum that the clinician needs to "do good" for the patient. As clinicians, our responsibility is to always act in the best interest of the patient.
- *Autonomy*, whereby informed patients have the right to determine what is in their own best interest.
- *Confidentiality*, meaning that we are obligated not to tell others what we learn from our patients. Note that some frameworks posit Justice as the fourth critical principle, namely that all patients be treated fairly with equitable distribution of health care resources.

The Tavistock Principles guide behavior in health care for both individuals and institutions.

The Tavistock Principles

Rights: People have a right to health and health care.
Balance: Care of individual patients is central, but the health of populations is also our concern.
Comprehensiveness: In addition to treating illness, we have an obligation to ease suffering, minimize disability, prevent disease, and promote health.
Cooperation: Health care succeeds only if we cooperate with those we serve, each other, and those in other sectors.
Improvement: Improving health care is a serious and continuing responsibility.
Safety: Do no harm.
Openness: Being open, honest, and trustworthy is vital in health care.

Beginning the Physical Examination: General Survey, Vital Signs, and Pain

The Health History

Common or Concerning Symptoms

- Fatigue and weakness
- Fever, chills, and night sweats
- Weight change
- Pain

Fatigue and Weakness. *Fatigue* is a nonspecific symptom with many causes. Use open-ended questions to explore the attributes of the patient's fatigue, and encourage the patient to fully describe what he or she is experiencing.

Weakness differs from fatigue. It denotes a demonstrable loss of muscle power and will be discussed later with other neurologic symptoms.

Fever, Chills, and Night Sweats. Ask about fever if the patient has an acute or chronic illness. Find out whether the patient has used a thermometer to measure the temperature. Distinguish between *feeling cold* and a *shaking chill*, with shivering throughout the body and chattering of teeth. *Night sweats* raise concerns about tuberculosis or malignancy.

Focus your questions on the timing of the illness and its associated symptoms. Become familiar with patterns of infectious diseases that may affect your patient. Inquire about travel, contact with sick people, or other unusual exposures. Be sure to inquire about medications, as they may cause fever. In contrast, recent ingestion of aspirin, acetaminophen, corticosteroids, and nonsteroidal anti-inflammatory drugs may mask fever.

Weight Change. Good opening questions include "How often do you check your weight?" and "How is it compared to a year ago?"

■ *Weight gain* occurs when caloric intake exceeds caloric expenditure over time. It also may reflect abnormal accumulation of body fluids.

■ *Weight loss* has many causes: decreased food intake, dysphagia, vomiting, and insufficient supplies of food; defective absorption of nutrients; increased metabolic requirements; and loss of nutrients through the urine, feces, or injured skin. Also consider chronic illnesses, malignancy, and abuse of alcohol, cocaine, amphetamines, or opiates, or withdrawal from marijuana. Be alert for signs of malnutrition.

Pain. Each year, approximately 100 million Americans report chronic pain, often underassessed. Adopt the comprehensive approach found on pp. 69–71.

Health Promotion and Counseling: Evidence and Recommendations

Important Topics for Health Promotion and Counseling

- Optimal weight, nutrition, and diet
- Blood pressure and dietary sodium
- Exercise

Optimal Weight, Nutrition, and Diet. Nearly 69% of U.S. adults are overweight (BMI ≥25 to 29 kg/m^2) or obese (BMI ≥30 kg/m^2). Obesity has increased in every segment of the population. More than 80% of people with type 2 diabetes and roughly 20% of those with hypertension or elevated cholesterol levels are overweight or obese. Increasing obesity in children contributes to rising rates of childhood diabetes. Reducing weight by even 5% to 10% can improve blood pressure, lipid levels, and glucose tolerance, and reduce the risk of diabetes and hypertension. Diet recommendations hinge on assessment of the patient's motivation and readiness to lose weight and individual risk factors.

Four Steps to Promote Optimal Weight and Nutrition

1. Measure BMI and waist circumference; adults with a BMI ≥25 kg/m², men with waist circumferences >40 inches, and women with waist circumferences >35 inches are at increased risk for heart disease and obesity-related diseases. Ratios >0.95 in men and >0.85 in women are considered elevated. Determine additional risk factors for cardiovascular diseases, including smoking, high blood pressure, high cholesterol, physical inactivity, and family history.
2. Assess dietary intake.
3. Assess the patient's motivation to change.
4. Provide counseling about nutrition and exercise.

Review the 2010 dietary guidelines of the U.S. Department of Agriculture and counsel patients to turn to its helpful *MyPlate icon and website.*

Blood Pressure and Dietary Sodium. The Institute of Medicine (IOM) recommends a maximum daily dietary intake of 2,300 mg of sodium for adults to reduce risk of hypertension. Advise patients to read the Nutrition Facts panel on food labels to help them adhere to the 2,300-mg/day guideline and to consider adopting the well-investigated Dietary Approaches to Stop Hypertension, or DASH Eating Plan (see Table 4-1, Patients with Hypertension: Recommended Changes in Diet, p. 72).

Exercise. Adults should do at least 150 minutes (2 hours and 30 minutes) of moderate-intensity cardiorespiratory activity, for example, walking briskly at a pace of 3 to 4.5 miles per hour, each week. Alternatively, adults can engage in vigorous-intensity aerobic activity, such as jogging or running, for 75 minutes (1 hour and 15 minutes) each week. Patients can increase exercise by such simple measures as parking further away from their place of work or using stairs instead of elevators.

Techniques of Examination

EXAMINATION TECHNIQUES

POSSIBLE FINDINGS

General Survey

Apparent State of Health

Acutely or chronically ill, frail, robust, vigorous

Level of Consciousness. Is the patient awake, alert, and interactive?

If not, promptly assess level of consciousness (see p. 332)

EXAMINATION TECHNIQUES	POSSIBLE FINDINGS

Signs of Distress

- Cardiac or respiratory distress

Clutching the chest, pallor, diaphoresis; labored breathing, wheezing, cough

- Pain

Wincing, sweating, protecting painful area

- Anxiety or depression

Anxious face, fidgety movements, cold and moist palms; inexpressive or flat affect, poor eye contact, psychomotor slowing

Skin Color and Obvious Lesions. See Chapter 6, *The Skin, Hair, and Nails*, for details.

Pallor, cyanosis, jaundice, rashes, bruises

Dress, Grooming, and Personal Hygiene

- How is the patient dressed? Is the clothing suitable for the temperature and weather? Is it clean and appropriate to the setting?

Body piercing or tattoos can be associated with alcohol and drug use.

- Note patient's hair, fingernails, and use of make-up.

These may be clues to the patient's personality, mood, lifestyle, and self-regard.

Facial Expression. Watch for eye contact. Is it natural? Sustained and unblinking? Averted quickly? Absent?

Stare of hyperthyroidism; flat or sad affect of depression. Decreased eye contact may be cultural or may suggest anxiety, fear, or sadness.

Odors of Body and Breath. Odors can be important diagnostic clues.

Breath odor of alcohol, acetone (diabetes), uremia, or liver failure. Fruity odor of diabetes. (Never assume that alcohol on a patient's breath explains changes in mental status or neurologic findings.)

Posture, Gait, and Motor Activity

Preference to sit up in left-sided heart failure and to lean forward with arms braced in chronic obstructive pulmonary disease (COPD).

POSSIBLE FINDINGS

Height and Weight

Height. Measure the patient's height in stocking feet. Note the build—muscular or deconditioned, tall or short. Observe the body proportions.

Short stature in Turner syndrome; elongated arms in Marfan syndrome; loss of height in osteoporosis.

Weight. Is the patient emaciated? Plump? If obese, is there central or dispersed distribution of fat? Weigh the patient with shoes off.

Obesity (BMI ≥30 kg/m²) increases risk of diabetes, heart disease, stroke, hypertension, osteoarthritis, sleep apnea syndrome, and some forms of cancer.

Calculate the *body mass index* (BMI), which incorporates estimated but more accurate measurements of body fat than weight alone.

Methods to Calculate Body Mass Index (BMI)

Unit of Measure	Method of Calculation
Weight in pounds, height in inches	(1) Standard BMI Chart
	(2) $\left(\dfrac{\text{Weight (lb)} \times 700^a}{\text{Height (inches)}} \right)$
Weight *in kilograms, height in meters squared*	(3) $\dfrac{\text{Weight (kg)}}{\text{Height (m}^2)}$
Either unit of measure	(4) "BMI Calculator" at http://www.nhlbi.nih.gov/health/educational/lose_wt/BMI/bmicalc.htm

^{a}Several organizations use 704.5, but the variation in BMI is negligible. Conversion formulas: 2.2 lb = 1 kg; 1 inch = 2.54 cm; 100 cm = 1 m.
Source: National Institutes of Health–National Heart, Lung, and Blood Institute: Calculate Your Body Mass Index. Available at: http://www.nhlbi.nih.gov/health/educational/lose_wt/BMI/bmicalc.htm. Accessed January 21, 2015.

If the BMI is *above* 25, engage the patient in a 24-hour dietary recall and compare the intake of food groups and number of servings per day with current recommendations. Or, choose a screening tool and provide appropriate counseling or referral (see Table 4-2, Nutrition Screening, p. 73, and Table 4-3, Nutrition Counseling, p. 74).

If the BMI falls *below* 17, be concerned about possible anorexia nervosa, bulimia, or other medical conditions (see Table 4-4, Eating Disorders and Excessively Low BMI, p. 75).

The Vital Signs: Blood Pressure, Heart Rate, Respiratory Rate, and Temperature

Blood Pressure

Methods for Measuring Blood Pressure. Office screening with *manual and automated cuffs* remains common, but elevated readings increasingly require confirmation with *home and ambulatory monitoring*, which are more predictive of cardiovascular disease and end-organ damage than manual and automated measurements in the office. Automated ambulatory blood pressure monitoring measures blood pressure at preset intervals over 24 to 48 hours, usually every 15 to 20 minutes during the day and 30 to 60 minutes during the night. Be familiar with these different methods of blood pressure measurement and their varying criteria for hypertension.

Types of Hypertension. Three types of hypertension are especially important to recognize, described below. Suspicion of these entities and assessing the effects of treatment are indications for ambulatory blood pressure monitoring.

Types of Hypertension

White coat hypertension (isolated clinic hypertension)	Blood pressure ≥140/90 in medical settings and mean awake ambulatory readings <135/85. Reported in up to 20% of patients with elevated office blood pressure Carries normal to slightly increased cardiovascular risk and does not require treatment; attributed to a conditioned anxiety response
Masked hypertension	Blood pressure <140/90, but an elevated daytime blood pressure of >135/85 on home or ambulatory testing Reported in an estimated 10% to 30% of the general population If untreated, it increases risk of cardiovascular disease and end-organ damage

(continued)

Types of Hypertension (Continued)

Nocturnal hypertension	Physiologic blood pressure "dipping" occurs in most patients as they shift from wakefulness to sleep A nocturnal fall of <10% of daytime values is associated with poor cardiovascular outcomes and can only be identified on 24-hour ambulatory blood pressure monitoring Two other patterns have poor cardiovascular outcomes, a nocturnal rising pattern and a marked nocturnal fall of >20% of daytime values

Selecting the Correct Size Blood Pressure Cuff

It is important for clinicians and patients to use a cuff that fits the patient's arm. Follow the guidelines outlined here for selecting the correct size:

- Width of the inflatable bladder of the cuff should be about 40% of upper arm circumference (about 12 to 14 cm in the average adult).
- Length of the inflatable bladder should be about 80% of upper arm circumference (almost long enough to encircle the arm).
- The standard cuff is 12 × 23 cm, appropriate for arm circumferences up to 28 cm.

Steps to Ensure Accurate Blood Pressure Measurement

1. The patient should avoid smoking or drinking caffeinated beverages for 30 minutes before the blood pressure is taken and rest for at least 5 minutes.
2. Make sure the examining room is quiet and comfortably warm.
3. Make sure the arm selected is *free of clothing*. There should be no arteriovenous fistulas for dialysis, scarring from prior brachial artery cutdowns, or signs of lymphedema (seen after axillary node dissection or radiation therapy).
4. Palpate the brachial artery to confirm that it has a viable pulse.
5. Position the arm so that the brachial artery, at the antecubital crease, is *at heart level*—roughly level with the 4th interspace at its junction with the sternum.
6. If the patient is seated, rest the arm on a table a little above the patient's waist; if standing, try to support the patient's arm at the midchest level.

Measuring Blood Pressure

- Center the inflatable bladder over the brachial artery. The lower border of the cuff should be about 2.5 cm above the antecubital crease. Secure the cuff snugly. Position the patient's arm so that it is slightly flexed at the elbow.
- To determine how high to raise the cuff pressure, first estimate the systolic pressure by palpation. As you feel the radial artery with the fingers of one hand, rapidly inflate the cuff until the radial pulse disappears. Read this pressure on the manometer and add 30 mm Hg to it. Use of this sum as the target for subsequent inflations prevents discomfort from unnecessarily high cuff pressures. It also avoids the occasional error caused by an auscultatory gap—a silent interval between the systolic and diastolic pressures.
- Deflate the cuff promptly.
- Now place the bell of a stethoscope lightly over the brachial artery, taking care to make an air seal with its full rim. Because the sounds to be heard *(Korotkoff sounds)* are relatively low in pitch, they are heard better with the *bell*.
- Inflate the cuff rapidly again to the level just determined, and then deflate it slowly, at a rate of about 2 to 3 mm Hg per second. Note the level at which you hear the sounds of at least two consecutive beats. This is the *systolic pressure.*
- Continue to lower the pressure slowly. The disappearance point, usually only a few mm Hg below the muffling point, is the best estimate of *diastolic pressure.*
- Read both the systolic and diastolic levels to the nearest 2 mm Hg. Wait 2 or more minutes and repeat. Average your readings. If the first two readings differ by more than 5 mm Hg, take additional readings.
- Take blood pressure in both arms at least once.
- In patients taking antihypertensive medications or with a history of fainting, postural dizziness, or possible depletion of blood volume, take the blood pressure in two positions—supine and standing (unless contraindicated). A fall in systolic pressure of 20 mm Hg or more within 3 minutes after standing up, especially when accompanied by symptoms, indicates *orthostatic (postural) hypotension.*

In 2013, the Joint National Committee on Detection, Evaluation, and Treatment of High Blood Pressure (JNC) updated the classification of systolic blood pressure (SBP) and diastolic blood pressure (DBP).

JNC 8 Blood Pressure Classification for Adults

Category	Systolic (mm Hg)	Diastolic (mm Hg)
Normal	<120	<80
Prehypertension	120–139	80–89
Stage 1 hypertension		
Ages ≥18 to <60 years; diabetes or renal disease	140–159	90–99
Age ≥60 years[a]	150–159	90–99
Stage 2 hypertension	≥160	≥100

[a]The American Society of Hypertension raises this cutoff to age ≥80 years.

When the systolic and diastolic levels fall in different categories, use the higher category. For example, 170/92 mm Hg is Stage 2 hypertension; 135/100 mm Hg is Stage 1 hypertension. In *isolated systolic hypertension*, SBP is ≥140 mm Hg, and DBP is <90 mm Hg.

Heart Rate. The radial pulse is used commonly to count the heart rate. With the pads of your index and middle fingers, compress the radial artery until you detect a maximal pulsation (Fig. 4-1). If the rhythm is regular, count the rate for 15 seconds and multiply by 4. If the rate is unusually fast or slow, count it for 60 seconds. When the rhythm is irregular, evaluate the rate by auscultation at the cardiac apex (the apical pulse).

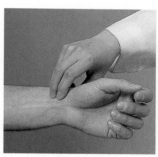
Figure 4-1 Palpate the radial pulse.

EXAMINATION TECHNIQUES	POSSIBLE FINDINGS
Rhythm. Palpate the radial pulse. Check the rhythm again by listening with your stethoscope at the cardiac apex. Is the rhythm regular or irregular? If irregular, try to identify a pattern: (1) Do early beats appear in a basically regular rhythm? (2) Does the irregularity vary consistently with respiration? (3) Is the rhythm totally irregular?	Palpation of an irregularly irregular rhythm reliably indicates *atrial fibrillation*. For all irregular patterns, an ECG is needed to identify the arrhythmia.
Respiratory Rate and Rhythm. Observe the *rate, rhythm, depth,* and *effort of breathing.* Count the number of respirations in 1 minute either by visual inspection or by subtly listening over the patient's trachea with your stethoscope during examination of the head and neck or chest. Normally, adults take 14 to 20 breaths per minute in a quiet, regular pattern.	See Table 8-4, p. 162, Abnormalities in Rate and Rhythm of Breathing.

EXAMINATION TECHNIQUES	POSSIBLE FINDINGS

Temperature. Average *oral temperature*, usually 37°C (98.6°F), fluctuates considerably from the early morning to the late afternoon or evening. *Rectal temperatures are higher* than oral temperatures by about 0.4 to 0.5°C (0.7 to 0.9°F) but also vary. *Axillary temperatures are lower* than oral temperatures by approximately 1°C but take 5 to 10 minutes to register and are considered less accurate than other measurements.

Tympanic membrane temperatures can be more variable than oral or rectal temperatures. Studies suggest that in adults, *oral and temporal artery temperatures* correlate more closely with the pulmonary artery temperature, but are about 0.5°C lower.

Oral temperatures: Choose either glass or electronic thermometer.

■ *Glass thermometer:* Shake the thermometer down to 35°C (96°F) or below, insert it under the tongue, instruct the patient to close both lips, and wait 3 to 5 minutes. Then read the thermometer, reinsert for 1 minute, and read it again. Avoid breakage.

■ *Electronic thermometer:* Carefully place the disposable cover over the probe and insert the thermometer under the tongue for about 10 seconds.

Rectal temperatures: Position the patient on one side with the hip flexed. Select a rectal thermometer with a stubby tip, lubricate it, and

Fever or pyrexia refers to an elevated body temperature. *Hyperpyrexia* refers to extreme elevation in temperature, above 41.1°C (106°F), while *hypothermia* refers to an abnormally low temperature, below 35°C (95°F) rectally.

Causes of *fever* include infection, trauma (such as surgery or crush injuries), malignancy, blood disorders (such as acute hemolytic anemia), drug reactions, and immune disorders such as collagen vascular disease.

The chief cause of *hypothermia* is exposure to cold. Other causes include reduced movement as in paralysis, interference with vasoconstriction as from sepsis or excess alcohol, starvation, hypothyroidism, and hypoglycemia. Older adults are especially susceptible to hypothermia and also less likely to develop fever.

Taking rectal temperatures is common practice in unresponsive patients or those at risk for biting down on the thermometer.

EXAMINATION TECHNIQUES	POSSIBLE FINDINGS

insert it about 3 to 4 cm
(1½ inches) into the anal canal,
in a direction pointing to the umbilicus. Remove it after 3 minutes,
then read. Alternatively, use an
electronic thermometer after lubri-
cating the probe cover. Wait about
10 seconds for the digital temperature recording to appear.

Tympanic membrane temperature:
Make sure the external auditory
canal is free of cerumen. Position
the probe in the canal. Wait 2 to
3 seconds until the digital reading
appears. This method measures
core body temperature, which is
higher than the normal oral temperature by approximately 0.8°C
(11.4°F).

Temporal artery temperature:
Place the probe against the center
of the forehead, depress the infra-
red scanning button, and brush the
device across the forehead, down
the cheek, and behind an earlobe.
Read the display, which records
the highest measure temperature.
Industry information suggests that
combined forehead and behind-
the-ear contact is more accurate
than scanning only the forehead.

Acute and Chronic Pain

The experience of pain is complex and multifactorial. It involves sensory,
emotional, and cognitive processing but may lack a specific physical
etiology.

Chronic pain is defined in several ways: pain not associated with cancer or
other clinical conditions that persists for more than 3 to 6 months; pain
lasting more than 1 month beyond the course of an acute illness or injury;
or pain recurring at intervals of months or years. Chronic noncancer pain
affects 5% to 33% of patients in primary care settings.

Adopt a multidisciplinary measurement-based approach to assessing pain, carefully listening to the patient's story, and any contributing factors. Pursue the seven features of pain, as you would with any symptom. Accept the patient's self-report, which experts state is the most reliable indicator of pain.

Location: Ask the patient to point to the pain. Lay terms may not be specific enough to localize the site of origin.

Severity: Use a consistent method to determine severity. Three scales are common: the Visual Analog Scale, and two scales using ratings from 1 to 10—the Numeric Rating Scale and the Faces Pain Scale.

Contributing Factors. Be sure to ask about any treatments that the patient has tried, including medications, physical therapy, and alternative medicines. A comprehensive medication history helps you to identify drugs that interact with analgesics and reduce their efficacy.

Identify any comorbid conditions such as arthritis, diabetes, HIV/AIDS, substance abuse, sickle cell disease, or psychiatric disorders. These can significantly affect the patient's experience of pain.

Health Disparities. Be aware of the well-documented health disparities in pain treatment and delivery of care, which range from lower use of analgesics in emergency rooms for African-American and Hispanic patients to disparities in use of analgesics for cancer, postoperative, and low back pain. Clinician stereotypes, language barriers, and unconscious clinician biases in decision making all contribute to these disparities. Critique your own communication style, seek information and best practice standards, and improve your techniques of patient education and empowerment.

Pain Management. Managing pain is a complex clinical challenge.

Experts recommend a stepped-care approach, with an emphasis on measurement and tracking tools to follow responses to treatment and referrals to specialists, summarized below.

Managing Chronic Pain: Steps for Measurement-Based Care

Step 1: *Measure pain intensity and pain interference.* A validated 2-item questionnaire is available for primary care asking patients to rate pain in the past month and interference with daily activities on a scale of 1 to 10.

Step 2: *Measure mood.* Treatable depression, anxiety, and posttraumatic stress disorder (PTSD) frequently accompany chronic pain. The PHQ-4 is a 4-item questionnaire for detecting anxiety and depression. The Primary Care-PTSD is a 4-question screen for PTSD.

(continued)

Managing Chronic Pain: Steps for Measurement-Based Care (Continued)

Step 3: *Measure the effect of pain on sleep.* Opioid doses correlate with sleep-disordered breathing and sleep apnea.

Step 4: Measure risk of co-occurring substance abuse, estimated at 18% to 30%.

Step 5: *Measure the opioid dose* and calculate the opioid dose equivalency using available web-based calculators.

Source: Tauben D. Chronic pain management: measurement-based stepped care solutions. Pain: Clinical Updates. International Association for the Study of Pain. December 2012. Available at http://www.iasp-pain.org/PublicationsNews/NewsletterIssue. aspx?ItemNumber=2064. Accessed January 28, 2015.

Recording Your Findings

Record the vital signs taken at the time of your examination. They are preferable to those taken earlier in the day by other providers. (Common abbreviations for blood pressure, heart rate, and respiratory rate are self-explanatory.)

Recording the Physical Examination—General Survey and Vital Signs

- "Mrs. Scott is a young, healthy-appearing woman, well-groomed, fit, and in good spirits. Height is 5′4″, weight 135 lb, BP 120/80, HR 72 and regular, RR 16, temperature 37.5°C."

OR

- "Mr. Jones is an elderly man who looks pale and chronically ill. He is alert, with good eye contact, but cannot speak more than two or three words at a time because of shortness of breath. He has intercostal muscle retraction when breathing and sits upright in bed. He is thin, with diffuse muscle wasting. Height is 6′2″, weight 175 lb, BP 160/95, HR 108 and irregular, RR 32 and labored, temperature 101.2°F." *(These findings suggest COPD exacerbation.)*

Aids to Interpretation

Table 4-1   Patients with Hypertension: Recommended Changes in Diet

Dietary Change	Food Source
Increase foods high in potassium	Baked white or sweet potatoes, white beans, beet greens, soybeans, spinach, lentils, kidney beans
	Yogurt
	Tomato paste, juice, puree, and sauce
	Bananas, plantains, many dried fruits, orange juice
Decrease foods high in sodium	Canned foods (soups, tuna fish)
	Pretzels, potato chips, pizza, pickles, olives
	Many processed foods (frozen dinners, ketchup, mustard)
	Batter-fried foods
	Table salt, including for cooking

Source: Adapted from: U.S. Department of Agriculture and U.S. Department of Health and Human Services. Dietary Guidelines for Americans, 2010. Washington, D.C.: U.S. Government Printing Office; 2010; Choose MyPlate.gov. Available at http://www.choosemyplate.gov/index.html. Accessed December 15, 2014; Office of Dietary Supplements, National Institutes of Health. Dietary Supplement Fact Sheets: Calcium; Vitamin D. Available at http://ods.od.nih.gov/factsheets/list-all/. Accessed December 15, 2014.

Table 4-2   Nutrition Screening

Mini Nutritional Assessment
MNA®

Nestlé
NutritionInstitute

Last name:			First name:	
Sex:	Age:	Weight, kg:	Height, cm:	Date:

Complete the screen by filling in the boxes with the appropriate numbers. Total the numbers for the final screening score.

Screening

A Has food intake declined over the past 3 months due to loss of appetite, digestive problems, chewing or swallowing difficulties?

0 = severe decrease in food intake
1 = moderate decrease in food intake
2 = no decrease in food intake   ☐

B Weight loss during the last 3 months

0 = weight loss greater than 3 kg (6.6 lbs)
1 = does not know
2 = weight loss between 1 and 3 kg (2.2 and 6.6 lbs)
3 = no weight loss   ☐

C Mobility

0 = bed or chair bound
1 = able to get out of bed / chair but does not go out
2 = goes out   ☐

D Has suffered psychological stress or acute disease in the past 3 months?

0 = yes   2 = no   ☐

E Neuropsychological problems

0 = severe dementia or depression
1 = mild dementia
2 = no psychological problems   ☐

F1 Body Mass Index (BMI) (weight in kg) / (height in m)^2

0 = BMI less than 19
1 = BMI 19 to less than 21
2 = BMI 21 to less than 23
3 = BMI 23 or greater   ☐

IF BMI IS NOT AVAILABLE, REPLACE QUESTION F1 WITH QUESTION F2.
DO NOT ANSWER QUESTION F2 IF QUESTION F1 IS ALREADY COMPLETED.

F2 Calf circumference (CC) in cm

0 = CC less than 31
3 = CC 31 or greater   ☐

Screening score (max. 14 points)

12 - 14 points: Normal nutritional status
8 - 11 points: At risk of malnutrition
0 - 7 points: Malnourished   ☐ ☐

Source: Vellas B, Villars H, Abellan G, et al. *Overview of the MNA—Its history and challenges. J Nutr Health Aging.* 2006;10:456.

Rubenstein LZ, Harker JO, Salva A, et al. Screening for undernutrition in geriatric practice: developing the short-form mini nutritional assessment (MNA-SF). *J Gerontol A Biol Sci Med Sci.* 2001;56(6):M366.

Guigoz Y. The Mini-Nutritional Assessment (MNA) Review of the Literature—What does it tell us? *J Nutr Health Aging.* 2006;10:466.

Kaiser MJ, Bauer JM, Ramsch C, et al. Validation of the Mini Nutritional Assessment Short-Form (MNA-SF): a practical tool for identification of nutritional status. *J Nutr Health Aging.* 2009; 13:782.

®Société des Produits Nestlé, S.A., Vevey, Switzerland, Trademark Owners
©Nestlé, 1994, Revision 2009. N67200 12/99 10M
For more information: www.mna-elderly.com

Table 4-3 Nutrition Counseling: Sources of Nutrients

Nutrient	Food Source
Calcium	Dairy foods such as milk, natural cheeses, and yogurt
	Calcium-fortified cereals, fruit juice, soy milk, and tofu
	Dark green leafy vegetables like collard, turnip, and mustard greens; bok choy
	Sardines
Iron	Lean meat, dark turkey meat, liver
	Clams, mussels, oysters, sardines, anchovies
	Iron-fortified cereals
	Enriched and whole grain bread
	Spinach, peas, lentils, turnip greens, and artichokes
	Dried prunes and raisins
Folate	Cooked dried beans and peas
	Oranges, orange juice
	Liver
	Spinach, mustard greens
	Black-eyed peas, lentils, okra, chickpeas, peanuts
	Folate-fortified cereals
Vitamin D	Vitamin D–fortified milk, orange juice, and cereals
	Cod liver oil; swordfish, salmon, herring, mackerel, tuna, trout
	Egg yolk
	Mushrooms

Source: Adapted from U.S. Department of Agriculture and U.S. Department of Health and Human Services. Dietary Guidelines for Americans, 2010. Washington, D.C.: U.S. Government Printing Office; 2010; Choose MyPlate.gov. Available at http://www.choosemyplate.gov/index.html. Accessed December 15, 2014; Office of Dietary Supplements, National Institutes of Health. Dietary Supplement Fact Sheets: Calcium; Vitamin D. Available at http://ods.od.nih.gov/factsheets/list-all/. Accessed December 15, 2014.

Table 4-4   Eating Disorders and Excessively Low BMI

Anorexia Nervosa	Bulimia Nervosa
Refusal to maintain minimally normal body weight (or BMI above 17.5 kg/m^2)	Repeated binge eating followed by self-induced vomiting, misuse of laxatives, diuretics, or other medications; fasting; or excessive exercise
Fear of appearing fat	
Frequently starving but in denial; lacking insight	
Often brought in by family members	Often with normal weight
May present as failure to make expected weight gains in childhood or adolescence, amenorrhea in women, loss of libido or potency in men	Overeating at least twice a week during 3-month period; large amounts of food consumed in short period (~2 hrs)
Associated with depressive symptoms such as depressed mood, irritability, social withdrawal, insomnia, decreased libido	Preoccupation with eating; craving and compulsion to eat; lack of control over eating; alternating with periods of starvation
Additional features supporting diagnosis: self-induced vomiting or purging, excessive exercise, use of appetite suppressants and/or diuretics	Dread of fatness but may be obese

Biologic complications

- *Neuroendocrine changes:* amenorrhea, hormonal alterations
- *Cardiovascular disorders:* bradycardia, hypotension, dysrhythmias, cardiomyopathy
- *Metabolic disorders:* hypokalemia, hypochloremic metabolic alkalosis, increased BUN, edema
- *Other:* dry skin, dental caries, delayed gastric emptying, constipation, anemia, osteoporosis

Subtypes of

- *Purging:* bulimic episodes accompanied by self-induced vomiting or use of laxatives, diuretics, or enemas
- *Nonpurging:* bulimic episodes accompanied by compensatory behavior such as fasting, exercise without purging

Biologic complications; see changes listed for anorexia nervosa.

Sources: World Health Organization. *The ICD-10 Classification of Mental and Behavioral Disorders: Diagnostic Criteria for Research.* Geneva: World Health Organization, 1993; American Psychiatric Association. *DSM-IV-TR: Diagnostic and Statistical Manual of Mental Disorders.* 4th ed. Text Revision. Washington, DC: American Psychiatric Association, 2000. Halmi KA: Eating disorders: In: Kaplan HI, Sadock BJ, eds. *Comprehensive Textbook of Psychiatry,* 7th ed. Philadelphia, PA: Lippincott Williams & Wilkins, 1663–1676, 2000. Mehler PS. Bulimia nervosa. *N Engl J Med.* 2003;349(9):875–880.

Behavior and
Mental Status

Clinicians are uniquely poised to detect clues to mental illness and harmful behavior through empathic listening and close observation. Nonetheless, these clues are often missed. Recognizing mental illness is especially important given its significant prevalence and morbidity, the high likelihood that it is treatable, the shortage of psychiatrists, and the increasing importance of primary care clinicians as the first to encounter the patient's distress. The prevalence of mental health disorders in U.S. adults in 2012 was 18%, affecting 43.7 million people; yet, only 41% received treatment. Even for those receiving care, adherence to treatment guidelines in primary care offices is <50% and disproportionately lower for ethnic minorities.

Mental health disorders are commonly masked by other clinical conditions. Look for the interaction of anxiety and depression in patients with substance abuse, termed "dual diagnosis," because both must be treated for the patient to achieve optimal function. Watch for underlying psychiatric conditions in "difficult encounters" and patients with unexplained symptoms. Explore the outlook of patients with chronic illness, a group that is especially vulnerable to depression and anxiety. Nearly half of those with any single mental disorder meet the criteria for one or more additional disorders, with severity strongly related to comorbidity.

Approximately 5% of somatic symptoms are acute, triggering immediate evaluation. Another 70% to 75% are minor or self-limited and resolve in 6 weeks. Nevertheless, approximately 25% of patients have persisting and recurrent symptoms that elude assessment and fail to improve. Overall, 30% of symptoms are *medically unexplained,* masking anxiety, depression, or even somatoform disorders (see Table 5-1, Somatoform Disorders: Types and Approach to Symptoms, p. 87). Depression and anxiety are highly correlated with substance abuse, for example, and clinicians are advised to look for overlap in these conditions. "Difficult patients" are frequently those with multiple unexplained symptoms and underlying psychiatric conditions that are amenable to therapy. Without better "dual diagnosis," patient health, function, and quality of life are at risk.

Mental Health Disorders and Unexplained Symptoms in Primary Care Settings

Mental Disorders in Primary Care

- Approximately 20% of primary care outpatients have mental disorders, but 50% to 75% of these disorders are undetected and untreated.
- Prevalence of mental disorders in primary care settings is roughly:
  - Anxiety—20%
  - Mood disorders including dysthymia, depressive, and bipolar disorders—25%
  - Depression—10%
  - Somatoform disorders—10% to 15%
  - Alcohol and substance abuse—15% to 20%

Explained and Unexplained Symptoms

- Physical symptoms account for approximately 50% of office visits.
- Roughly one third of physical symptoms are unexplained; in 20% to 25% of patients, physical symptoms become chronic or recurring.
- In patients with *unexplained symptoms,* the prevalence of depression and anxiety exceeds 50% and increases with the total number of reported physical symptoms making detection and "dual diagnosis" important clinical goals.

Common Functional Syndromes

- Co-occurrence rates for *common functional syndromes* such as irritable bowel syndrome, fibromyalgia, chronic fatigue, temporomandibular joint disorder, and multiple chemical sensitivity reach 30% to 90%, depending on the disorders compared.
- The prevalence of *symptom overlap* is high in the common functional syndromes: namely, complaints of fatigue, sleep disturbance, musculoskeletal pain, headache, and gastrointestinal problems.
- The common functional syndromes also overlap in rates of functional impairment, psychiatric comorbidity, and response to cognitive and antidepressant therapy.

Personality Disorders. Difficult patients may have personality disorders resulting in problematic office behaviors that escape diagnosis. The *DSM-5* characterizes these disorders as "an enduring pattern of inner experience and behavior that deviates markedly from the expectations of the individual's culture, is pervasive and inflexible, has an onset in adolescence or early adulthood, is stable over time, and leads to distress or impairment." These patients have dysfunctional interpersonal coping styles that disrupt and destabilize their relationships, including those with health care providers.

For unexplained conditions lasting beyond 6 weeks, experts recommend brief screening questions with high sensitivity and specificity, followed by more detailed investigation when indicated due to high rates of coexisting depression and anxiety.

Mental Health Screening. Unexplained conditions lasting more than 6 weeks are increasingly recognized as chronic disorders that should prompt screening for depression, anxiety, or both. Because screening all patients is time consuming and expensive, experts recommend a two-tiered approach: brief screening questions with high sensitivity and specificity for patients at risk, followed by more detailed investigation when indicated.

Patient Identifiers for Mental Health Screening

- Medically unexplained physical symptoms—more than half have a depressive or anxiety disorder
- Multiple physical or somatic symptoms or "high symptom count"
- High severity of the presenting somatic symptom
- Chronic pain
- Symptoms for more than 6 weeks
- Physician rating as a "difficult encounter"
- Recent stress
- Low self-rating of overall health
- High use of health care services
- Substance abuse

The Health History

Common or Concerning Symptoms

- Changes in attention, mood, or speech
- Changes in insight, orientation, or memory
- Anxiety, panic, ritualistic behavior, and phobias
- Delirium or dementia

Your assessment of mental status begins with the patient's first words. As you gather the health history, you will quickly observe the patient's level of *alertness* and *orientation, mood, attention,* and *memory.* You will learn about the patient's *insight* and *judgment,* as well as any *recurring or unusual thoughts or perceptions.* For some, you will need to conduct a more formal evaluation of mental status.

Many of the terms used to describe the mental status examination are familiar to you from social conversation. Take the time to learn their precise meanings in the context of the formal evaluation of mental status (see below).

Terminology: The Mental Status Examination

Level of Consciousness	Alertness or State of Awareness of the Environment
Attention	The ability to focus or concentrate over time on one task or activity
Memory	The process of registering or recording information. Recent or short-term memory covers minutes, hours, or days; remote or long-term memory refers to intervals of years.
Orientation	Awareness of personal identity, place, and time; requires both memory and attention
Perceptions	Sensory awareness of objects in the environment and their interrelationships; also refers to internal stimuli (e.g., dreams)
Thought processes	The logic, coherence, and relevance of the patient's thoughts, or how people think
Thought content	What the patient thinks about, including level of insight and judgment
Insight	Awareness that symptoms or disturbed behaviors are normal or abnormal
Judgment	Process of comparing and evaluating alternatives; reflects values that may or may not be based on reality and social conventions or norms
Affect	An observable, usually episodic, feeling tone expressed through voice, facial expression, and demeanor
Mood	A more sustained emotion that may color a person's view of the world (affect is to mood as weather is to climate)
Language	A complex symbolic system for expressing, receiving, and comprehending words; essential for assessing other mental functions
Higher cognitive functions	Assessed by vocabulary, fund of information, abstract thinking, calculations, construction of objects with two or three dimensions

Assess level of consciousness, general appearance and mood, and ability to pay attention, remember, understand, and speak.

Assess the patient's responses to illness and life circumstances, which often tell you about his or her insight and judgment. Test orientation and memory.

Explore any unusual thoughts, preoccupations, beliefs, or perceptions as they arise during the interview (see Table 20-2, Delirium and Dementia, pp. 418–419).

Health Promotion and Counseling: Evidence and Recommendations

Important Topics for Health Promotion and Counseling

- Screening for depression and suicidality
- Screening for substance use disorders, including alcohol and prescription drugs

Mood Disorders and Depression. Depressive and bipolar disorders affect over 9% of the U.S. population. About 16 million adult Americans, or almost 7%, have major depression, often with coexisting anxiety disorders and substance abuse. Depression is nearly twice as common in women as men, and frequently accompanies chronic clinical illness, yet is frequently underdiagnosed. Look closely for early clues of depression in primary care settings such as low self-esteem, loss of pleasure in daily activities (*anhedonia*), sleep disorders, and difficulty concentrating or making decisions.

Failure to diagnose depression can have fatal consequences—suicide rates in patients with major depression are eight times higher than in the general population. Ask, "Over the past 2 weeks, have you felt down, depressed, or hopeless?" and "Over the past 2 weeks, have you felt little interest or pleasure in doing things?"

Suicide. Suicide ranks as the 10th leading cause of death in the United States, accounting for nearly 40,000 deaths annually, and is the second leading cause of death among 15- to 24-year olds. Suicide rates are highest among those ages 45 to 54 years, followed by elderly adults ≥age 85 years. Men have suicide rates nearly four times higher than women, though women are three times more likely to attempt suicide. Risk factors include suicidal or homicidal ideation, intent, or plan; access to the means for suicide; current symptoms of psychosis or severe anxiety; any history of psychiatric illness (especially linked to a hospital admission); substance abuse; personality disorder; and prior history or family history of suicide. Patients at high risk should be referred immediately for psychiatric evaluation and possible hospitalization.

Substance Use Disorders, Including Alcohol and Prescription Drugs. The overlap of substance abuse and mental health disorders is extensive. The 2013 National Survey on Drug Use and Health showed that 23% of the U.S. population ages 12 years or older (60.1 million people) reported binge drinking, and over 6% reported heavy drinking. Over 24 million Americans, or 9.4% of the population, reported use of an illicit drug during the month before the survey, including nearly 20 million marijuana users, 1.6 million cocaine users, and 6.5 million users of prescription drugs for nonmedical indications. Prescription drug abuse now kills more people than illicit substances. Because screening for alcohol and drug use is part of *every* patient history, review the screening questions recommended in Chapter 3, Interviewing and the Health History.

Techniques of Examination

The Mental Status Examination

- Appearance and behavior
- Speech and language
- Mood
- Thoughts and perceptions
- Cognition, including memory, attention, information and vocabulary, calculations, abstract thinking, and constructional ability

Observe the patient's mental status throughout your interaction. Test specific functions if indicated during the interview or physical examination. The Mental Status Examination consists of five components: *appearance and behavior; speech and language; mood; thoughts and perceptions;* and *cognitive function.*

POSSIBLE FINDINGS

Appearance and Behavior

Assess the following:

- *Level of Consciousness.* Observe alertness and response to verbal and tactile stimuli.

  Normal consciousness, lethargy, obtundation, stupor, coma (see pp. 331–332)

- *Posture and Motor Behavior.* Observe pace, range, character, and appropriateness of movements.

  Restlessness, agitation, bizarre postures, immobility, involuntary movements

- *Dress, Grooming, and Personal Hygiene*

  Fastidiousness, neglect

- *Facial Expressions.* Assess during rest and interaction.

  Anxiety, depression, elation, anger, and facial immobility of parkinsonism

- *Manner, Affect, and Relation to People and Things*

  Anger, hostility, suspiciousness, or evasiveness in patients with *paranoia*; the elation and euphoria of *mania*; the flat affect and remoteness of *schizophrenia*; the apathy and dulled affect of depression and *dementia*

Speech and Language

Note quantity, rate, loudness, clarity, and fluency of speech. If indicated, test for aphasia. A person who can write a correct sentence does not have aphasia.

Aphasia, dysphonia, dysarthria, changes with mood disorders

Testing for Aphasia

Word Comprehension	Ask patient to follow a one-stage command, such as "Point to your nose." Try a two-stage command: "Point to your mouth, then your knee."
Repetition	Ask patient to repeat a phrase of one-syllable words (the most difficult repetition task): "No ifs, ands, or buts."
Naming	Ask patient to name the parts of a watch.
Reading Comprehension	Ask patient to read a paragraph aloud.
Writing	Ask patient to write a sentence.

POSSIBLE FINDINGS

Mood

Ask about the patient's spirits. Note nature, intensity, duration, and stability of any abnormal mood. If indicated, assess risk of suicide.

Happiness, elation, depression, anxiety, anger, indifference

Thought and Perceptions

Thought Processes. Assess logic, relevance, organization, and coherence.

Derailments, flight of ideas, incoherence, confabulation, blocking

Thought Content. Ask about and explore any unusual or unpleasant thoughts.

Obsessions, compulsions, delusions, feelings of unreality

Perceptions. Ask about any unusual perceptions (e.g., seeing or hearing things).

Illusions, hallucinations

Insight and Judgment. Assess patient's insight into the illness and level of judgment used in making decisions or plans.

Recognition or denial of mental cause of symptoms; bizarre, impulsive, or unrealistic judgment

Cognitive Functions

If indicated, assess:

Orientation to time, place, and person

Disorientation

Attention

■ *Digit span*—ability to repeat a series of numbers forward and then backward

Poor performance of digit span, serial 7s, and spelling backward are common in dementia and delirium but have other causes, too.

■ *Serial 7s*—ability to subtract 7 repeatedly, starting with 100

■ *Spelling backward* of a five-letter word, such as W-O-R-L-D

Remote Memory (e.g., birthdays, anniversaries, social security number, schools, jobs, wars)

Impaired in late stages of dementia

EXAMINATION TECHNIQUES	POSSIBLE FINDINGS

Recent Memory (e.g., events of the day)

New Learning Ability—ability to repeat three or four words after a few minutes of unrelated activity

Recent memory and new learning ability impaired in dementia, delirium, and amnestic disorders

Higher Cognitive Functions

If indicated, assess:

Information and Vocabulary. Note range and depth of patient's information, complexity of ideas expressed, and vocabulary used. For the fund of information, ask names of presidents, other political figures, or large cities.

These attributes reflect intelligence, education, and cultural background. They are limited by mental retardation but are fairly well preserved in early dementia.

Calculating Abilities, such as addition, subtraction, and multiplication

Poor calculation in mental retardation and dementia

Abstract Thinking—ability to respond abstractly to questions about

Concrete responses (observable details rather than concepts) are common in mental retardation, dementia, and delirium. Responses are sometimes bizarre in schizophrenia.

- The meaning of *proverbs,* such as "A stitch in time saves nine."

- The *similarities* of beings or things, such as a cat and a mouse or a piano and a violin

Constructional Ability. Ask patient:

Impaired ability common in dementia and with parietal lobe damage

- To copy figures such as circle, cross, diamond, and box, and two intersecting pentagons, or

- To draw a clock face with numbers and hands

Special Technique

Mini-Mental State Examination (MMSE). This brief test is useful in screening for cognitive dysfunction and dementia and following their course over time. For more detailed information regarding the MMSE, contact the Publisher, Psychological Assessment Resources, Inc., 16204 North Florida Avenue, Lutz, Florida 33549. Some sample questions are given on the next page.

MMSE Sample Items

Orientation to Time	"What is the date?"
Registration	"Listen carefully. I am going to say three words. You say them back after I stop. Ready? Here they are . . . APPLE (pause), PENNY (pause), TABLE (pause). Now repeat those words back to me." (Repeat up to five times, but score only the first trial.)
Naming	"What is this?" (Point to a pencil or pen.)
Reading	"Please read this and do what it says." (Show examinee the words on the stimulus form.) CLOSE YOUR EYES

Recording Your Findings

Recording the Behavior and Mental Status Examination

"*Mental Status:* The patient is alert, well-groomed, and cheerful. Speech is fluent and words are clear. Thought processes are coherent, insight is good. The patient is oriented to person, place, and time. Serial 7s accurate; recent and remote memory intact. Calculations intact."

OR

"*Mental Status:* The patient appears sad and fatigued; clothes are wrinkled. Speech is slow and words are mumbled. Thought processes are coherent, but insight into current life reverses is limited. The patient is oriented to person, place, and time. Digit span, serial 7s, and calculations accurate, but responses delayed. Clock drawing is good." (*These findings suggest depression.*)

Aids to Interpretation

Table 5-1	Somatoform Disorders: Types and Approach to Symptoms
Type of Disorder	**Diagnostic Features**
Somatic symptom disorder	Somatic symptoms are either very distressing or result in significant disruption of functioning, as well as excessive and disproportionate thoughts, feelings, and behaviors related to those symptoms. Symptoms should be specific if with predominant pain.
Illness anxiety disorder	Preoccupation with having or acquiring a serious illness where somatic symptoms, if present, are only mild in intensity.
Conversion disorder	Syndrome of symptoms of deficits mimicking neurologic or clinical illness in which psychological factors are judged to be of etiologic importance.
Psychological factors affecting other clinical conditions	Presence of one or more clinically significant psychological or behavioral factors that adversely affect a clinical condition by increasing the risk for suffering, death, or disability
Factitious disorder	Falsification of physical or psychological signs or symptoms, or induction of injury or disease, associated with identified deception. The individual presents himself or herself as ill, impaired, or injured even in the absence of external rewards.
Other Related Disorders or Behaviors	
Body dysmorphic disorder	Preoccupation with one or more perceived defects or flaws in physical appearance that are not observable or appear only slight to others
Dissociative disorder	Disruption of and/or discontinuity in the normal integration of consciousness, memory, identity, emotion, perception, body representation, motor control, and behavior

Note to readers: Regarding tables in past editions on mood, anxiety, and psychotic disorders, per current *DSM-5* copyright, readers are referred to the *DSM-5* for further diagnostic information.

The Skin, Hair, and Nails

This edition provides a helpful new approach that features careful history taking; thorough inspection and palpation of benign and suspicious lesions to better detect the three major skin cancers—*basal cell carcinoma, squamous cell carcinoma,* and *melanoma;* focused techniques for assessing changes in the hair and nails; accurate use of terminology to describe your findings; and visual familiarity with important common benign and malignant skin conditions.

The Health History

Common or Concerning Symptoms

- Growths
- Rash
- Hair loss

Growths. Ask about any new growths or rashes: "Have you noticed any changes in your skin? . . . your hair? . . . your nails?" "Have you had any rashes? . . . sores? . . . lumps? . . . itching?" Pursue the personal and family history of skin cancer and note the type, location, and date of occurrence. Ask about regular self-skin examination and use of sunscreen.

Rashes. Ask about itching, the most important symptom when assessing rashes. Does itching precede the rash or follow the rash? For itchy rashes, ask about seasonal allergies with itching and watery eyes, asthma, and *atopic dermatitis.* Can the patient sleep all night or does itching wake up the patient?

Causes of generalized itching, without apparent rash, include dry skin; pregnancy; uremia; jaundice; lymphomas and leukemia; drug reactions; and, less commonly, *polycythemia vera* and thyroid disease.

Hair Loss or Nail Changes.
Ask if there is hair thinning or
hair shedding and, if so, where. If
shedding, does the hair come out
at the roots or break along the hair
shafts? Be familiar with common
nail changes such as onychomycosis, habit tic deformity, and
melanonychia, shown in Table 6-8,
pp. 113–114.

Hair shedding at the roots is common in
telogen effluvium and alopecia areata.
Hair breaks along the shaft suggest
damage from hair care or *tinea capitis.*

Health Promotion and Counseling: Evidence and Recommendations

Important Topics for Health Promotion and Counseling

- Skin cancer prevention
- Skin cancer screening

Skin Cancer Prevention. Skin cancers affect an estimated one in five
Americans during their lifetime. The most common skin cancer is *BCC,*
followed by *SCC,* and *melanoma.*

Melanoma. Although it is the least common skin cancer, *melanoma* is
the most lethal due to its high rate of metastasis and high mortality at
advanced stages, causing over 70% of skin cancer deaths. The incidence of
melanoma has the most rapid increase of any cancer and is now the fifth
most frequently diagnosed cancer in men and the seventh most frequently
diagnosed in women.

Use of the *Melanoma Risk Assessment Tool* developed by the National
Cancer Institute, available at http://www.cancer.gov/melanomarisktool/
to assess an individual's 5-year risk of melanoma based on geographic
location, gender, race, age, history of blistering sunburns, complexion,
number and size of moles, freckling, and sun damage.

Avoiding Ultraviolet Radiation and Tanning Beds. Increasing
lifetime sun exposure correlates directly with increasing risk of skin cancer. Intermittent sun exposure appears to be more harmful than chronic
exposure. The best defense against skin cancers is to avoid ultraviolet
radiation exposure by limiting time in the sun, avoiding midday sun, using
sunscreen, and wearing sun-protective clothing with long sleeves and
hats with wide brims. Advise patients to avoid indoor tanning, especially

children, teens, and young adults. Use of indoor tanning beds, especially before age 35 years, increases risk of melanoma by as much as 75%. In 2009, the International Agency for Research on Cancer classified ultraviolet-emitting tanning devices as "carcinogenic to humans."

Regular Use of Sunscreen Prevents Skin Cancer. A landmark study in 2011 demonstrated that the regular use of sunscreen decreases the incidence of melanoma. Advise patients to use at least sun-protective factor (SPF) 30 and broad-spectrum protection. For water exposure, patients should use water-resistant sunscreens.

Skin Cancer Screening. Although the USPSTF found insufficient evidence (grade I) to recommend routine skin cancer screening, it does advise clinicians to "remain alert for skin lesions with malignant features" during routine physical examinations and reference the ABCDE criteria. The American Cancer Society (ACS) and the AAD recommend full-body examinations for patients over age 50 years or at high risk, because melanoma can appear in any location. High-risk patients are those with a personal or family history of multiple or dysplastic nevi or previous melanoma. Both new and changing nevi should be closely examined, as at least half of melanomas arise de novo from isolated melanocytes rather than pre-existing nevi.

Screening for Melanoma: The ABCDEs. Clinicians should apply the ABCDE-EFG method when screening moles for melanoma (this does not apply for nonmelanocytic lesions like seborrheic keratoses). The sensitivity of this tool for detecting melanoma ranges from 43% to 97%, and specificity from 36% to 100%; diagnostic accuracy depends on how many criteria are used to define abnormality.

The ABCDE Rule

If two or more of the ABCDE criteria are present, risk of melanoma increases and biopsy should be considered. Some have suggested adding EFG to help detect aggressive nodular melanomas.

	Melanoma	Benign Nevus
Asymmetry Of one side of mole compared to the other		

(continued)

The ABCDE Rule (Continued)

	Melanoma	Benign Nevus
Border irregularity Especially if ragged, notched, or blurred		
Color variations[a] More than two colors, especially blue-black, white (loss of pigment due to regression), or red (inflammatory reaction to abnormal cells)		
Diameter >6 mm[b] Approximately the size of a pencil eraser		
Evolving[c] Or changing rapidly in size, symptoms, or morphology		

- Elevated
- Firm to palpation
- Growing progressively over several weeks

[a]With the exception of a homogeneous blue color in a blue nevus, blue or black color within a larger pigmented lesion is especially concerning for melanoma.
[b]Early melanomas may be <6 mm, and many benign lesions are >6 mm.
[c]Evolution, or change, is the most sensitive of these criteria. A reliable history of change may prompt biopsy of a benign-appearing lesion.

Patient Screening: The Self-Skin Examination. The AAD and the ACS recommend regular self-skin examination. Instruct patients with risk factors for skin cancer and melanoma, especially those with a history of high sun exposure, prior or family history of melanoma, and ≥50 moles or >5 to 10 atypical moles, to perform regular self-skin examinations.

Techniques of Examination

Full-Body and Integrated Skin Examinations

Perform a *full-body skin examination* in the context of the overall physical examination. *Inspect and palpate all skin lesions*, focusing on key features that help distinguish if lesions are benign or suspicious for malignancy. Are they raised, flat, or fluid-filled? Are they rough or smooth? What about color? Is the lesion pink or brown? Measure the size. Is the size changing? Learn to describe each lesion accurately, using the terminology specified below. Changing moles, a history of skin cancer, and other risk factors all warrant a full-body skin examination.

See Tables 6-1 to 6-5, pp. 100–108, for examples of primary lesions (flat, raised, and fluid-filled; pustules, furuncles, nodules, cysts, wheals, and burrows); and rough, pink, and brown lesions.

Even during routine examinations, you can pursue an integrated skin examination as you examine areas on the head and neck, arms and hands, and over the back as you listen to the lungs that are already easily accessible.

Integrating the skin examination into the physical examination and routinely recording your findings as part of the general write-up saves time and contributes to earlier detection of skin cancers, when they are easier to treat. Systemic illnesses also have many associated skin findings.

Preparing for the Examination

Make sure there is good overhead ambient lighting or natural light from windows. Add a strong light source if the room is dark. You will also need a small ruler or tape measure and a small magnifying glass to help you document important features of skin lesions, such as size, shape, color, and texture. *Dermoscopy* provides cross-polarized or unpolarized light to visualize patterns of pigmentation or vascular structures and improves the sensitivity and specificity of differentiating melanomas from benign lesions.

Ask the patient to change into a gown with the opening in the back and clothes removed except for underwear. Before beginning the examination, cleanse your hands thoroughly. It is important for you to palpate lesions for texture, firmness, and scaliness.

Important Terms for Describing Skin Lesions. It is important to use specific terminology. Good descriptions include each of the following elements: type of primary lesion, number, size, shape, color, texture, location, and configuration.

Describing Skin Findings

Primary lesions are *flat* or *raised*.

- *Flat:* You cannot palpate the lesion with your eyes closed.
  - *Macule:* Lesion is flat and <1 cm.
  - *Patch:* Lesion is flat and >1 cm.
- *Raised:* You can palpate the lesion with eyes closed.
  - *Papule:* Lesion is raised, <1 cm, and not fluid-filled.
  - *Plaque:* Lesion is raised, >1 cm, but not fluid-filled.
  - *Vesicle:* Lesion is raised, <1 cm, and filled with fluid.
  - *Bulla:* Lesion is raised, >1 cm, and fluid-filled.
- *Other primary lesions* include erosions, ulcers, nodules, ecchymoses, petechiae, and palpable purpura.

Number: Lesions can be solitary or multiple. If multiple, record how many. Also consider estimating the total number of the type of lesion you are describing.

Size: Measure with a ruler in millimeters or centimeters. For oval lesions, measure in the long axis then perpendicular to the axis.

Shape: Some good words to learn are "circular," "oval," "annular" (ring-like, with central clearing), "nummular" (coin-like, no central clearing), and "polygonal."

Color: Be creative. Refer to a color wheel if needed. There are many shades of brown, but you can start with tan, light brown, and dark brown.

- Use "skin-colored" when appropriate.
- For red lesions or rashes, blanch the lesion by pressing it firmly with your finger or a glass slide to see if the redness temporarily lightens then refills.

Blanching lesions are *erythematous* and suggest inflammation. Nonblanching lesions, petechiae, purpura, and vascular structures are red, purple, and violaceous but not erythematous. See Table 6-6, Vascular and Purpuric Lesions of the Skin, pp. 109–110.

Texture: Palpate the lesion to see if it is smooth, fleshy, verrucous, warty, or scaly (fine, keratotic, or greasy scale).

Scaling can be greasy, like *seborrheic dermatitis* or *seborrheic keratoses,* dry and fine like *tinea pedis,* or hard and keratotic like *actinic keratoses* or *SCC.*

(continued)

EXAMINATION TECHNIQUES

POSSIBLE FINDINGS

Describing Skin Findings (Continued)

Location: Be as specific as possible. For single lesions, measure their distance from other landmarks (e.g., 1 cm lateral to left oral commissure).

Configuration: Describing patterns is often very helpful.

For more information and additional illustrations of each of these elements, LearnDerm is a free and very helpful website.

Examples are *herpes zoster* with unilateral and dermatomal vesicles; *herpes simplex,* with grouped vesicles or pustules on an erythematous base; *tinea pedis* with annular lesions; and *poison ivy allergic contact dermatitis* with linear lesions.

Techniques of Examination— Patient Seated. Choose one of two patient positions for performing the full-body skin examination. The patient can be seated or lie supine then prone. Plan to *examine the skin in the same order every time,* so you are less likely to skip part of the examination.

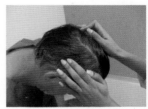

Figure 6-1 Part the hair on the scalp.

Stand in front of the patient and adjust the table to a comfortable height. Start by examining the *hair and scalp* (Fig. 6-1).

Alopecia, or hair loss, can be diffuse, patchy, or total. Male and female pattern hair loss are normal with aging. Focal patches may be lost suddenly in *alopecia areata.* Refer scarring alopecia to a dermatologist.

Sparse hair is seen in hypothyroidism; fine, silky hair in hyperthyroidism.

See Table 6-7, Hair Loss, pp. 111–112.

Inspect the *head and neck,* including the forehead; eyes including eyelids, conjunctivae, sclerae, eyelashes, and eyebrows; nose, cheeks, lips, oral cavity, and chin; and anterior neck (Figs. 6-2 to 6-4).

Look for signs of basal cell carcinoma on the face. See Table 6-4, Pink Lesions: Basal Cell Carcinoma and Its Mimics, p. 106.

Move the gown to see each area. Ask permission first.

EXAMINATION TECHNIQUES	POSSIBLE FINDINGS

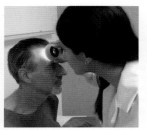

Figure 6-2 Inspect the forehead.

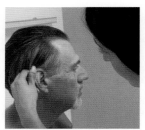

Figure 6-3 Inspect the face, eyes, and ears.

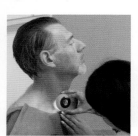

Figure 6-4 Inspect the anterior neck.

Inspect the *shoulders, arms,* and *hands* (Fig. 6-5). Inspect and palpate the *fingernails.* Note their color, shape, and any lesions.

See Table 6-8, Findings in or near the Nails, pp. 113–114.

Inspect the *chest and abdomen* (Fig. 6-6). Lower or raise the gown to expose these areas and cover up when you are finished.

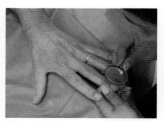

Figure 6-5 Inspect the arms, hands, and nails.

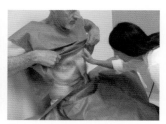

Figure 6-6 Inspect the chest and abdomen.

EXAMINATION TECHNIQUES

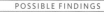

Inspect the *thighs* and *lower legs* (Fig. 6-7). Inspect and palpate the toenails, and inspect the soles and between the toes (Fig. 6-8).

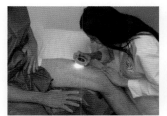

Figure 6-7 Inspect the thighs and lower legs.

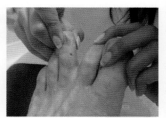

Figure 6-8 Inspect the soles of the feet and between the toes.

Ask the patient to stand so that you inspect the *lower back* and *posterior legs* (Fig. 6-9). If needed, uncover the buttocks. Examination of the breasts and genitalia may be saved for last.

Techniques of Examination—Patient Supine and Prone. Some clinicians prefer this positioning for more thorough examinations (Fig. 6-10). With the patient *supine,* inspect the *scalp, face,* and *anterior neck;* the *shoulders, arms,* and *hands;* the *chest* and *abdomen; anterior thighs;* and *lower legs, feet,* and, if appropriate, the *genitalia.* Ask permission when moving the gown to expose different areas, and let the patient know which areas you will be examining next.

Ask the patient to turn over to the *prone* position, lying face down. Look at the *posterior scalp, posterior neck, back, posterior thighs, legs, soles of the feet,* and *buttocks* (if appropriate).

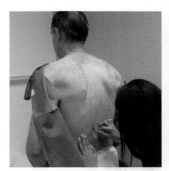

Figure 6-9 Inspect the back, buttocks, and posterior legs.

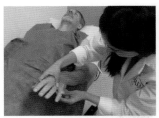

Figure 6-10 Inspect the scalp, arms, hands, chest, abdomen, anterior and posterior thighs, and feet.

EXAMINATION TECHNIQUES	POSSIBLE FINDINGS

Special Techniques

The Patient Self-Skin Examination. The patient will need a full-length mirror, a hand-held mirror, and a well-lit room that provides privacy. Teach the patient the *ABCDE-EFG method* for assessing moles. Help them and to identify melanomas by looking at photographs of benign and malignant nevi on easy-to-access websites, handouts, or tables in this chapter.

Examining the Patient with Hair Loss. Examine the hair to determine the overall pattern of hair loss or hair thinning. Inspect the scalp for erythema, scaling, pustules, tenderness, bogginess, and scarring. Look at the width of the hair part in various sections of the scalp. For shedding from the roots, perform a *hair pull test* by gently grasping 50 to 60 hairs with your thumb and index and middle fingers, pulling firmly away from the scalp (Fig. 6-11). If all the hairs have telogen bulbs, the most likely diagnosis is *telogen effluvium.* For fragility, perform the *tug test* by holding a group of hairs in one hand, pulling along the hair shafts with the other (Fig. 6-12); if any hairs break, it is abnormal.

Possible internal causes of diffuse nonscarring hair shedding in young women are *iron-deficiency anemia* and *hyper-* or *hypothyroidism.*

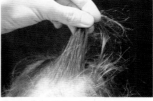

Figure 6-11 Hair pull test.

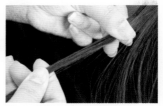

Figure 6-12 Tug test.

Evaluating the Bedbound Patient. People confined to bed, especially when they are emaciated, elderly, or neurologically impaired, are particularly susceptible to *pressure sores.* Carefully inspect the skin that overlies the sacrum, buttocks, greater trochanters, knees, and heels. Roll the patient onto one side to see the low back and gluteal area best.

Local redness of the skin warns of impending necrosis, although some deep pressure sores develop without antecedent redness. Inspect closely for skin breaks and ulcers.

Recording Your Findings

As stated on p. 94, use specific terms to describe skin lesions and rashes, including number of lesions, size, color, shape, texture, location, configuration, and whether a primary lesion.

Recording the Skin, Hair, and Nails Examination

"Skin warm and dry. Nails without clubbing or cyanosis. Approximately 20 brown, round macules on upper back, chest, and arms, are all symmetric in pigmentation, none suspicious. No rash, petechiae, or ecchymoses." *(These findings suggest normal nevi and perfusion without any rashes or suspicious lesions.)*

OR

"Scattered stuck-on verrucous plaques on back and abdomen. Over 30 small round brown macules with symmetric pigmentation on back, chest, and arms. Single 1.2 × 1.6 cm asymmetric dark brown and black plaque with erythematous, uneven border, on left upper arm." *(These findings suggest normal seborrheic keratoses and benign nevi, but also a possible malignant melanoma.)*

Aids to Interpretation

Table 6-1 Describing Primary Skin Lesions: Flat, Raised, and Fluid-Filled

Describe skin lesions accurately, including number, size, color, texture, shape, primary lesion, location, and configuration. This table identifies common primary skin lesions and includes classic descriptions of each lesion with the diagnosis in italics.

Flat spots: If you run your finger over the lesion but do not feel the lesion, the lesion is flat. If a flat spot is small (<1 cm), it is a **macule**. If a flat spot is larger (>1 cm), it is a patch.

Macules (flat, small)

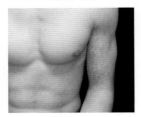

Multiple 3–8-mm erythematous confluent round **macules** on chest, back, and arms; *morbilliform drug eruption*

Patches (flat, large)

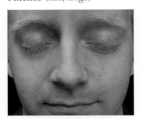

Bilaterally symmetric erythematous **patches** on central cheeks and eyebrows, some with overlying greasy scale; *seborrheic dermatitis*

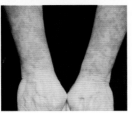

Large confluent completely depigmented patches on dorsal hands and distal forearms; *vitiligo*

Table 6-1 Describing Primary Skin Lesions: Flat, Raised, and Fluid-Filled (*continued*)

Raised spots: If you run your finger over the lesion and it is palpable above the skin, it is *raised*. If a raised spot is small (<1 cm), it is a **papule**. If a raised spot is larger (>1 cm), it is a **plaque**.

Papules (raised, small)

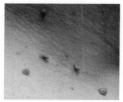

Multiple 2–4-mm soft, fleshy skin-colored to light brown **papules** on lateral neck and axillae in skin folds; *skin tags*

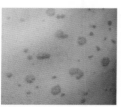

Scattered erythematous round drop-like, flat-topped well-circumscribed scaling **papules** and plaques on trunk; *guttate psoriasis*

Plaques (raised, large)

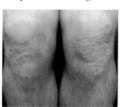

Scattered erythematous to bright pink well-circumscribed flat-topped **plaques** on extensor knees and elbows, with overlying silvery scale; *plaque psoriasis*

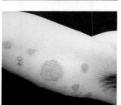

Multiple round coin-like eczematous **plaques** on arms, legs, and abdomen, with overlying dried transudate crust; *nummular dermatitis*

(table continues on page 102)

Table 6-1 Describing Primary Skin Lesions: Flat, Raised, and Fluid-Filled (*continued*)

Fluid-filled lesions: If the lesion is raised, filled with fluid, and small (<1 cm), it is a **vesicle**. If a fluid-filled spot is larger (>1 cm), it is a **bulla**.

Vesicles (fluid-filled, small)

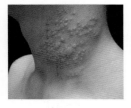

Multiple 2–4-mm **vesicles** and pustules on erythematous base, grouped together on left neck; *herpes simplex virus*

Bullae (fluid-filled, large)

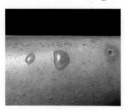

Several tense bullae on lower legs; *insect bites*

Table 6-2   Additional Primary Lesions: Pustules, Furuncles, Nodules, Cysts, Wheals, Burrows

Pustule: Small palpable collection of neutrophils or keratin that appears white

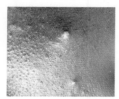

~15–20 **pustules** and acneiform papules on buccal and parotid cheeks bilaterally; *acne vulgaris*

Furuncle: Inflamed hair follicle; multiple furuncles together form a carbuncle

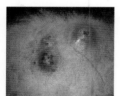

Two large (2-cm) **furuncles** on forehead, without fluctuance; *furunculosis* (Note: fluctuant deep infections are *abscesses*)

Nodule: Larger and deeper than a papule

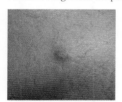

Solitary blue-brown 1.2-cm firm **nodule** with positive dimple sign and hyperpigmented rim on left lateral thigh; *dermatofibroma*

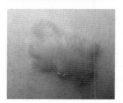

Solitary 4-cm pink and brown scar-like **nodule** on central chest at site of previous trauma; *keloid*

(table continues on page 104)

Table 6-2 Additional Primary Lesions: Pustules, Furuncles, Nodules, Cysts, Wheals, Burrows *(continued)*

Subcutaneous mass/cyst: Whether mobile or fixed, cysts are encapsulated collections of fluid or semisolid

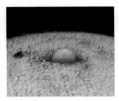

Three 6–8-mm mobile subcutaneous **cysts** on vertex scalp, that on excision reveal pearly white balls; *pilar cysts*

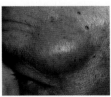

Solitary 9-cm mobile rubbery subcutaneous **mass** on left temple; *lipoma*

Wheal: Area of localized dermal edema that evanesces (comes and goes) within a period of 1–2 days; this is the essential primary lesion of *urticaria*

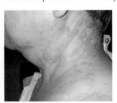

Many variably sized (1–10-cm) **wheals** on lateral neck, shoulders, abdomen, arms, and legs; *urticaria*

Burrow: Small linear or serpiginous pathways in the epidermis created by the scabies mite

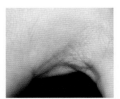

Multiple small (3–6-mm) erythematous papules on abdomen, buttocks, scrotum, and shaft and head of penis, with four **burrows** noted on interdigital web spaces; *scabies*

Table 6-3 Rough Lesions: Actinic Keratoses and Squamous Cell Carcinoma

Patients commonly report feeling rough lesions. Many are benign, like *seborrheic keratoses* or *warts*, but *squamous cell carcinoma (SCC)* and its precursor *actinic keratosis* can also feel rough or keratotic.

Actinic keratosis

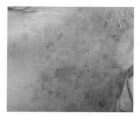

- Often easier to feel than to see
- *Superficial keratotic papules* that "come and go," on sun-damaged skin

Warts

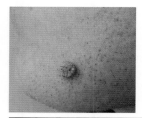

- Usually skin-colored to pink, texture more verrucous than keratotic
- May be filiform
- Often have hemorrhagic punctate that can be seen with a magnifying glass or dermatoscope

Squamous cell carcinoma

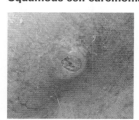

- Keratoacanthomas are SCCs that arise rapidly and have a crateriform center
- Often have a *smooth but firm border*
- SCCs can become quite large if left untreated (Note: *highest sites of metastasis are the scalp, lips, and ears*)

Table 6-4	Pink Lesions: Basal Cell Carcinoma and its Mimics

Basal cell carcinoma (BCC) is the most common cancer in the world. Fortunately, it rarely spreads to other parts of the body. Nonetheless, it can invade and destroy local tissues, causing significant morbidity to the eye, nose, or brain.

Basal Cell Carcinoma
Superficial basal cell carcinoma

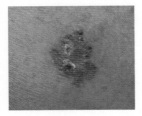

- Pink patch *that does not heal*
- May have *focal scaling*

Nodular basal cell carcinoma

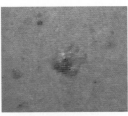

- Pink papule, often with *translucent or pearly appearance* and *overlying telangiectasias*
- May have *focal pigmentation*
- Dermoscopy shows arborizing vessels, focal pigment globules, and other specific patterns

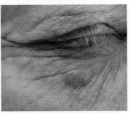

Table 6-5 Brown Lesions: Melanoma and Its Mimics

Most patients have brown spots on their body surface. Although these are usually freckles, benign nevi, solar lentigines, or seborrheic keratoses, you and the patient must look closely for any that stand out as a possible melanoma. With enough practice, when you see a *melanoma*, it will stick out as the "ugly duckling." Review the ABCDE rule and photographs on pp. 91–92.

Melanoma	Mimics
Amelanotic melanoma	**Skin tags or intradermal nevi**

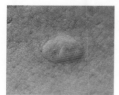

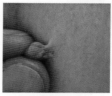

- Usually in very fair-skinned people
- *Evolution or rapid change* is the most important feature, because variegation or dark pigment is missing in this type

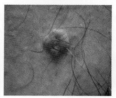

- Soft and fleshy
- Often around neck, axillae, or back
- Sessile nevi may have a hint of brown pigmentation

Melanoma in situ

Solar lentigo

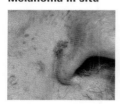

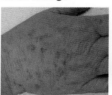

- *On sun-exposed or sun-protected skin*
- Look for ABCDE features

- On sun-exposed skin
- Light brown and uniform in color but may be asymmetric

(table continues on page 108)

Table 6-5 Brown Lesions: Melanoma and Its Mimics (*continued*)

Melanoma	Mimics
Melanoma	**Dysplastic nevus**

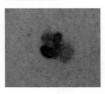 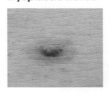

- *May arise de novo or in existing nevi* and exhibits ABCDEs
- Patients with many dysplastic nevi have increased risk of melanoma

- May have macular base and papular central "fried egg" component
- Compare to the patient's other nevi and monitor changes

Melanoma **Inflamed seborrheic keratosis**

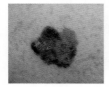 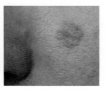

- May have *variegated color* (browns, red)
- Has melanocytic features on dermoscopy

- Can sometimes mimic a melanoma if it has an erythematous base
- Dermoscopy helps the trained eye distinguish these

Melanoma **Seborrheic keratosis**

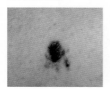 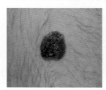

- May be uniform in color but *asymmetric;* key feature is *rapid change or evolution*

- Stuck-on and verrucous, may be darkly pigmented

Table 6-6   Vascular and Purpuric Lesions of the Skin

Lesions	Features: Appearance, Distribution, Significance
Cherry Angioma 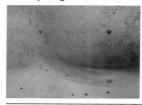	■ Bright or ruby red, may become purplish with age; 1–3 mm; round, flat, sometimes raised; may be surrounded by a pale halo ■ Found on trunk or extremities ■ Not significant; increase in size and number with aging
Spider Angioma[a] 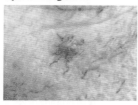	■ Fiery red; very small to 2 cm; central body, sometimes raised, radiating with erythema ■ Face, neck, arms, and upper trunk, but almost never below the waist ■ Seen in liver disease, pregnancy, vitamin B deficiency; normal in some people
Spider Vein[a] 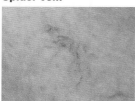	■ Bluish; varies from very small to several inches; may resemble a spider or be linear, irregular, or cascading ■ Most often on the legs, near veins; also on anterior chest ■ Often accompanies increased pressure in the superficial veins, as in varicose veins

(table continues on page 110)

Table 6-6 Vascular and Purpuric Lesions of the Skin (*continued*)

Lesions	Features: Appearance, Distribution, Significance
Petechia/Purpura 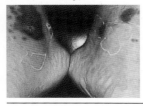	▪ Deep red or reddish purple; fades over time; 1–3 mm or larger; rounded, sometimes irregular, flat ▪ Varied distribution ▪ Seen if blood outside the vessels; may suggest a bleeding disorder or, if petechiae, emboli to skin
Ecchymosis 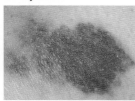	▪ Purple or purplish blue, fading to green, yellow, and brown over time; larger than petechiae; rounded, oval, or irregular ▪ Varied distribution ▪ Seen if blood outside the vessels; often secondary to bruising or trauma; also seen in bleeding disorders

*a*These are telangiectasias, or dilated small vessels that look red or bluish.

Sources of photos: *Spider Angioma*—Marks R. *Skin Disease in Old Age*. Philadelphia, PA: JB Lippincott; 1987; *Petechia/Purpura*—Kelley WN. *Textbook of Internal Medicine*. Philadelphia, PA: JB Lippincott; 1989.

Table 6-7   Hair Loss

Generalized or Diffuse Hair Loss

In men, look for frontal hairline regression and thinning on the posterior vertex; in women look for thinning that spreads from the crown down without hairline regression.

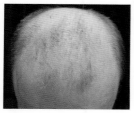

Male pattern hair loss (MPHL)

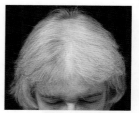

Female pattern hair loss (FPHL)

Telogen Effluvium and Anagen Effluvium

In *telogen effluvium* overall the patient's scalp and hair distribution appear normal, but a positive *hair pull test* reveals most hairs have telogen bulbs. In *anagen effluvium* there is diffuse hair loss from the roots. The *hair pull test* shows few if any hairs with telogen bulbs.

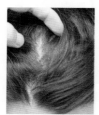

Normal hair part width in telogen effluvium

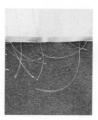

Positive hair pull test in telogen effluvium showing all hairs have telogen bulbs

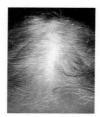

Anagen effluvium

(table continues on page 112)

Table 6-7 Hair Loss (*continued*)

Focal Hair Loss
Alopecia Areata
There is sudden onset of clearly demarcated, usually localized, round or oval patches of hair loss leaving smooth skin without hairs, in children and young adults. There is no visible scaling or erythema.

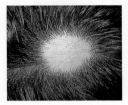

Tinea Capitis ("Ringworm")
There are round scaling patches of alopecia, usually caused by *Trichophyton tonsurans* from humans, and less commonly, *Microsporum canis* from dogs or cats.

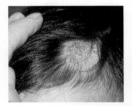 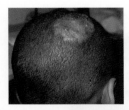

References: For a complete guide to evaluation of hair loss, review Mubki T, Rucnicka L, Olszewska M, et al. Evaluation and diagnosis of the hair loss patient. *J Am Acad Dermatol.* 2014;71:415.
aSee also Hair Loss Help. Hair loss classifications. Available at http://www.hairlosshelp.com/hair_loss_research/hair_loss_charts.cfm. Accessed February 13, 2015.

Table 6-8 Findings in or near the Nails

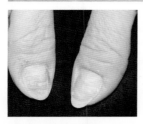

Paronychia

A superficial infection of the proximal and lateral nail folds adjacent to the nail plate. The nail folds are often red, swollen, and tender. Represents the most common infection of the hand, usually from *Staphylococcus aureus* or *Streptococcus*. Creates a felon if it extends into the pulp space of the finger.

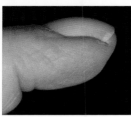

Clubbing of the Fingers

Clinically a bulbous swelling of the soft tissue at the nail base, with loss of the normal angle between the nail and the proximal nail fold. The angle increases to 180 degrees or more, and the nail bed feels spongy or floating. The mechanism is still unknown. Seen in congenital heart disease, interstitial lung disease and lung cancer, inflammatory bowel diseases, and malignancies.

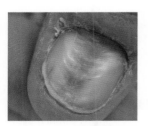

Habit Tic Deformity

There is depression of the central nail with a "Christmas tree" appearance from small horizontal depressions, resulting from repetitive trauma from rubbing the index finger over the thumb or vice versa.

Melanonychia

Caused by increased pigmentation in the nail matrix, leading to a streak as the nail grows out. This may be a normal ethnic variation if found in multiple nails. A wide streak, especially if growing or irregular, could represent a *subungual melanoma*.

(table continues on page 114)

Table 6-8 Findings in or near the Nails (*continued*)

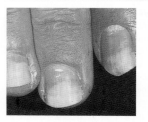

Onycholysis
A painless separation of the whitened opaque nail plate from the pinker translucent nail bed.

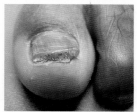

Onychomycosis
The most common cause of nail thickening and subungual debris is *onychomycosis,* most often from the dermatophyte *Trichophyton rubrum.*

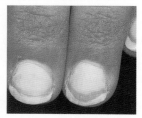

Terry Nails
Nail plate turns white with a ground-glass appearance, a distal band of reddish brown, and obliteration of the lunula. Seen in liver disease, usually cirrhosis, heart failure, and diabetes.

Sources of photos: *Clubbing of the Fingers, Paronychia, Onycholysis, Terry Nails*—Habif TP. *Clinical Dermatology: A Color Guide to Diagnosis and Therapy.* 2nd ed. St. Louis, MO: CV Mosby; 1990.

The Head and Neck

The Health History

Common or Concerning Symptoms

- Headache
- Change in vision: blurred vision, loss of vision, floaters, flashing lights
- Eye pain, redness, or tearing
- Double vision (diplopia)
- Hearing loss, earache, ringing in the ears (tinnitus)
- Dizziness and vertigo
- Nosebleed (epistaxis)
- Sore throat, hoarseness
- Swollen glands
- Goiter

The Head

Headache is a common symptom that always requires careful evaluation because a small fraction of headaches arise from life-threatening conditions. Elicit a full description of the headache and all seven attributes of the patient's pain (see p. 3).

See Table 7-1, Primary Headaches, p. 128, and Table 7-2, Secondary Headaches, pp. 129–131. *Tension* and *migraine headaches* are the most common recurring headaches.

Is the headache one sided or bilateral? Severe with sudden onset, like a thunderclap? Steady or throbbing? Continuous or comes and goes? Ask the patient to *point to the area of pain or discomfort.* Assess *chronologic pattern* and *severity.*

Tension headaches often arise in the temporal areas; cluster headaches may be retro-orbital.

Changing or progressively severe headaches increase the likelihood of *tumor, abscess,* or other *mass lesion.* Extremely severe headaches suggest *subarachnoid hemorrhage* or *meningitis.*

Headache Warning Signs for Immediate Investigation

- Progressively frequent or severe over a 3-month period
- Sudden onset like a "thunderclap" or "the worst headache of my life"
- New onset after age 50 years
- Aggravated or relieved by change in position
- Precipitated by Valsalva maneuver
- Associated symptoms of fever, night sweats, or weight loss
- Presence of cancer, HIV infection, or pregnancy
- Change in pattern from past headaches
- Lack of a similar headache in the past
- Recent head trauma
- Associated papilledema, neck stiffness, or focal neurologic deficits

Ask about associated symptoms, such as nausea and vomiting, and neurologic symptoms, such as change in vision or motor-sensory deficits.

Visual aura or scintillating scotomas may accompany *migraine*. Nausea and vomiting are common with migraine but also occur with *brain tumor* and *subarachnoid hemorrhage*.

Ask if coughing, sneezing, or changing the position of the head affects (better, worse, or none) the headache.

Such maneuvers may increase pain from brain tumor and acute sinusitis.

Ask about family history.

Family history is often positive in patients with migraine.

The Eyes

Ask "How is your vision?" If the patient reports a change in vision, pursue the related details:

Gradual blurring, often from refractive errors; also occurs in hyperglycemia.

Is the problem worse during close work or at distances?

Difficulty with close work suggests *hyperopia* (farsightedness) or *presbyopia* (aging vision); difficulty with distances suggests *myopia* (nearsightedness).

Is the onset sudden or gradual?

Sudden visual loss suggests retinal detachment, vitreous hemorrhage, or occlusion of the central retinal artery.

Is there blurring of the entire field of vision or only parts? Is blurring central, peripheral, or only on one side?

Slow central loss occurs in *nuclear cataract* and *macular degeneration*; peripheral loss in advanced *open-angle glaucoma*; one-sided loss in *hemianopsia* and quadrantic defects (p. 132).

■ Has the patient seen lights flashing across the field of vision? Vitreous floaters?

These symptoms suggest detachment of vitreous from the retina. Prompt eye consultation is indicated.

Ask about *pain* in or around the eyes, *redness*, and *excessive tearing* or *watering*.

Eye pain in acute glaucoma and optic neuritis.

Check for *diplopia*, or double vision.

Diplopia in brainstem or cerebellum lesions, also from weakness or paralysis of one or more extraocular muscles.

The Ears

Ask "How is your hearing?"

Does the patient have special difficulty understanding people as they talk? Does a noisy environment make a difference?

Sensorineural loss (inner ear) leads to difficulty understanding speech, often complaining that others mumble; noisy environments worsen hearing. In *conductive loss* (external or middle ear), noisy environments may help.

For complaints of *earache*, or *pain in the ear*, ask about associated fever, sore throat, cough, and concurrent upper respiratory infection.

Consider *otitis externa* if pain in the ear canal; *otitis media* if pain associated with respiratory infection.

Tinnitus is an internal musical ringing or rushing or roaring noise, often unexplained.

When associated with hearing loss and vertigo, tinnitus suggests *Ménière* disease.

Ask about *vertigo*, the perception that the patient or the environment is rotating or spinning.

Vertigo in *labrynthitis* (inner ear), CN VII lesions, brainstem lesions

The Nose and Sinuses

Rhinorrhea, or drainage from the nose, frequently accompanies *nasal congestion*. Ask further about *sneezing*, watery eyes, throat discomfort, and *itching* in the eyes, nose, and throat.

Causes include viral infections, *allergic rhinitis* ("hay fever"), and *vasomotor rhinitis*. Itching favors an allergic cause.

For *epistaxis,* or bleeding from the nose, identify the source carefully—is bleeding actually from the nose, or has the patient coughed up or vomited blood? Assess the site of bleeding, its severity, and associated symptoms.

Local causes of epistaxis include trauma (especially nose-picking), inflammation, drying and crusting of the nasal mucosa, tumors, and foreign bodies. Anticoagulants, NSAIDs, and coagulopathies may contribute.

The Mouth, Throat, and Neck

Sore throat or pharyngitis is a frequent complaint. Ask about fever, swollen glands, and any associated cough.

Fever, pharyngeal exudates, and anterior cervical lymphadenopathy, especially without cough, suggest *streptococcal pharyngitis,* or *"strep throat"* (p. 142).

Hoarseness may arise from overuse of the voice, allergies, smoking, or inhaled irritants.

If present more than 2 weeks, refer for laryngoscopy; consider hypothyroidism, reflux, vocal cord nodules, head and neck cancers, thyroid masses, and neurologic disorders (*Parkinson disease, amyotrophic lateral sclerosis,* or *myasthenia gravis*).

Assess thyroid function. Ask about goiter, temperature intolerance, and sweating.

With goiter, thyroid function may be increased, decreased, or normal. Cold intolerance in *hypothyroidism;* heat intolerance, palpitations, and involuntary weight loss in *hyperthyroidism*

Health Promotion and Counseling: Evidence and Recommendations

Important Topics for Health Promotion and Counseling

- Loss of vision: cataracts, macular degeneration, glaucoma
- Hearing loss
- Oral health

Disorders of vision shift with age. Healthy young adults generally have refractive errors. Older adults have refractive errors, *cataracts, macular degeneration,* and *glaucoma.* Glaucoma is the leading cause of blindness in African Americans and the U.S. population overall. Glaucoma causes gradual vision loss, with damage to the optic nerve, loss of visual fields, beginning usually at the periphery, and pallor and increasing size of the optic cup (enlarging to more than half the diameter of the optic disc).

More than a third of adults older than 65 years have *detectable hearing deficits.* Questionnaires and handheld audioscopes work well for periodic screening.

Be sure to promote *oral health:* 19% of children aged 2 to 19 years have untreated cavities, and about 5% of adults aged 40 to 59 years and 25% of those older than age 60 years have no teeth at all. Inspect the oral cavity for decayed or loose teeth, inflammation of the gingiva, signs of periodontal disease (bleeding, pus, receding gums, and bad breath), and oral cancers. Counsel patients to use fluoride-containing toothpastes, brush, floss, and seek dental care at least annually.

Techniques of Examination

EXAMINATION TECHNIQUES	POSSIBLE FINDINGS

⚷The Head

Examine the:

- Hair, including quantity, distribution, and texture

  Coarse and sparse in hypothyroidism, fine in *hyperthyroidism*

- Scalp, including lumps or lesions

  Pilar cysts, psoriasis, seborrheic dermatitis, pigmented nevi

- Skull, including size and contour

  Hydrocephalus, skull depression from trauma

- Face, including symmetry and facial expression

  Facial paralysis; flat affect of depression, moods such as anger, sadness

- Skin, including color, texture, hair distribution, and lesions

  Pale, fine, hirsute, acne, skin cancer

The Eyes

Test visual acuity in each eye with a Snellen wall chart or handheld card.

Vision of 20/200 means that at 20 feet, the patient can read print that a person with normal vision could read at 200 feet.

Assess visual fields by confrontation with the *static finger wiggle test* and the *kinetic red target test*, if indicated (Fig. 7-1).

Hemianopsia, quadrantic defects in cerebrovascular accidents (CVAs). See Table 7-3, Visual Field Defects, p. 132.

EXAMINATION TECHNIQUES	POSSIBLE FINDINGS

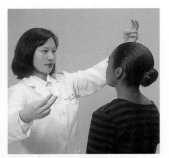

Figure 7-1 Static finger wiggle test.

Inspect the:

See Table 7-4, Physical Findings in and Around the Eye, pp. 133–134.

■ Position and alignment of eyes

Exophthalmos, strabismus

■ Eyebrows

Seborrheic dermatitis

■ Eyelids

Sty, chalazion, ectropion, ptosis, xanthelasma, blepharitis

■ Lacrimal apparatus

Swollen lacrimal sac, excessive tearing

■ Conjunctiva and sclera

Red eye, conjunctivitis, jaundice, episcleritis

■ Cornea, iris, and lens

Cataract, crescentic shadow of acute angle glaucoma

Inspect pupils for:

■ Size, shape, and symmetry

Miosis, mydriasis, anisocoria

■ Reactions to light, direct and consensual

Absent in paralysis of CN III

■ The near reaction, namely pupillary constriction with gaze shift to near object; note the accompanying convergence of the eyes and accommodation of the lens (becomes more convex) (Fig. 7-2)

Constriction slows in tonic (Adie) pupil and is absent in Argyll Robertson pupils of syphilis; poor convergence in hyperthyroidism

EXAMINATION TECHNIQUES

POSSIBLE FINDINGS

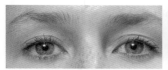 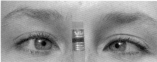

Figure 7-2 The pupils constrict when the focus shifts to a close object.

Assess the extraocular muscles by observing:

■ The symmetry of corneal reflections from a midline light

Asymmetric reflection if deviation in ocular alignment

■ The six cardinal directions of gaze (Fig. 7-3)

Cranial nerve palsy, strabismus, nystagmus, lid lag of hyperthyroidism

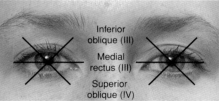

Superior rectus (III)
Lateral rectus (VI)
Inferior rectus (III)

Inferior oblique (III)
Medial rectus (III)
Superior oblique (IV)

Superior rectus (III)
Lateral rectus (VI)
Inferior rectus (III)

Figure 7-3 The six cardinal directions of gaze.

Inspect the fundi with an ophthalmoscope.

Steps for Using the Ophthalmoscope

● Darken the room. Switch on the ophthalmoscope light and turn the lens disc until you see the large round beam of white light.* Shine the light on the back of your hand to check the type of light, its desired brightness, and the electrical charge of the ophthalmoscope.

 *Some clinicians like to use the large round beam for large pupils, and the small round beam for small pupils. The other beams are rarely helpful. The slit-like beam is sometimes used to assess elevations or concavities in the retina, the green (or red-free) beam to detect small red lesions, and the grid to make measurements. Ignore the last three lights and practice with the large or small round white beam.

(continued)

EXAMINATION TECHNIQUES	POSSIBLE FINDINGS

Steps for Using the Ophthalmoscope (Continued)

- Turn the lens disc to the 0 diopter. (A diopter is a unit that measures the power of a lens to converge or diverge light.) At this diopter, the lens neither converges nor diverges light. Keep your finger on the edge of the lens disc so you can turn the disc to focus the lens when you examine the fundus.
- Hold the ophthalmoscope *in your right hand and use your right eye* to examine *the patient's right eye;* hold it *in your left hand and use your left eye to examine the patient's left eye.* This keeps you from bumping the patient's nose and gives you more mobility and closer range for visualizing the fundus. With practice, you will become accustomed to using your nondominant eye.
- Hold the ophthalmoscope firmly braced against the medial aspect of your bony orbit, with the handle tilted laterally at about a 20-degree slant from the vertical. Check to make sure you can see clearly through the aperture. *Instruct the patient to look* slightly up and *over your shoulder at a point directly ahead on the wall.*
- Place yourself about 15 inches away from the patient and at an angle *15-degree lateral to the patient's line of vision.* Shine the light beam on the pupil and look for the orange glow in the pupil— the *red reflex.* Note any opacities interrupting the red reflex.
- Now *place the thumb of your other hand across the patient's eyebrow,* which steadies your examining hand. Keeping the light beam focused on the red reflex, move in with the ophthalmoscope on the 15-degree angle toward the pupil until you are very close to it, almost touching the patient's eyelashes and the thumb of your other hand.

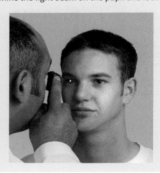

Inspect the fundi for the following:

- Red reflex

  Cataracts, artificial eye

- Optic disc (Fig. 7-4)

  Papilledema, glaucomatous cupping, optic atrophy. See Table 7-5, Abnormalities of the Optic Disc, p. 135, and Table 7-6, Ocular Fundi: Diabetic Retinopathy, p. 136.

| EXAMINATION TECHNIQUES | POSSIBLE FINDINGS |

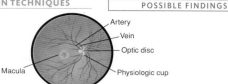

Figure 7-4 The optic disc.

▨ Arteries, veins, and AV crossings

AV nicking, copper wiring in hypertensive changes

▨ Adjacent retina (note any lesions)

Hemorrhages, exudates, cotton-wool patches, microaneurysms, pigmentation

▨ Macular area

Macular degeneration

▨ Anterior structures

Vitreous floaters, cataracts

Tips for Examining the Optic Disc and Retina

- *Locate the optic disc.* Look for the round yellowish-orange structure.
- Now, *bring the optic disc into sharp focus* by adjusting the lens of your ophthalmoscope.
- *Inspect the optic disc.* Note the following features:
  - *The sharpness or clarity of the disc outline*
  - *The color of the disc*
  - *The size of the central physiologic cup* (an enlarged cup suggests chronic open-angle glaucoma)
  - *Venous pulsations* in the retinal veins as they emerge from the central portion of the disc (loss of venous pulsations from elevated intracranial pressure may occur in head trauma, meningitis)
- *Inspect the retina.* Distinguish arteries from veins based on the features listed below.

	Arteries	**Veins**
Color	Light red	Dark red
Size	Smaller (2/3 to 3/4 the diameter of veins)	Larger
Light Reflex (reflection)	Bright	Inconspicuous or absent

- *Follow the vessels peripherally in each of four directions.*
- Inspect the *fovea* and surrounding *macula*. Macular degeneration types include *dry atrophic* (more common but less severe) and *wet exudative* (neovascular). Undigested cellular debris, called drusen, may be hard or soft.
- Assess for any *papilledema* from increased intracranial pressure leading to swelling of the optic nerve head.

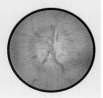

EXAMINATION TECHNIQUES	POSSIBLE FINDINGS

The Ears

Examine on each side:

The Auricle. Inspect the auricle.   Keloid, epidermoid cyst

If you suspect otitis:

- Move the auricle up and down, and press on the tragus.   Pain in otitis externa ("the tug test")

- Press firmly behind the ear.   Possible tenderness in otitis media and mastoiditis

Ear Canal and Drum. Pull the auricle up, back, and slightly out. Inspect, through an otoscope with speculum:

- The canal   Cerumen; swelling and erythema in otitis externa

- The eardrum (Fig. 7-5)   Red bulging drum in acute otitis media; serous otitis media, tympanosclerosis, perforations. See Table 7-7, Abnormalities of the Eardrum, p. 137.

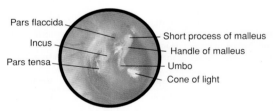

Pars flaccida — Short process of malleus
Incus — Handle of malleus
Pars tensa — Umbo — Cone of light

Figure 7-5 Anatomy of middle and inner ear.

Hearing. "Do you feel you have a hearing loss or difficulty hearing?" is a sensitive screening question. Assess auditory acuity to spoken or whispered voice or with a hand-held audiometer.

EXAMINATION TECHNIQUES	POSSIBLE FINDINGS

If hearing is diminished, use a 512-Hz tuning fork to:

- Test *lateralization* (Weber test), but only in patients with unilateral hearing loss. Place vibrating and tuning fork on vertex of skull and check hearing.

In unilateral *conductive hearing loss*, sound is heard in (lateralized to) the impaired ear. See Table 7-8, Patterns of Hearing Loss, p. 138.

- Compare *air and bone conduction* (Rinne test). Place vibrating and tuning fork on mastoid bone, then remove and check hearing.

In *conductive hearing loss*, sound is heard through bone longer than through air (BC = AC or BC > AC). In *sensorineural hearing loss*, sound is heard longer through air (AC > BC).

The Nose and Sinuses

Inspect the external nose.

Inspect, through a speculum, the:

- Nasal mucosa that covers the septum and turbinates, noting its color and any swelling

Swollen and red in viral rhinitis, swollen and pale in allergic rhinitis; polyps (Fig. 7-6); ulcer from cocaine use

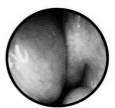

Figure 7-6 Nasal polyps.

- Nasal septum for position and integrity

Deviation, perforation

Palpate the frontal and maxillary sinuses.

Tender in acute sinusitis

EXAMINATION TECHNIQUES | POSSIBLE FINDINGS

The Mouth and Pharynx

Inspect the:

■ Lips

Cyanosis, pallor, cheilosis. See also Table 7-9, Abnormalities of the Lips, p. 139.

■ Oral mucosa

Aphthous ulcers (canker sores)

■ Gums

Gingivitis, periodontal disease

■ Teeth

Dental caries, tooth loss

■ Roof of the mouth

Torus palatinus (benign)

■ Tongue, including:

See Table 7-10, Abnormalities of the Tongue, pp. 140–141.

■ Papillae

Glossitis

■ Symmetry

Deviation to one side from paralysis of CN XII from CVA

■ Any lesions

Erythroplakia, leukoplakia (precancerous); squamous cell or other carcinomas

■ Floor of the mouth

Lesions suspicious for cancer

■ Pharynx, including:

See Table 7-11, Abnormalities of the Pharynx, p. 142.

■ Color or any exudate

Pharyngitis

■ Presence and size of tonsils

Exudates, tonsillitis, peritonsillar abscess

■ Symmetry of the soft palate as patient says "ah"

Soft palate fails to rise, uvula deviates to opposite side in CN X paralysis from CVA.

The Neck

Inspect the neck.

Scars, masses, torticollis

Palpate superficial and deep anterior, posterior cervical, and supraclavicular lymph nodes.

Cervical lymphadenopathy from HIV or AIDS, infectious mononucleosis, lymphoma, leukemia, and sarcoidosis. Enlarged supraclavicular node from possible abdominal malignancy

Inspect and palpate the position of the trachea.

Deviated trachea from neck mass or pneumothorax

EXAMINATION TECHNIQUES

POSSIBLE FINDINGS

Inspect the thyroid gland:

▪ At rest

Goiter, nodules. See Table 7-12, Abnormalities of the Thyroid Gland, p. 143.

▪ As patient swallows water

From behind patient, palpate the thyroid gland, including the isthmus, and first one then the opposite lobe:

Goiter, nodules, tenderness of thyroiditis

▪ At rest

▪ As patient swallows water (Fig. 7-7)

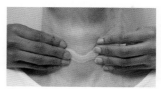

Figure 7-7 Thyroid gland with goiter while swallowing.

Alternative Examination Sequence—After examining the thyroid gland, you may proceed to musculoskeletal examination of the neck and upper back and check for costovertebral angle tenderness.

Recording Your Findings

Recording the Head, Eyes, Ears, Nose, and Throat (HEENT) Examination

Head—The skull is normocephalic/atraumatic. Frontal balding. *Eyes*—Visual acuity 20/100 bilaterally. Sclera white; conjunctiva injected. Pupils constrict from 3 to 2 mm, equally round and reactive to light and accommodation. Disc margins sharp; no hemorrhages or exudates. Arteriolar-to-venous ratio (AV ratio) 2:4; no AV nicking. *Ears*—Acuity diminished to whispered voice; intact to spoken voice. TMs clear. *Nose*—Mucosa swollen with erythema and clear drainage. Septum midline. Tender over maxillary sinuses. *Throat*—Oral mucosa pink, dental caries in lower molars, pharynx erythematous, no exudates.

Neck—Trachea midline. Neck supple; thyroid isthmus midline, lobes palpable but not enlarged.

Lymph Nodes—Submandibular and anterior cervical lymph nodes tender, 1 × 1 cm, rubbery and mobile; no posterior cervical, epitrochlear, axillary, or inguinal lymphadenopathy.

(These findings suggest myopia and mild arteriolar narrowing as well as upper respiratory infection.)

Aids to Interpretation

Table 7-1   Primary Headaches

Problem	Common Characteristics	Associated Symptoms, Provoking and Relieving Factors
Tension	**Location:** variable **Quality:** pressing or tightening pain; mild-to-moderate intensity **Onset:** gradual **Duration:** minutes to days	Sometimes photophobia, phonophobia; nausea absent ↑ by sustained muscle tension, as in driving or typing ↓ possibly by massage, relaxation
Migraine ■ *With aura* ■ *Without aura* ■ *Variants*	**Location:** unilateral in ~70%; bifrontal or global in ~30% **Quality:** throbbing or aching, variable in severity **Onset:** fairly rapid, peaks in 1–2 hours **Duration:** 4–72 hours	Nausea, vomiting, photophobia, phonophobia, visual auras (flickering zig-zagging lines), motor auras affecting hand or arm, sensory auras (numbness, tingling usually precede headache) ↑ by alcohol, certain foods, tension, noise, bright light. More common premenstrually ↓ by quiet dark room, sleep
Cluster	**Location:** unilateral, usually behind or around the eye **Quality:** deep, continuous, severe **Onset:** abrupt, peaks within minutes **Duration:** up to 3 hours	Lacrimation, rhinorrhea, miosis, ptosis, eyelid edema, conjunctival infection ↑ sensitivity to alcohol during some episodes

Table 7-2   Secondary Headaches

Problem	Common Characteristics	Associated Symptoms, Provoking and Relieving Factors
Analgesic Rebound	**Location:** previous headache pattern **Quality:** variable **Onset:** variable **Duration:** depends on prior headache pattern	Depends on prior headache pattern ↑ by fever, carbon monoxide, hypoxia, withdrawal of caffeine, other headache triggers ↓—depends on cause
Headaches from Eye Disorders *Errors of Refraction (farsightedness and astigmatism, but not nearsightedness)*	**Location:** around and over the eyes; may radiate to the occipital area **Quality:** steady, aching, dull **Onset:** gradual **Duration:** variable	Eye fatigue, "sandy" sensation in eyes, redness of the conjunctiva ↑ by prolonged use of the eyes, particularly for close work ↓ by resting the eyes
Acute Glaucoma	**Location:** in and around one eye **Quality:** steady, aching, often severe **Onset:** often rapid **Duration:** variable, may depend on treatment	Diminished vision, sometimes nausea and vomiting ↑—sometimes by drops that dilate the pupils
Headache from Sinusitis	**Location:** usually above eye (frontal sinus) or over maxillary sinus **Quality:** aching or throbbing, variable in severity; consider possible migraine **Onset:** variable **Duration:** often several hours at a time, recurring over days or longer	Local tenderness, nasal congestion, tooth pain, discharge, and fever ↑ by coughing, sneezing, or jarring the head ↓ by nasal decongestants, antibiotics

(table continues on page 130)

Table 7-2	Secondary Headaches (*continued*)	
Problem	**Common Characteristics**	**Associated Symptoms, Provoking and Relieving Factors**
Meningitis	**Location:** generalized	Fever, stiff neck, photophobia, change in mental status
	Quality: steady or throbbing, very severe	
	Onset: fairly rapid	Can ↓ from immediate antibiotics until viral versus bacterial cause identified
	Duration: variable, usually days	
Subarachnoid Hemorrhage— "Thunderclap Headache"	**Location:** generalized	Nausea, vomiting, possibly loss of consciousness, neck pain
	Quality: severe, "the worst of my life"	
	Onset: usually abrupt; prodromal symptoms may occur	↑ rebleeding, ↑ intracranial pressure, cerebral edema
	Duration: variable, usually days	↓ by subspecialty treatments
Brain Tumor	**Location:** varies with the location of the tumor	↑ by coughing, rebleeding, ↑ intracranial pressure, cerebral edema
	Quality: aching, steady, variable in intensity	↓ by subspecialty treatments
	Onset: variable	
	Duration: often brief	
Giant Cell (Temporal) Arteritis	**Location:** near the involved artery, often the temporal, also the occipital; age related	Tenderness of the adjacent scalp; fever (in ~50%), fatigue, weight loss; new headache (~60%), jaw claudication (~50%), visual loss or blindness (~15–20%), polymyalgia rheumatica (~50%)
	Quality: throbbing, generalized, persistent, often severe	
	Onset: gradual or rapid	↑ by movement of neck and shoulders
	Duration: variable	Often ↓ by steroids

Table 7-2   Secondary Headaches (*continued*)

Problem	Common Characteristics	Associated Symptoms, Provoking and Relieving Factors
Postconcussion Headache	**Location:** often but not always localized to the injured area **Quality:** generalized, dull, aching, constant **Onset:** within hours to 1–2 days of the injury **Duration:** weeks, months, or even years	Drowsiness, poor concentration, confusion, memory loss, blurred vision, dizziness, irritability, restlessness, fatigue ↑ by mental and physical exertion, straining, stooping, emotional excitement, alcohol ↓ by rest
Cranial Neuralgias: Trigeminal Neuralgia (CN V)	**Location:** cheek, jaws, lips, or gums; trigeminal nerve divisions 2 and 3 >1 **Quality:** shocklike, stabbing, burning, severe **Onset:** abrupt, paroxysmal **Duration:** each jab lasts seconds but recurs at intervals of seconds or minutes	Exhaustion from recurrent pain ↑ by touching certain areas of the lower face or mouth; chewing, talking, brushing teeth ↓ by medication; neurovascular decompression

Table 7-3   Visual Field Defects

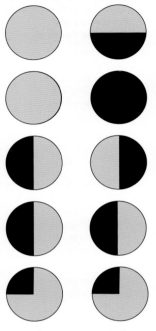

Altitudinal (horizontal) defect, usually resulting from a vascular lesion of the retina

Unilateral blindness, from a lesion of the retina or optic nerve

Bitemporal hemianopsia, from a lesion at the optic chiasm

Homonymous hemianopsia, from a lesion of the optic tract or optic radiation on the side contralateral to the blind area

Homonymous quadrantic defect, from a partial lesion of the optic radiation on the side contralateral to the blind area

Left   **Right**
(*from patient's viewpoint*)

Table 7-4   Physical Findings in and Around the Eye

Eyelids

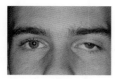

Ptosis. A drooping upper eyelid that narrows the palpebral fissure from a muscle or nerve disorder

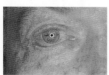

Ectropion. Outward turning of the margin of the lower lid, exposing the palpebral conjunctiva

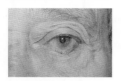

Entropion. Inward turning of the lid margin, causing irritation of the cornea or conjunctiva

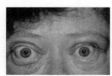

Lid retraction and exophthalmos. A wide-eyed stare suggests hyperthyroidism. Note the rim of sclera between the upper lid and the iris. Retracted lids and "lid lag" when eyes move from up to down markedly increase the likelihood of hyperthyroidism, especially when accompanied by fine tremor, moist skin, and heart rate >90 beats per minute. Exophthalmos describes protrusion of the eyeball, a common feature of Graves ophthalmopathy, triggered by autoreactive T lymphocytes

(table continues on page 134)

| Table 7-4 | **Physical Findings in and Around the Eye** (*continued*) |

In and Around the Eye

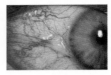

Pinguecula. Harmless yellowish nodule in the bulbar conjunctiva on either side of the iris; associated with aging

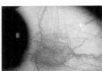

Episcleritis. A localized ocular redness from inflammation of the episcleral vessels. Seen in rheumatoid arthritis, Sjögren syndrome, and herpes zoster

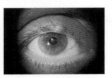

Sty. A pimple-like infection around a hair follicle near the lid margin, usually from *Staphylococcus aureus*

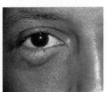

Chalazion. A beady nodule in either eyelid caused by a chronically inflamed meibomian gland

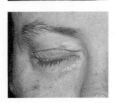

Xanthelasma. Yellowish plaque seen in lipid disorders. Half of affected patients have *hyperlipidemia;* also common in *primary biliary cirrhosis*

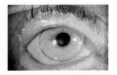

Blepharitis. Chronic inflammation of the eyelids at the base of the hair follicles, often from *S. aureus.* Also a scaling seborrheic variant

Table 7-5   Abnormalities of the Optic Disc

	Process	Appearance
Normal 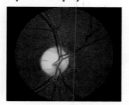	Tiny disc vessels give normal color to the disc	Disc is yellowish orange to creamy pink Disc vessels are tiny Disc margins are sharp (except perhaps nasally)
Papilledema	Venous stasis leads to engorgement and swelling	Disc is pink, hyperemic Disc vessels are more visible, more numerous, and curve over the borders of the disc Disc is swollen, with margins blurred
Glaucomatous Cupping	Increased pressure within the eye leads to increased cupping (backward depression of the disc) and atrophy	The base of the enlarged cup is pale
Optic Atrophy	Death of optic nerve fibers leads to loss of the tiny disc vessels	Disc is white Disc vessels are absent

Table 7-6　Ocular Fundi: Diabetic Retinopathy

Nonproliferative Retinopathy, Moderately Severe 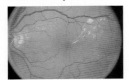	Note tiny red dots or microaneurysms, also the ring of hard exudates (white spots) located superotemporally. Retinal thickening or edema in the area of hard exudates can impair visual acuity if it extends to center of macula. Detection requires specialized stereoscopic examination
Nonproliferative Retinopathy, Severe 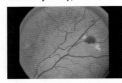	In superior temporal quadrant, note large retinal hemorrhage between two cotton-wool patches, beading of the retinal vein just above, and tiny tortuous retinal vessels above the superior temporal artery, termed *intraretinal microvascular abnormalities*
Proliferative Retinopathy, with Neovascularization 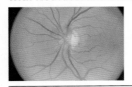	Note new preretinal vessels arising on disc and extending across disc margins. Visual acuity is still normal, but the risk of severe visual loss is high. Photocoagulation can reduce this risk by >50%
Proliferative Retinopathy, Advanced 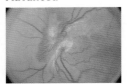	Same eye as above, but 2 years later and without treatment. Neovascularization has increased, now with fibrous proliferations, distortion of the macula, and reduced visual acuity

Source of photos: Nonproliferative Retinopathy, Moderately Severe; Proliferative Retinopathy, With Neovascularization; Nonproliferative Retinopathy, Severe; Proliferative Retinopathy, Advanced—Early Treatment Diabetic Retinopathy Study Research Group. Courtesy of MF Davis, MD, University of Wisconsin, Madison. Source: Frank RB. Diabetic retinopathy. *N Engl J Med* 2004;350:48.

Table 7-7   Abnormalities of the Eardrum

Perforation

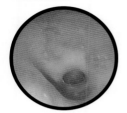

Hole in the eardrum that may be central or marginal

Usually from *otitis media* or trauma

Tympanosclerosis

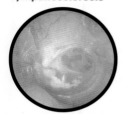

A chalky white patch

Scarring process of the middle ear from otitis media with deposition of hyaline and calcium and phosphate crystals in the eardrum and middle ear. When severe, it may entrap the ossicles and cause conductive hearing loss

Serous Effusion

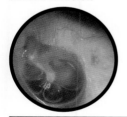

Amber fluid behind the eardrum, with or without air bubbles

Associated with viral upper respiratory infections or sudden changes in atmospheric pressure (diving, flying)

Acute Otitis Media with Purulent Effusion

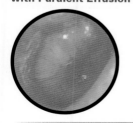

Red, bulging drum, loss of landmarks

Painful hemorrhagic vesicles appear on the tympanic membrane and/or ear canal causing earache, blood-tinged discharge from the ear, and conductive hearing loss. Seen in mycoplasma and viral infections and bacterial otitis media

Table 7-8 Patterns of Hearing Loss

	Conductive Loss	**Sensorineural Loss**
Impaired Understanding of Words	Minor	Often troublesome
Effects	Noisy environment may improve hearing	Noisy environment worsens hearing
	Voice remains soft since cochlear nerve intact	Voice may be loud due to nerve damage
Usual Age of Onset	Childhood, young adulthood	Middle and later years
Ear Canal and Drum	Often a visible abnormality	Problem not visible
Weber Test (in Unilateral Hearing Loss)	Lateralizes to the impaired ear	Lateralizes to the good ear
Rinne Test	BC ≥ AC	AC > BC
Causes Include	Plugged ear canal, *otitis media,* immobile or perforated drum, otosclerosis, foreign body	Sustained loud noise, drugs, inner ear infections, trauma, hereditary disorder, aging, acoustic neuroma

Table 7-9   Abnormalities of the Lips

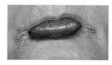 **Angular cheilitis.** Softening and cracking of the angles of the mouth

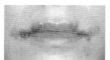 **Herpes simplex.** Painful vesicles, followed by crusting; also called **cold sore** or **fever blister**

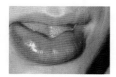 **Angioedema.** Diffuse, tense, subcutaneous swelling, usually allergic in cause

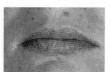 **Hereditary hemorrhagic telangiectasia.** Small red spots. Autosomal dominant disorder causing vascular fragility and arteriovascular malformations (AVMs), including in the brain and lungs. Associated bleeding in nose and GI tract

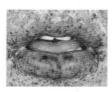 **Peutz–Jeghers syndrome.** Brown spots of the lips and buccal mucosa, significant because of associated intestinal polyposis and high risk of GI cancer

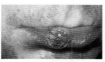 **Syphilitic chancre.** A firm lesion that ulcerates and may crust

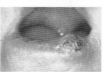 **Carcinoma of the lip.** A thickened plaque or irregular nodule that may ulcerate or crust; malignant

Table 7-10   Abnormalities of the Tongue

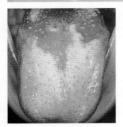

Geographic tongue. Scattered areas in which the papillae are lost, giving a map-like appearance; benign

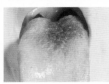

Hairy tongue. Results from elongated papillae that may look yellowish, brown, or black; benign

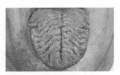

Fissured tongue. May appear with aging; benign

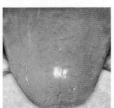

Smooth tongue. Results from loss of papillae; seen in deficiency of riboflavin, niacin, folic acid, vitamin B12, pyridoxine, or iron, and treatment with chemotherapy

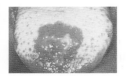

Candidiasis. May show a thick, white coat, which, when scraped off, leaves a raw red surface; tongue may also be red; antibiotics, corticosteroids, AIDS may predispose

Table 7-10 Abnormalities of the Tongue (*continued*)

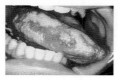

Hairy leukoplakia. White raised, feathery areas, usually on sides of tongue. Seen in HIV/AIDS

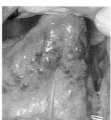

Varicose veins. Dark round spots in the undersurface of the tongue, associated with aging; also called **caviar lesions**

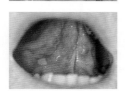

Aphthous ulcer (canker sore). Painful, small, whitish ulcer with a red halo; heals in 7–10 days

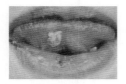

Mucous patch of syphilis. Slightly raised, oval lesion, covered by a grayish membrane

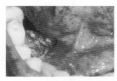

Carcinoma of the tongue or floor of the mouth. Malignancy should be considered in any nodule or nonhealing ulcer at the base or edges of the mouth

Table 7-11 Abnormalities of the Pharynx

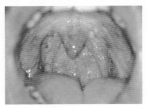

Pharyngitis, mild to moderate. Note redness and vascularity of the pillars and uvula

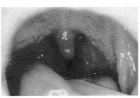

Pharyngitis, diffuse. Note redness is diffuse and intense. Cause may be viral or, if patient has fever, bacterial. If patient has no fever, exudate, or cervical lymphadenopathy, viral infection is more likely

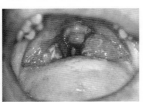

Exudative pharyngitis. A sore red throat with patches of white exudate on the tonsils is associated with streptococcal pharyngitis and some viral illnesses

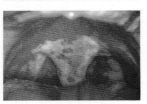

Diphtheria. An acute infection caused by *Corynebacterium diphtheriae*. The throat is dull red, and a gray exudate appears on the uvula, pharynx, and tongue

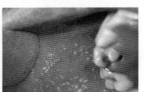

Koplik spots. These small white specks that resemble grains of salt on a red background are an early sign of measles

Table 7-12 Abnormalities of the Thyroid Gland

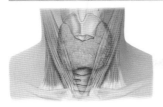

Diffuse enlargement. May result from Graves disease, Hashimoto thyroiditis, endemic goiter (iodine deficiency), or sporadic goiter

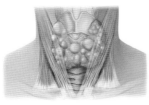

Multinodular goiter. An enlargement with two or more identifiable nodules, usually metabolic in cause

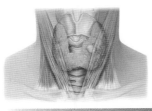

Single nodule. May result from a cyst, a benign tumor, or cancer of the thyroid, or may be one palpable nodule in a clinically unrecognized multinodular goiter

The Thorax and Lungs

The Health History

Common or Concerning Symptoms

- Chest pain
- Shortness of breath (dyspnea)
- Wheezing
- Cough
- Blood-streaked sputum (hemoptysis)
- Daytime sleepiness or snoring and disordered sleep

Complaints of *chest pain* or *chest discomfort* raise the specter of heart disease but often arise from conditions in the thorax and lungs. For this important symptom, keep the possible causes below in mind. Also see Table 8-1, Chest Pain, pp. 155–156.

Sources of Chest Pain and Related Causes

The myocardium	*Angina pectoris, myocardial infarction, myocarditis*
The pericardium	*Pericarditis*
The aorta	*Aortic dissection*
The trachea and large bronchi	*Bronchitis*
The parietal pleura	*Pericarditis, pneumonia, pneumothorax, pleural effusion, pulmonary embolus*
The chest wall, including the musculo-skeletal and neurologic systems	*Costochondritis, herpes zoster*
The esophagus	*Gastroesophageal reflux disease, esoph-ageal spasm, esophageal tear*
Extrathoracic structures such as the neck, gallbladder, and stomach	*Cervical arthritis, biliary colic, gastritis*

For patients who are *short of breath*, focus on *pulmonary complaints*:

■ Dyspnea and wheezing See Table 8-2, Dyspnea, pp. 157–158.

■ Cough and hemoptysis See Table 8-3, Cough and Hemoptysis, pp. 159–161.

■ Daytime sleepiness or snoring and disordered sleep

Snoring, witnessed apneas ≥10 seconds, awakening with a choking sensation, or morning headache point to obstructive sleep apnea.

Health Promotion and Counseling: Evidence and Recommendations

Important Topics for Health Promotion and Counseling

- Tobacco cessation
- Lung cancer
- Immunizations—influenza and streptococcal pneumonia vaccines

Despite declines in smoking over the past several decades, 19% of Americans still smoke. Regularly counsel all adults, pregnant women, parents, and adolescents who smoke to stop. Use "the five **As**" and the Stages of Change Model to assess readiness to quit.

Assessing Readiness to Quit Smoking: Brief Interventions Models

5 As Model	Stages of Change Model
Ask about tobacco use	**Precontemplation**—"I don't want to quit."
Advise to quit	**Contemplation**—"I am concerned but not ready to quit now."
Assess willingness to make a quit attempt	**Preparation**—"I am ready to quit."
Assist in quit attempt	**Action**—"I just quit."
Arrange follow-up	**Maintenance**—"I quit 6 months ago."

Counsel patients to never smoke or quit smoking. The U.S. Preventive Services Task Force recommends annual low-dose computed tomography (LDCT) screening for current smokers (or those who have quit within the last 15 years) ages 55 to 79 years (grade B recommendation).

Provide *flu shots* to everyone age 6 months or older and especially to those with chronic pulmonary conditions, nursing home residents, household contacts, and health care personnel.

Recommend *pneumococcal vaccine* to adults 65 years and older, smokers between the ages of 16 and 64 years, and those with increased risk of pneumococcal infection.

Techniques of Examination

EXAMINATION TECHNIQUES

POSSIBLE FINDINGS

Initial Inspection of Thorax

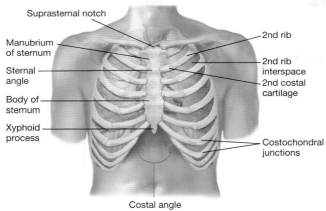

Suprasternal notch

Manubrium of sternum

Sternal angle

Body of sternum

Xyphoid process

2nd rib

2nd rib interspace

2nd costal cartilage

Costochondral junctions

Costal angle

Figure 8-1 Chest wall anatomy.

Inspect the thorax (Fig. 8-1) and its respiratory movements for signs of distress and note:

- Facial color

  Cyanosis and pallor in lips and oral mucosa signal hypoxia.

- Rate, rhythm, depth, and effort of breathing

  Tachypnea, hyperpnea, Cheyne–Stokes breathing. Normally 14 to 20 breaths/minute in adults. See Table 8-4 Abnormalities in Rate and Rhythm of Breathing, p. 162.

- Inspiratory retraction of the supraclavicular areas

  Occurs in chronic obstructive pulmonary disease (COPD), asthma, upper airway obstruction

- Inspiratory contraction of the sternocleidomastoids

  Indicates severe breathing difficulty

| **EXAMINATION TECHNIQUES** | POSSIBLE FINDINGS |

If distress, auscultate the neck and lungs for:

- Stridor

    Stridor in upper airway obstruction from foreign body or epiglottitis

- Wheezes

    Expiratory wheezing in asthma and COPD

Observe shape of patient's chest.

Normal or barrel chest (see Table 8-5, Deformities of the Thorax, pp. 163–164)

The Posterior Chest

Inspect the chest for:

- Deformities or asymmetry

    Kyphoscoliosis

- Abnormal inspiratory retraction of the interspaces

    Retraction in asthma, COPD, upper airway obstruction

- Impairment or unilateral lag in respiratory movement

    Disease of the underlying lung or pleura, phrenic nerve palsy

Palpate the chest for:

- Tender areas

    Fractured ribs

- Assessment of visible abnormalities

    Masses, sinus tracts

- Chest expansion (Fig. 8-2)

    Impairment, both sides in COPD and restrictive lung disease; unilateral decrease or delay in chronic fibrosis of the underlying lung or pleura, pleural effusion, lobar pneumonia, pleural pain with associated splinting, unilateral bronchial obstruction, and paralysis of the hemidiaphragm

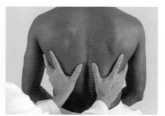

Figure 8-2 Assess lung expansion.

- Tactile fremitus as the patient says "aa" or "blue moon"

    Decreased or absent fremitus when transmission of vibrations to the chest is impeded by a thick chest wall, obstructed bronchus, COPD, or pleural effusion, fibrosis, air (pneumothorax), or an infiltrating tumor.

EXAMINATION TECHNIQUES

POSSIBLE FINDINGS

Asymmetric decreased fremitus in uni-lateral pleural effusion, pneumothorax, or neoplasm; asymmetric increased fremitus occurs in unilateral pneumonia, which increases transmission through consolidated tissue.

Percuss the chest, comparing one side with the other at each level, using the side-to-side "ladder pattern," as shown in Figures 8-3 and 8-4.

Dullness when fluid or solid tissue replaces normally air-filled lung; *hyper-resonance* in emphysema or pneumo-thorax

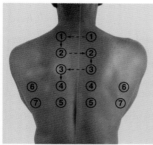

Figure 8-3 Percuss and auscultate in a "ladder" pattern.

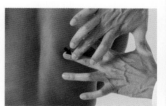

Figure 8-4 Strike the pleximeter finger with the right middle finger.

Percussion Notes and Their Characteristics

	Relative Intensity, Pitch, and Duration	Examples
Flat	Soft/high/short	Large pleural effusion
Dull	Medium/medium/medium	Lobar pneumonia
Resonant	Loud/low/long	Healthy lung, simple chronic bronchitis
Hyperresonant	Louder/lower/longer	Emphysema, pneumothorax
Tympanitic	Loud/high (timbre is musical)	Large pneumothorax

Percuss level of diaphragmatic dullness on each side and estimate diaphragmatic descent after patient takes full inspiration (Fig. 8-5).

Pleural effusion or a *paralyzed diaphragm* raises level of dullness.

EXAMINATION TECHNIQUES | POSSIBLE FINDINGS

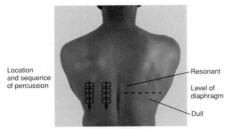

Location and sequence of percussion

Resonant

Level of diaphragm

Dull

Figure 8-5 Identify the extent of diaphragmatic excursion.

Auscultate the chest with stethoscope in the "ladder" pattern, again comparing sides.

See Table 8-6, Physical Findings in Selected Chest Disorders, p. 165.

■ Evaluate the breath sounds.

Vesicular, bronchovesicular, or bronchial breath sounds; decreased breath sounds from decreased airflow.

■ Note any adventitious (added) sounds.

Crackles (fine and coarse) and continuous sounds (wheezes and rhonchi)

Observe qualities of breath sound, timing in the respiratory cycle, and location on the chest wall. Do they clear with deep breathing or coughing?

Clearing after cough suggests atelectasis.

Characteristics of Breath Sounds

	Duration	Intensity and Pitch of Expiratory Sound	Example Locations
Vesicular	Insp > Exp	Soft/low	Most of the lungs
Bronchovesicular	Insp = Exp	Medium/medium	1st and 2nd interspaces, interscapular area
Bronchial	Exp > Insp	Loud/high	Over the manubrium
Tracheal	Insp = Exp	Very loud/high	Over the trachea

Duration is indicated by the length of the line, intensity by the width of the line, and pitch by the slope of the line.

EXAMINATION TECHNIQUES

POSSIBLE FINDINGS

Adventitious or Added Breath Sounds

Crackles (or Rales)

Discontinuous
- Intermittent, *nonmusical,* and brief

- Like dots in time
- *Fine crackles:* soft, high-pitched (~650 Hz), very brief (5–10 ms)

  • • • • •

- *Coarse crackles:* somewhat louder, lower in pitch (~350 Hz), brief (15–30 ms)

  • • • • •

Wheezes and Rhonchi

Continuous
- Sinusoidal, *musical,* prolonged (but not necessarily persisting throughout the respiratory cycle)

- Like dashes in time
- *Wheezes:* relatively high-pitched (≥400 Hz) with hissing or shrill quality (>80 ms)

- *Rhonchi:* relatively low-pitched (150–200 Hz) with snoring quality (>80 ms)

Source: Loudon R, Murphy LH. Lung sounds. *Am Rev Respir Dis.* 1994;130:663; Bohadana A, Izbicki G, Kraman SS. Fundamentals of lung auscultation. *N Engl J Med.* 2014;370:744.

Assess transmitted voice sounds and bronchial breath sounds heard in abnormal places. Ask patient to:

▪ Say "ninety-nine" and "ee."

Bronchophony if sounds become louder; egophony if "ee" to "A" change from lobar consolidation

▪ Whisper "ninety-nine" or "one-two-three."

Whispered pectoriloquy if whispered sounds transmit louder and more clearly

Transmitted Voice Sounds

Through Normally Air-Filled Lung	Through Airless Lung[a]
Usually accompanied by vesicular breath sounds and normal tactile fremitus	Usually accompanied by bronchial or bronchovesicular breath sounds and increased tactile fremitus
Spoken words muffled and indistinct	Spoken words louder, clearer (*bronchophony*)
Spoken "ee" heard as "ee"	Spoken "ee" heard as "ay" (*egophony*)
Whispered words faint and indistinct, if heard at all	Whispered words louder, clearer (*whispered pectoriloquy*)

[a]As in lobar pneumonia and toward the top of a large pleural effusion.

|

Alternative Examination Sequence—While the patient is still sitting, you may inspect the breasts and examine the axillary and epitrochlear lymph nodes, and examine the temporomandibular joint and the musculoskeletal system of the upper extremities.

๑ The Anterior Chest

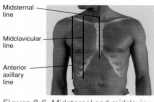

Midsternal line
Midclavicular line
Anterior axillary line

Figure 8-6 Midsternal and midclavicular lines.

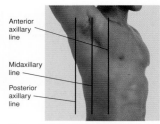

Anterior axillary line
Midaxillary line
Posterior axillary line

Figure 8-7 Anterior, posterior, and midaxillary lines.

Inspect the chest (Figs. 8-6 and 8-7) for:

- Deformities or asymmetry

  Pectus excavatum

- Intercostal retraction

  From obstructed airways

- Impaired or lagging respiratory movement

  Disease of the underlying lung or pleura, phrenic nerve palsy

Palpate the chest for:

- Tender areas

  Tender pectoral muscles, costochondritis

- Assessment of visible abnormalities

  Flail chest

- Respiratory expansion

- Tactile fremitus

EXAMINATION TECHNIQUES

| POSSIBLE FINDINGS |

Percuss the chest in the areas illustrated in Figure 8-8.

Normal cardiac dullness may disappear in emphysema.

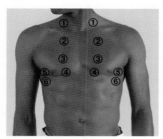

Figure 8-8 Palate and percuss in a "ladder" pattern.

Auscultate the chest. Assess breath sounds, adventitious sounds, and if indicated transmitted voice sounds.

Special Techniques

⚕ Clinical Assessment of Pulmonary Function. Walk
with patient down the hall or up a flight of stairs. Observe the rate, effort, and sound of breathing, and inquire about symptoms. Or learn to do a standardized "6-minute walk test."

Older adults walking 8 feet in <3 seconds are less likely to be disabled than those taking >5 to 6 seconds.

⚕ Forced Expiratory
Time. Ask the patient to take a deep breath in and then breathe out as quickly and completely as possible, with mouth open. Listen over trachea with diaphragm of stethoscope, and time audible expiration. Try to get three consistent readings, allowing rests as needed.

Patients age ≥60 years with a forced expiratory time of ≥9 seconds are four times more likely to have COPD.

Recording Your Findings

Recording the Thorax and Lungs Examination

"Thorax is symmetric with good expansion. Lungs resonant. Breath sounds vesicular; no rales, wheezes, or rhonchi. Diaphragms descend 4 cm bilaterally."

OR

"Thorax symmetric with moderate kyphosis and increased anteroposterior (AP) diameter, decreased expansion. Lungs are hyperresonant. Breath sounds distant with delayed expiratory phase and scattered expiratory wheezes. Fremitus decreased; no bronchophony, egophony, or whispered pectoriloquy. Diaphragms descend 2 cm bilaterally." *(These findings suggest COPD.)*

Aids to Interpretation

Table 8-1   Chest Pain

Problem and Location	Quality, Severity, Timing, and Associated Symptoms
Cardiovascular	
Angina Pectoris Retrosternal or across the anterior chest, sometimes radiating to the shoulders, arms, neck, lower jaw, or upper abdomen	■ Pressing, squeezing, tight, heavy, occasionally burning ■ Mild to moderate severity, sometimes perceived as discomfort rather than pain ■ Usually 1–3 min but up to 10 min; prolonged episodes up to 20 min ■ Sometimes with dyspnea, nausea, swelling
Myocardial Infarction Same as in angina	■ Same as in angina ■ Often but not always a severe pain ■ 20 min to several hours ■ Associated with nausea, vomiting, sweating, weakness
Pericarditis *Retrosternal or Precordial:* May radiate to the tip of the shoulder and to the neck	■ Sharp, knifelike quality ■ Often severe ■ Persistent timing ■ Relieved by leaning forward ■ Seen in autoimmune disorders, postmyocardial infarction, viral infection, chest irradiation
Dissecting Aortic Aneurysm Anterior chest, radiating to the neck, back, or abdomen	■ Ripping, tearing quality ■ Very severe ■ Abrupt onset, early peak, persistent for hours or more ■ Associated syncope, hemiplegia, paraplegia

(table continues on page 156)

Table 8-1   Chest Pain (*continued*)

Problem and Location	Quality, Severity, Timing, and Associated Symptoms
Pulmonary	
Pleuritic Pain Chest wall overlying the process	▪ Sharp, knifelike quality ▪ Often severe ▪ Persistent timing ▪ Associated symptoms of the underlying illness (often pneumonia, pulmonary embolism)
Gastrointestinal and Other	
Gastrointestinal Reflux Disease Retrosternal, may radiate to the back	▪ Burning quality, may be squeezing ▪ Mild to severe ▪ Variable timing ▪ Associated with regurgitation, dysphagia; also cough, laryngitis, asthma
Diffuse Esophageal Spasm Retrosternal, may radiate to the back, arms, and jaw	▪ Usually squeezing quality ▪ Mild to severe ▪ Variable timing ▪ Associated dysphagia
Chest Wall Pain, Costochondritis Often below the left breast or along the costal cartilages; also elsewhere	▪ Stabbing, sticking, or dull aching quality ▪ Variable severity ▪ Fleeting timing, hours or days ▪ Often with local tenderness
Anxiety, Panic Disorder	▪ Pain may be stabbing, sticking, or dull, aching ▪ Can mimic angina ▪ Associated with breathlessness, palpitations, weakness, anxiety

Table 8-2 Dyspnea

Problem	Timing	Provoking/Relieving Factors; Associated Symptoms
Left-Sided Heart Failure (*Left Ventricular Failure or Mitral Stenosis*)	Dyspnea may progress slowly or suddenly, as in acute pulmonary edema	↑ by exertion, lying down ↓ by rest, sitting up, though dyspnea may become persistent *Associated Symptoms:* Often cough, orthopnea, paroxysmal nocturnal dyspnea; sometimes wheezing
Chronic Bronchitis (*may be seen with COPD*)	Chronic productive cough followed by slowly progressive dyspnea	↑ by exertion, inhaled irritants, respiratory infections ↓ by expectoration, rest though dyspnea may become persistent *Associated Symptoms:* Chronic productive cough, recurrent respiratory infections; wheezing possible
Chronic Obstructive Pulmonary Disease (COPD)	Slowly progressive; relatively mild cough later	↑ by exertion ↓ by rest, though dyspnea may become persistent *Associated Symptoms:* Cough with scant mucoid sputum

(table continues on page 158)

Table 8-2 Dyspnea *(continued)*

Problem	Timing	Provoking/Relieving Factors; Associated Symptoms
Asthma	Acute episodes, then symptom-free periods; nocturnal episodes common	↑ by allergens, irritants, respiratory infections, exercise, emotion ↓ by separation from aggravating factors *Associated Symptoms:* Wheezing, cough, tightness in chest
Diffuse Interstitial Lung Diseases *(Sarcoidosis, Neoplasms, Asbestosis, Idiopathic Pulmonary Fibrosis)*	Progressive; varies in rate of development depending on cause	↑ by exertion ↓ by rest, though dyspnea may become persistent *Associated Symptoms:* Often weakness, fatigue; cough less common than in other lung diseases
Pneumonia	Acute illness; timing varies with causative agent	*Associated Symptoms:* Pleuritic pain, cough, sputum, fever, though not necessarily present
Spontaneous Pneumothorax	Sudden onset of dyspnea	*Associated Symptoms:* Pleuritic pain, cough
Acute Pulmonary Embolism	Sudden onset of dyspnea	*Associated Symptoms:* Often none; retrosternal oppressive pain if massive occlusion; pleuritic pain, cough, syncope, hemoptysis, and/or unilateral leg swelling and pain from instigating deep vein thrombosis; anxiety

Table 8-3   Cough and Hemoptysis

Problem	Cough, Sputum, Associated Symptoms, and Setting
Acute Inflammation	
Laryngitis	*Cough and Sputum:* Dry, or with variable amounts of sputum
	Associated Symptoms and Setting: Acute, fairly minor illness with hoarseness. Associated with viral nasopharyngitis
Acute Bronchitis	*Cough and Sputum:* Dry or productive of sputum
	Associated Symptoms and Setting: An acute, often viral illness, with burning retrosternal discomfort
Mycoplasma and Viral Pneumonias	*Cough and Sputum:* Dry and hacking often with mucoid sputum
	Associated Symptoms and Setting: Acute febrile illness, often with malaise, headache, and possibly dyspnea
Bacterial Pneumonias	*Cough and Sputum:* Sputum is mucoid or purulent; may be blood-streaked, diffusely pinkish, or rusty
	Associated Symptoms and Setting: Acute illness with chills, often high fever, dyspnea, and chest pain. Commonly from *Streptococcus pneumonia, Haemophilus influenza, Moraxella catarrhalis; Klebsiella* in alcoholism
Chronic Inflammation	
Postnasal Drip	*Cough and Sputum:* Chronic cough with mucoid or mucopurulent sputum
	Associated Symptoms and Setting: Repeated attempts to clear the throat. Postnasal drip, discharge in posterior pharynx. Associated with chronic rhinitis, with or without sinusitis

(table continues on page 160)

Table 8-3   Cough and Hemoptysis (*continued*)

Problem	Cough, Sputum, Associated Symptoms, and Setting
Chronic Bronchitis	*Cough:* Chronic
	Sputum: Mucoid to purulent; may be blood-streaked or even bloody
	Associated Symptoms and Setting: Often long history of cigarette smoking. Recurrent superimposed infections; often wheezing and dyspnea
Bronchiectasis	*Cough and Sputum:* Chronic cough; sputum mucoid to purulent, may be blood-streaked or even bloody
	Associated Symptoms and Setting: Recurrent bronchopulmonary infections common; sinusitis may coexist
Pulmonary Tuberculosis	*Cough and Sputum:* Dry, mucoid or purulent; may be blood-streaked or bloody
	Associated Symptoms and Setting: Early, no symptoms. Later, anorexia, weight loss, fatigue, fever, and night sweats
Lung Abscess	*Cough and Sputum:* Sputum purulent and foul-smelling; may be bloody
	Associated Symptoms and Setting: Often from aspiration pneumonia from oral anaerobes and poor dental hygiene; often with dysphagia, impaired consciousness
Asthma	*Cough and Sputum:* Thick and mucoid, especially near end of an attack
	Associated Symptoms and Setting: Episodic wheezing and dyspnea, but cough may occur alone. Often a history of allergy

Table 8-3   Cough and Hemoptysis (*continued*)

Problem	Cough, Sputum, Associated Symptoms, and Setting
Gastroesophageal Reflux	*Cough and Sputum:* Chronic cough, especially at night or early morning
	Associated Symptoms and Setting: Wheezing, especially at night (often mistaken for asthma), early morning hoarseness, repeated attempts to clear throat. Often with history of heartburn and regurgitation
Neoplasm	*Cough:* Dry to productive
Lung Cancer	*Sputum and Cough:* Cough, dry to productive; sputum may be blood-streaked or bloody
	Associated symptoms and setting: Commonly with dyspnea, weight loss, and history of tobacco abuse
Cardiovascular Disorders	
Left Ventricular Failure or Mitral Stenosis	*Cough and Sputum:* Cough often dry, especially on exertion or at night. Sputum may progress to pink and frothy, as in pulmonary edema, or to frank hemoptysis
	Associated Symptoms and Setting: Dyspnea, orthopnea, paroxysmal nocturnal dyspnea.
Pulmonary Embolism	*Cough and Sputum:* Dry cough, at times with hemoptysis
	Associated Symptoms and Setting: Tachypnea, chest or pleuritic pain, dyspnea, fever, syncope, anxiety; factors that predispose to deep venous thrombosis
Irritating Particles, Chemicals, or Gases	*Cough and Sputum:* Variable. May be a latent period between exposure and symptoms
	Associated Symptoms and Setting: Exposure to irritants; eye, nose, and throat symptoms

Table 8-4 Abnormalities in Rate and Rhythm of Breathing

Inspiration Expiration

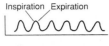

Normal. In adults, 14–20 per min; in infants, up to 44 per min.

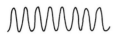

Rapid Shallow Breathing (*Tachypnea*). Many causes, including salicylate intoxication, restrictive lung disease, pleuritic chest pain, and an elevated diaphragm.

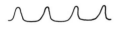

Rapid Deep Breathing (*Hyperpnea, Hyperventilation*). Many causes, including exercise, anxiety, metabolic acidosis, brainstem injury. Kussmaul breathing, due to metabolic acidosis, is deep, but rate may be fast, slow, or normal.

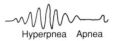

Slow Breathing (*Bradypnea*). May be secondary to diabetic coma, drug-induced respiratory depression.

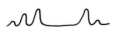

Hyperpnea Apnea

Cheyne–Stokes Breathing. Rhythmically alternating periods of hyperpnea and apnea. In infants and the aged, may be normal during sleep; also accompanies brain damage, heart failure, uremia, drug-induced respiratory depression.

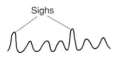

Ataxic (*Biot*) Breathing. Unpredictable irregularity of depth and rate. Causes include meningitis, respiratory depression, and brain injury.

Sighs

Sighing Breathing. Breathing punctuated by frequent sighs. When associated with other symptoms, it suggests the hyperventilation syndrome. Occasional sighs are normal.

Prolonged expiration

Obstructive Breathing. In obstructive lung disease, expiration is prolonged due to narrowed airways increase the resistance to air flow. Causes include asthma, chronic bronchitis, and COPD.

Table 8-5 Deformities of the Thorax

Cross-Section of Thorax

Normal Adult

The thorax is wider than it is deep; lateral diameter is greater than anteroposterior (AP) diameter.

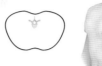

Barrel Chest

Has increased AP diameter, seen in normal infants and normal aging; also in COPD.

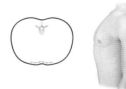

Traumatic Flail Chest

If multiple ribs are fractured, can see paradoxical movements of the thorax. Descent of the diaphragm decreases intrathoracic pressure on inspiration. The injured area may cave inward; on expiration, it moves outward.

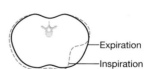

— Expiration

— Inspiration

Funnel Chest
(*Pectus Excavatum*)

Depression in the lower portion of the sternum. Related compression of the heart and great vessels may cause murmurs.

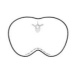

(table continues on page 164)

Table 8-5 Deformities of the Thorax (*continued*)

Cross-Section of Thorax
Pigeon Chest
(*Pectus Carinatum*)

Sternum is displaced anteriorly, increasing the AP diameter; costal cartilages adjacent to the protruding sternum are depressed.

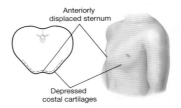

Anteriorly displaced sternum

Depressed costal cartilages

Thoracic Kyphoscoliosis

Abnormal spinal curvatures and vertebral rotation deform the chest, making interpretation of lung findings difficult.

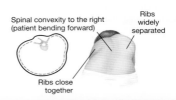

Spinal convexity to the right (patient bending forward)

Ribs widely separated

Ribs close together

Table 8-6 Physical Findings in Selected Chest Disorders

	Trachea	Percussion Note	Breath Sounds	Transmitted Voice Sounds	Adventitious Sounds
Chronic Bronchitis	Midline	Resonant	Normal	Normal	None, or wheezes, rhonchi, crackles
Left Heart Failure (Early)	Midline	Resonant	Normal	Normal	Late inspiratory crackles in lower lungs; possible wheezes
Consolidation[a]	Midline	Dull	Bronchial	Increased[b]	Late inspiratory crackles
Atelectasis (Lobar Obstruction)	May be shifted *toward* involved side	Dull	Usually absent	Usually absent	None
Pleural Effusion	May be shifted *away*	Dull	Decreased to absent	Decreased to absent	Usually none, possible pleural rub
Pneumothorax	May be shifted *away*	Hyperresonant or tympanitic	Decreased to absent	Decreased to absent	Possible pleural rub
COPD	Midline	Hyperresonant	Decreased to absent	Decreased	None or the wheezes and rhonchi of chronic bronchitis
Asthma	Midline	Resonant to hyperresonant	May be obscured by wheezes	Decreased	Wheezes, perhaps crackles

[a]As in lobar pneumonia, pulmonary edema, or pulmonary hemorrhage.
[b]With increased tactile fremitus, bronchophony, egophony, whispered pectoriloquy.

The Cardiovascular System

The Health History

Common or Concerning Symptoms

- Chest pain
- Palpitations
- Shortness of breath: dyspnea, orthopnea, or paroxysmal nocturnal dyspnea
- Swelling or edema
- Fainting (syncope)

As you assess reports of *chest pain or discomfort,* keep serious adverse events in mind, such as *angina pectoris, myocardial infarction,* or even a *dissecting aortic aneurysm.* Ask about any palpitations, shortness of breath from orthopnea or paroxysmal nocturnal dyspnea (PND), swelling from edema, and fainting. Be systematic as you think through the range of possible cardiac, pulmonary, and extrathoracic etiologies. Know the presentations of *chest pain, dyspnea, wheezing, cough,* and even *hemoptysis,* because these symptoms can be cardiac as well as pulmonary in origin. Also, when assessing cardiac symptoms, it is important to *quantify the patient's baseline level of activity compared to the symptomatic episode.*

Common Cardiac Symptoms

- *Chest pain* refers to classic exertional pain, pressure, or discomfort in the chest, shoulder, back, neck, or arm in angina pectoris, occurs in 18% of patients with acute MI; atypical descriptors also are common, such as cramping, grinding, pricking or, rarely, tooth or jaw pain.
- *Palpitations* are an unpleasant awareness of the heartbeat.
- *Shortness of breath* may represent dyspnea, orthopnea, or PND.
  - *Dyspnea* is an uncomfortable awareness of breathing that is inappropriate for a given level of exertion.

(continued)

Common Cardiac Symptoms *(Continued)*

- *Orthopnea* is dyspnea that occurs when the patient is lying down and improves when the patient sits up. It suggests *left ventricular heart failure* or *mitral stenosis;* it also may accompany *obstructive pulmonary disease.*
- PND describes episodes of sudden dyspnea and orthopnea that awaken the patient from sleep, usually 1 to 2 hours after going to bed, prompting the patient to sit up, stand up, or go to a window for air.
- *Edema* refers to the accumulation of excessive fluid in the interstitial tissue spaces; it appears as swelling. *Dependent edema* appears in the feet and lower legs when sitting or in the sacrum when bedridden.
- *Fainting* ("blacking out") or *syncope,* is a transient loss of consciousness followed by recovery.

Health Promotion and Counseling: Evidence and Recommendations

Important Topics for Health Promotion and Counseling

- Special populations at risk
- Screening for cardiovascular risk factors
  - *Step 1:* Screen for global risk factors
  - *Step 2:* Calculate 10-year and lifetime cardiovascular disease (CVD) risk using an online calculator
  - *Step 3:* Track individual risk factors—hypertension, diabetes, dyslipidemias, metabolic syndrome, smoking, family history, and obesity
- Promoting lifestyle changes and risk factor modification

CVD, which consists primarily of hypertension (the vast majority of diagnoses), coronary heart disease (CHD), heart failure, and stroke, affects nearly 84 million U.S. adults. CVD is the leading cause of death for both men and women in the United States. *Primary prevention,* in those without evidence of CVD, and *secondary prevention,* in those with known cardiovascular events, remain important clinical priorities. Provide education and counseling to promote optimal levels of blood pressure, cholesterol, weight, exercise, and smoking cessation and to reduce risk factors for CVD and stroke.

The American Heart Association recommends important goals for ideal cardiovascular health.

AHA 2020 Goals for Ideal Cardiovascular Health

1. Total cholesterol <200 mg/dL (untreated)
2. Lean body mass
3. BP <120/<80 (untreated)
4. Fasting glucose <100 mg/dL (untreated)
5. Abstinence from smoking
6. Physical activity goal: ≥150 min/wk moderate intensity, ≥75 min/wk vigorous intensity, or combination
7. Healthy diet

Special Populations at Risk

Virtually no U.S. adults have optimal health behaviors for all seven goals. Women and African Americans are groups at especially high risk.

Screening for Cardiovascular Risk Factors

Step 1: Screen for Global Risk Factors. Begin routine screening at age 20 for combined individual risk factors or "global" risk of CVD and any family history or premature heart disease, defined as onset at age <55 years in first-degree male relatives and <60 years in first-degree female relatives. See the recommended screening intervals listed below.

Major Cardiovascular Risk Factors and Screening Frequency

Risk Factor	Screening Frequency	Goal
Family history of premature CVD	Update regularly	
Cigarette smoking	At each visit	Cessation
Poor diet	At each visit	Improved overall eating pattern
Physical inactivity	At each visit	30 minutes moderate intensity daily
Obesity, especially central adiposity	At each visit	BMI 20–25 kg/m²; waist circumference: ≤40 inches for men, ≤35 inches for women
Hypertension	At each visit	<140/90 for adults <60 years, adults >60 years with diabetes or chronic kidney disease; <150/90 for all other adults ≥60 years
Dyslipidemias	Every 5 years if low risk Every 2 years if strong risk	Initiate statin therapy if meeting ACC/AHA guidelines

(continued)

Major Cardiovascular Risk Factors and Screening Frequency (Continued)

Risk Factor	Screening Frequency	Goal
Diabetes	Every 3 years (if normal) beginning at age 45 years; more frequently at any age if risk factors	Prevent/delay diabetes for those with HbA_{1c} of 5.7–6.4%
Pulse	At each visit	Identify and treat atrial fibrillation

Sources: see p. 186.

Step 2: Calculate 10-year and Long-Term CVD Risk Using Online Calculators.
Use the CVD risk calculators to establish 10-year and lifetime risk for ages 40 to 79 years. The most recent ACC/AHA Cholesterol Guideline provides a new risk-assessment calculator.

CVD Risk Calculators

- http://my.americanheart.org/cvriskcalculator
- http://www.acc.org/tools-and-practice-support/mobile-resources/features/2013-prevention-guidelines-ascvd-risk-estimator?w_nav=S.

Step 3: Track Individual Risk Factors—Hypertension, Diabetes, Dyslipidemias, Metabolic Syndrome, Smoking, Family History, and Obesity

Hypertension. The U.S. Preventive Services Task Force recommends *screening all people age ≥18 years for high blood pressure.* Use the blood pressure classification of the Seventh Report of the Joint National Committee on Prevention, Detection, Evaluation, and Treatment of High Blood Pressure (JNC 7).

Blood Pressure Classification for Adults—JNC 7, American Society of Hypertension

Category	Systolic (mm Hg)	Diastolic (mm Hg)
Normal	<120	<80
Prehypertension	120–139	80–89
Stage 1 hypertension		
Age ≥18 to <60 years	140–159	90–99
Age ≥60 years[a]	150–159	90–99

(continued)

Blood Pressure Classification for Adults—JNC 7, American Society of Hypertension (Continued)

Category	Systolic (mm Hg)	Diastolic (mm Hg)
Stage 2 hypertension	≥160	≥100
If diabetes or renal disease (including age ≥60 years)	<140	<90

[a]The American Society of Hypertension raises this cutoff to age ≥80 years.

Sources: Weber MA, Schiffrin EL, White WB, et al. Clinical practice guidelines for the management of hypertension in the community: a statement by the American Society of Hypertension and the International Society of Hypertension. *J Clin Hypertens*. 2014;16:14; Chobanian AV, Bakris GL, Black HR, et al. The Seventh Report of the Joint National Committee on Prevention, Detection, Evaluation, and Treatment of High Blood Pressure—The JNC 7 Report. *JAMA*. 2003;289:2560. Available at http://www.nhlbi.nih.gov/health-pro/guidelines/current/.

Diabetes. Use the screening and diagnostic criteria below.

American Diabetes Association 2015: Classification and Diagnosis of Diabetes

Screening Criteria

Healthy adults with no risk factors: begin at age 45 years, repeat at 3-year intervals

Adults with BMI ≥25 kg/m² and additional risk factors:

- Physical inactivity
- First-degree relative with diabetes
- Members of a high-risk ethnic population—African American, Hispanic/Latino American, Asian American, Pacific Islander
- Mothers of infants ≥4.08 kg (9 lb) at birth or diagnosed with GDM
- Hypertension ≥140/90 mm Hg or on therapy for hypertension
- HDL cholesterol <35 mg/dL and/or triglycerides >250 mg/dL
- Women with polycystic ovary syndrome
- HbA$_{1c}$ ≥5.7%, impaired glucose tolerance, or impaired fasting glucose on previous testing
- Other conditions associated with insulin resistance such as severe obesity, acanthosis nigricans
- History of CVD

Diagnostic Criteria	Diabetes[a]	Prediabetes
HbA$_{1c}$	≥6.5%	5.7%–6.4%
Fasting plasma glucose (on at least 2 occasions)	≥126 mg/dL	100–125 mg/dL

(continued)

American Diabetes Association 2015: Classification and Diagnosis of Diabetes (Continued)

Diagnostic Criteria	Diabetes[a]	Prediabetes
2-Hour plasma glucose (oral glucose tolerance test)	≥200 mg/dL	140–199 mg/dL
Random glucose if classic symptoms	≥200 mg/dL	

[a]In the absence of classic symptoms, an abnormal test must be repeated to confirm the diagnosis. However, if two different tests are both abnormal then no additional testing is necessary.
Source: American Diabetes Association. Classification and diagnosis of diabetes. *Diabetes Care.* 2015;38(Suppl):S8.

Dyslipidemias. LDL is the primary target of cholesterol-lowering therapy. The USPSTF has issued a grade A recommendation for routine lipid screening for all men of age >35 years and women >45 years who are at increased risk for CHD; and a grade B recommendation to screen for lipid disorders beginning at age 20 years for men and women who have diabetes, hypertension, obesity, tobacco use, noncoronary atherosclerosis, or family history of early CVD. In 2014 the ACC/AHA published "a guideline on the treatment of blood cholesterol to reduce atherosclerotic cardiovascular risk in adults." *Use the CVD risk calculator to establish 10-year risk* and lifetime gender and race-specific risks for CHD and stroke events to guide statin use for primary prevention (ACC/AHA Risk Calculator: http://tools.cardiosource.org/ASCVD-Risk-Estimator). The most recent ACC/AHA Cholesterol Guideline provides evidence-based recommendations for initiating statin therapy based on high, moderately high, and low risk level.

ATP III Guidelines: 10-Year Risk and LDL Goals

10-Year Risk Category	LDL Goal (mg/dL)	Consider Drug Therapy if LDL (mg/dL)
High risk (>20%)	<100 *Optional goal:* <70	>100 (<100: consider drug options, including further 30%–40% reduction in LDL)
Moderately high risk (10%–20%)	<130 *Optional goal:* <100	≥130 100–129: consider drug options to achieve goal of <100
Moderate risk (<10%)	<130	≥160
Lower risk (0–1 risk factor)	<160	>190 (160–189: drug therapy *optional*)

Source: Adapted from National Cholesterol Education Panel Report. Implications of recent clinical trials for the National Cholesterol Education Program Adult Treatment Panel III Guidelines. Grundy SM, Cleeman JI, Merz NB, et al., for the Coordinating Committee of the National Cholesterol Education Program. *Circulation.* 2004;119:227–239.

Metabolic Syndrome. The *metabolic syndrome* consists of a cluster of risk factors which confer and increased risk of both CVD and diabetes. In 2009, the International Diabetes Association and other societies harmonized diagnostic criteria as the presence of three or more of the five risk factors listed below.

Metabolic Syndrome: 2009 Diagnostic Criteria

Waist circumference	Men ≥102 cm, women ≥88 cm
Fasting plasma glucose	≥100 mg/dL or being treated for elevated glucose
HDL cholesterol	Men <40 mg/dL, women <50 mg/dL, or being treated
Triglycerides	≥150 mg/dL, or being treated
Blood pressure	≥130/≥85, or being treated

Source: Alberti K, Eckel RH, Grundy SM, et al. Harmonizing the metabolic syndrome: a joint interim statement of the Internal Diabetes Federation Task Force on Epidemiology and Prevention; National Heart, Lung and Blood Institute; American Heart Association; World Heart Federation; Internal Atherosclerosis Society; and International Association for the Study of Obesity. *Circulation*. 2009;120:1620–1645.

Other Risk Factors: Smoking, Family History, and Obesity. *Smoking* increases the risk of CHD and stroke by two- to fourfold compared to nonsmokers or past smokers who quit >10 years previously; about 14% of U.S. cardiovascular deaths are attributed to smoking annually. Among adults, 13% report a *family history* of heart attack or angina before age 50 years. Along with a family history of premature revascularization, this risk factor is associated with about a 50% increased lifetime risk for CHD and for CVD mortality. Obesity, or BMI over 30 kg/m², contributed to 112,000 excess adult deaths compared to those of normal weight, and was associated with 13% of CVD deaths in 2004.

Promoting Lifestyle Change and Risk Factor Modification

Motivating behavior change is challenging, but it is an essential clinical skill for promoting risk factor reduction. Encourage the ACC/AHA recommendations below.

Lifestyle Modifications for Cardiovascular Health

- Optimal weight, or BMI of 18.5–24.9 kg/m²
- Intake of <6 g of sodium chloride or 2.3 g of sodium per day
- Regular aerobic exercise such as brisk walking three to four times a week, averaging 40 minutes per session

(continued)

Lifestyle Modifications for Cardiovascular Health (*Continued*)
• Moderate alcohol consumption per day of ≤2 drinks for men and ≤1 drink for women (2 drinks = 1 oz ethanol, 24 oz beer, 10 oz wine, or 2–3 oz whiskey) Diet rich in fruits, vegetables, whole grains, and low-fat dairy products with reduced intake of saturated and total fat, sweets, and red meats.

Source: Eckel RH, Jakicic JM, Ard JD, et al. 2013 AHA/ACC guideline on lifestyle management to reduce cardiovascular risk: a report of the American College of Cardiology/American Heart Association Task Force on Practice Guidelines. *Circulation.* 2014;129:S76.

Techniques of Examination

EXAMINATION TECHNIQUES | POSSIBLE FINDINGS

Heart Rate and Blood Pressure

If not already done, count the radial or apical pulse.

Estimate systolic blood pressure by palpation and **add** 30 mm Hg. Use this sum as the target for further cuff inflations.

This step helps you to detect an auscultatory gap and avoid recording an inappropriately low systolic blood pressure.

Measure blood pressure with a sphygmomanometer. If indicated, **recheck** it.

Orthostatic (postural) hypotension within 3 minutes of position change from supine to standing is SBP↓ ≥20 mm Hg; HR↑ ≥20 beats/min.

✎ Jugular Veins

Jugular venous pulsations: In the right internal jugular vein identify their highest point in the neck. Start with head of the bed at 30 degrees; adjust the head of the bed as necessary, giving consideration to volume status.

Jugular venous pressure (JVP)— Measure the vertical distance between this highest point and the sternal angle, normally <3 to 4 cm (Fig. 9-1).

Elevated JVP in right-sided heart failure; decreased JVP in hypovolemia from dehydration or gastrointestinal bleeding.

EXAMINATION TECHNIQUES

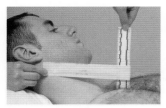

Figure 9-1 Measure the height of the JVP.

Study the waves of venous pulsation. Note the *a* wave of atrial contraction and the *v* wave of venous filling.

Abnormally prominent a waves in tricuspid stenosis, pulmonary hypertension, and pulmonic stenosis; absent a waves in atrial fibrillation. Increased v waves in tricuspid regurgitation, atrial septal defects, and constrictive pericarditis.

Carotid Pulse

Palpate the amplitude and contour of the carotid upstroke.

A delayed upstroke in aortic stenosis; a bounding upstroke in aortic insufficiency.

Pulsus Alternans. Palpate for alteration in carotid pulse amplitude. Lower pressure of blood pressure cuff slowly to systolic level while you listen with your stethoscope over the brachial artery.

Alternating amplitude of pulse or sudden doubling of Korotkoff sounds indicates *pulsus alternans*—a sign of left ventricular heart failure.

Paradoxical Pulse. Lower pressure of BP cuff slowly and note two pressure levels: (1) where Korotkoff sounds are first heard and (2) where they first persist through the respiratory cycle. These levels are normally not more than 3 to 4 mm Hg apart.

A drop of >10 mm Hg during inspiration signifies a paradoxical pulse. Consider obstructive pulmonary disease, asthma, COPD, pericardial tamponade, or constrictive pericarditis.

Listen for bruits.

Carotid bruits suggest atherosclerotic narrowing and increase stroke risk.

The Heart

Sequence of the Cardiac Examination

Patient Position	Examination
Supine, with the head elevated 30 degrees	After examining the JVP and carotid pulse, inspect and palpate the precordium: the 2nd right and left interspaces; the right ventricle; and the left ventricle, including the apical impulse (diameter, location, amplitude, duration).
Left lateral decubitus	Palpate the apical impulse to assess its diameter. Listen at the apex with the *bell* of the stethoscope.
Supine, with the head elevated 30 degrees	Listen at the six areas with the *diaphragm* then the *bell*: the 2nd right and left interspaces, down the left sternal border to the 4th and 5th interspaces, and across to the apex (see p. 177). As indicated, listen at the lower right sternal border for right-sided murmurs and sounds, often accentuated with inspiration, with the *diaphragm* and *bell*.
Sitting, leaning forward, after full exhalation	Listen down the left sternal border and at the apex with the *diaphragm* for the soft decrescendo murmur of aortic insufficiency.

Inspection and Palpation.
Inspect and palpate the anterior
chest for heaves, lifts, or thrills.

Inspect and palpate the *apical
impulse* (Fig. 9-2). Turn patient to
left as necessary. Note:

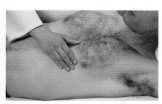

Figure 9-2 Palpate the apical impulse.

■ Location of impulse

Displaced to left in pregnancy.

■ Diameter

Increased diameter, amplitude, and
duration in left ventricular dilatation from
heart failure or *ischemic cardiomyopathy*.

EXAMINATION TECHNIQUES

POSSIBLE FINDINGS

■ Amplitude—usually *tapping*

Sustained in left ventricular hypertrophy; *diffuse* in CHF.

■ Duration

Feel for a right ventricular impulse in left parasternal and epigastric areas.

Prominent impulses suggest right ventricular enlargement.

Palpate left and right second interspaces close to sternum. Note any thrills in these areas.

Pulsations of great vessels; accentuated S_2; thrills of *aortic* or *pulmonic stenosis*.

Auscultation. Listen to the heart by "inching" your stethoscope from the base to the apex (or apex to base) in the areas illustrated in Figure 9-3.

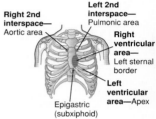

Figure 9-3 Auscultate the heart from the base to the apex.

Use the *diaphragm* to detect the relatively *high-pitched sounds* like S_1, S_2.

Also murmurs of aortic and mitral regurgitation, pericardial friction rubs.

Use the *bell* for *low-pitched sounds* at the lower left sternal border and apex.

S_3, S_4, murmur of *mitral stenosis*.

Listen at each area for:

■ S_1

See Table 9-1, Heart Sounds, p. 181; Table 9-2, Variations in the First Heart Sound—S_1, p. 182; Table 9-3, Variations in the Second Heart Sound—S_2 During Inspiration and Expiration, pp. 183–184.

■ S_2. Is splitting normal in left 2nd and 3rd interspaces?

Physiologic (inspiratory) or pathologic (expiratory) splitting

■ Extra sounds in systole

Systolic clicks

■ Extra sounds in diastole

S_3, S_4

EXAMINATION TECHNIQUES	POSSIBLE FINDINGS
■ Systolic murmurs	Midsystolic, pansystolic, late systolic murmurs
■ Diastolic murmurs	Early, mid-, or late diastolic murmurs

Use two maneuvers as needed to help identify the murmurs of mitral stenosis and aortic regurgitation.

Listen at the apex with patient turned toward left side for low-pitched sounds (Fig. 9-4).

Left-sided S_3, and diastolic murmur of *mitral stenosis*.

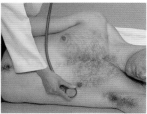

Figure 9-4 Listen at the apex for low-pitched sounds.

Listen down the left sternal border to the apex as patient sits, leaning forward, with breath held after exhalation (Fig. 9-5).

Diastolic decrescendo murmur of *aortic regurgitation*.

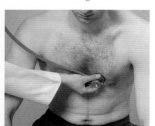

Figure 9-5 Listen at the lower left sternal border for aortic insufficiency.

Assessing and Describing Murmurs. Identify, if murmurs are present, their:

■ Timing in the cardiac cycle (systole, diastole). It is helpful to

See Table 9-4, Heart Murmurs, p. 185.

EXAMINATION TECHNIQUES

	POSSIBLE FINDINGS

palpate the carotid upstroke while listening to any murmur—murmurs occurring simultaneously with the upstroke are systolic.

- Shape

Plateau, crescendo, decrescendo

S₁   S₂

A *crescendo–decrescendo murmur* first rises in intensity, then falls (e.g., aortic stenosis).

S₁   S₂

A *plateau murmur* has the same intensity throughout (e.g., mitral regurgitation).

S₂   S₁

A *crescendo murmur* grows louder (e.g., mitral stenosis).

S₂   S₁

A *decrescendo murmur* grows softer (e.g., aortic regurgitation).

- Location of maximal intensity

Murmurs loudest at the *base* are often aortic; at the *apex,* they are often mitral.

- Radiation

- Pitch

High, medium, low

- Quality

Blowing, harsh, musical, rumbling

- Intensity on a six-point scale (see "Gradations of Murmurs" below)

Gradations of Murmurs

Grade	Description
Grade 1	Very faint, heard only after listener has "tuned in"; may not be heard in all positions
Grade 2	Quiet, but heard immediately after placing the stethoscope on the chest
Grade 3	Moderately loud
Grade 4	Loud, with *palpable thrill*
Grade 5	Very loud, *with thrill.* May be heard when the stethoscope is partly off the chest
Grade 6	Very loud, *with thrill.* May be heard with stethoscope entirely off the chest

EXAMINATION TECHNIQUES	POSSIBLE FINDINGS

Special Techniques

Aids to Identify Systolic Murmurs

Valsalva Maneuver. Ask patient to strain down.

In suspected *mitral valve prolapse* (*MVP*), listen to the timing of click and murmur.

Ventricular filling decreases, the systolic click of MVP is earlier, and the murmur lengthens.

To distinguish *aortic stenosis* (*AS*) from *hypertrophic cardiomyopathy* (*HCM*), listen to the intensity of the murmur.

In AS, the murmur decreases; in HCM, it often increases.

🧍 ***Squatting and Standing.*** In suspected *MVP*, listen for the click and murmur in both positions.

Squatting increases ventricular filling and delays the click and murmur. Standing reverses the changes.

Try to distinguish *AS* from *HCM* by listening to the murmur in both positions.

Squatting increases murmur of AS and decreases murmur of HCM. Standing reverses the changes.

Recording Your Findings

Recording the Cardiovascular Examination

"The jugular venous pulse is 3 cm above the sternal angle with the head of the bed elevated to 30 degrees. Carotid upstrokes are brisk, without bruits. The point of maximal impulse (PMI) is tapping, 7 cm lateral to the midsternal line in the 5th intercostal space. Crisp S_1 and S_2. At the base, S_2 is greater than S_1 and physiologically split, with $A_2 > P_2$. At the apex, S_1 is greater than S_2 and constant. No murmurs or extra sounds."

OR

"The JVP is 5 cm above the sternal angle with the head of the bed elevated to 50 degrees. Carotid upstrokes are brisk; a bruit is heard over the left carotid artery. The PMI is diffuse, 3 cm in diameter, palpated at the anterior axillary line in the 5th and 6th intercostal spaces. S_1 and S_2 are soft. S_3 present at the apex. High-pitched, harsh 2/6 holosystolic murmur best heard at the apex, radiating to the axilla. No S_4 or diastolic murmurs." *(These findings suggest CHF with possible left carotid stenosis and mitral regurgitation.)*

Aids to Interpretation

Table 9-1   Heart Sounds

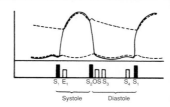

Finding	Possible Causes
S_1 accentuated	Tachycardia, states of high cardiac output; mitral stenosis
S_1 diminished	First-degree heart block; reduced left ventricular contractility; immobile mitral valve, as in mitral regurgitation
Systolic click(s)	Mitral valve prolapse (as in E_1 above)
S_2 accentuated in right 2nd interspace	Systemic hypertension, dilated aortic root
S_2 diminished or absent in right 2nd interspace	Immobile aortic valve, as in calcific aortic stenosis
P_2 accentuated	Pulmonary hypertension, dilated pulmonary artery, atrial septal defect
P_2 diminished or absent	Aging, pulmonic stenosis
Opening snap	Mitral stenosis
S_3	Physiologic (usually in children and young adults); volume overload of ventricle, as in mitral regurgitation or heart failure
S_4	Excellent physical conditioning (trained athletes); resistance to ventricular filling because of decreased compliance, left ventricular hypertrophy from pressure overload, as in hypertensive heart disease or aortic stenosis

Table 9-2 Variations in the First Heart Sound—S₁

Normal Variations

S_1 is softer than S_2 at the *base* (right and left 2nd interspaces).

S_1 S_2

S_1 is often but not always louder than S_2 at the *apex*.

S_1 S_2

Accentuated S₁

Occurs in (1) tachycardia, rhythms with a short PR interval, and high cardiac output states (e.g., exercise, anemia, hyperthyroidism), and (2) mitral stenosis.

S_1 S_2

Diminished S₁

Occurs in first-degree heart block, calcified mitral valve of mitral regurgitation, and ↓ left ventricular contractility in heart failure or coronary heart disease.

S_1 S_2

Varying S₁

S_1 varies in complete heart block and any totally irregular rhythm (e.g., atrial fibrillation).

S_1 S_2 S_1 S_2

Split S₁

Normally heard along the *lower left sternal border* if audible tricuspid component. If S_1 sounds split at apex, consider an S_4, an aortic ejection sound, an early systolic click, right bundle branch block, and premature ventricular contractions.

S_1 S_2

Table 9-3   Variations in the Second Heart Sound—S_2 During Inspiration and Expiration

Physiologic Splitting

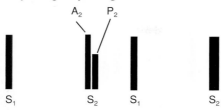

Heard in the 2nd or 3rd left interspace: the pulmonic component of S_2 is usually too faint to be heard at the apex or aortic area, where S_2 is single and derived from aortic valve closure alone. Accentuated by inspiration; usually disappears on exertion.

Pathologic Splitting

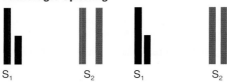

Wide splitting of S_2 persists throughout respiration; arises from delayed closure of the pulmonic valve (e.g., by pulmonic stenosis or right bundle branch block); also from early closure of the aortic valve, as in mitral regurgitation.

Fixed Splitting

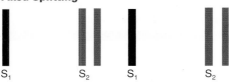

Does not vary with respiration, as in atrial septal defect, right ventricular failure.

(table continues on page 184)

Table 9-3 Variations in the Second Heart Sound— S₂ During Inspiration and Expiration *(continued)*

Paradoxical or Reversed Splitting

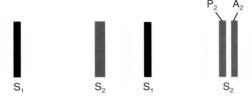

Appears on expiration and disappears on inspiration. Closure of the aortic valve is abnormally delayed, so A_2 follows P_2 on expiration, as in left bundle branch block.

More on A₂ and P₂

Increased Intensity of A_2, 2nd Right Interspace (where only A_2 can usually be heard) occurs in systemic hypertension because of the increased ejection pressure. It also occurs when the aortic root is dilated, probably because the aortic valve is then closer to the chest wall.

Decreased or Absent A_2, 2nd Right Interspace is noted in calcific aortic stenosis because of immobility of the valve. If A_2 is inaudible, no splitting is heard.

Increased Intensity of P_2. When P_2 is equal to or louder than A_2, pulmonary hypertension may be suspected. Other causes include a dilated pulmonary artery and an atrial septal defect. When a split S_2 is heard widely, even at the apex and the right base, P_2 is accentuated.

Decreased or Absent P_2 is most commonly due to the increased anteroposterior diameter of the chest associated with aging. It can also result from pulmonic stenosis. If P_2 is inaudible, no splitting is heard.

Table 9-4   Heart Murmurs

	Likely Causes
Midsystolic	Innocent murmurs (no valve abnormality)
	Physiologic murmurs (from ↑ flow across a semilunar valve, as in pregnancy, fever, anemia)
	Aortic stenosis
	Murmurs that mimic aortic stenosis—aortic sclerosis, bicuspid aortic valve, dilated aorta, and pathologically ↑ systolic flow across aortic valve
	Hypertrophic cardiomyopathy
	Pulmonic stenosis
Pansystolic	Mitral regurgitation
	Tricuspid regurgitation
	Ventricular septal defect
Late Systolic	Mitral valve prolapse, often with click (C)
Early Diastolic	Aortic regurgitation
Middiastolic and Presystolic	Mitral stenosis—note opening snap (OS)
Continuous Murmurs and Sounds	Patent ductus arteriosus—harsh, machinery-like
	Pericardial friction rub—a scratchy sound with 1–3 components
	Venous hum—continuous, above midclavicles, loudest in diastole

Sources for Major Cardiovascular Risk Factors and Screening Frequency Box on p. 170

Sources: Adapted from: Goff DC, Jr., Lloyd-Jones DM, Bennett G, et al. 2013 ACC/AHA guideline on the assessment of cardiovascular risk: a report of the American College of Cardiology/American Heart Association Task Force on Practice Guidelines. *J Am Coll Cardiol.* 2014;63(25 Pt B):2935; Stone NJ, Robinson JG, Lichtenstein AH, et al. 2013 ACC/AHA guideline on the treatment of blood cholesterol to reduce atherosclerotic cardiovascular risk in adults: a report of the American College of Cardiology/American Heart Association Task Force on Practice Guidelines. *Circulation.* 2014;129:S1; James PA, Oparil S, Carter BL, et al. 2014 evidence-based guideline for the management of high blood pressure in adults: report from the panel members appointed to the Eighth Joint National Committee (JNC 8). *JAMA.* 2014;311:507; Meschia JF, Bushnell C, Boden-Albala B, et al. Guidelines for the primary prevention of stroke: a statement for healthcare professionals from the American Heart Association/American Stroke Association. *Stroke.* 2014;45:3754; Flack JM, Sica DA, Bakris G, et al. Management of high blood pressure in Blacks: an update of the International Society on Hypertension in Blacks consensus statement. *Hypertension.* 2010;56:780; American Diabetes A. Executive summary: Standards of medical care in diabetes—2014. *Diabetes Care.* 2014;37 Suppl 1:S5.

The Breasts and Axillae

The Health History

Common or Concerning Symptoms

- Breast lump or mass
- Breast pain or discomfort
- Nipple discharge

Ask, "Do you examine your breasts?" ... "How often?" Ask about any discomfort, pain, or lumps in the breasts. Also ask about any discharge from the nipples, change in breast contour, dimpling, swelling, or puckering of the skin over the breasts.

Health Promotion and Counseling: Evidence and Recommendations

Important Topics for Health Promotion and Counseling

- Palpable masses of the breast
- Assessing risk of breast cancer
- Breast cancer screening

Palpable Masses of the Breast. Breast masses show marked variation in etiology, from fibroadenomas and cysts seen in younger women, to abscess or mastitis, to primary breast cancer. *All breast masses warrant careful evaluation, and definitive diagnostic measures should be pursued.*

Palpable Masses of the Breast

Age	Common Lesion	Characteristics
15–25	Fibroadenoma	Usually smooth, rubbery, round, mobile, nontender
25–50	Cysts	Usually soft to firm, round, mobile; often tender
	Fibrocystic changes	Nodular, rope-like
	Cancer	Irregular, firm, may be mobile or fixed to surrounding tissue
Over 50	Cancer until proven otherwise	As above
Pregnancy/ lactation	Lactating adenomas, cysts, mastitis, and cancer	As above

Adapted from Schultz MZ, Ward BA, Reiss M. Breast diseases. In: Noble J, Greene HL, Levinson W, et al. (eds). *Primary Care Medicine*. 2nd ed. St. Louis: MO; 1996; Venet L, Strax P, Venet W, et al. Adequacies and inadequacies of breast examinations by physicians in mass screenings. *Cancer*. 1971;28(6):1546–1551.

Assessing Risk of Breast Cancer. About 50% of affected women have no known predisposing risk factors; however, selected risk factors are well established.

Breast Cancer Risk Factors

Nonmodifiable risk factors:
- Age (most important)
- Family history of breast and ovarian cancers
- Inherited genetic mutations
- Personal history of breast cancer or lobular carcinoma in situ
- High levels of endogenous hormones
- Breast tissue density
- Proliferative lesions with atypia on breast biopsy
- Duration of unopposed estrogen exposure related to early menarche
- Age of first full-term pregnancy
- Late menopause
- Breast density on mammograms (commands increasing importance as a strong independent risk factor)
- History of radiation to the chest
- History of diethylstilbestrol (DES) exposure

Modifiable risk factors:
- Breastfeeding for <1 year
- Postmenopausal obesity
- Use of hormone replacement therapy (HRT)
- Cigarette smoking
- Alcohol ingestion
- Physical inactivity
- Type of contraception

See also Table 10-1, Breast Cancer in Women: Factors That Increase Relative Risk, p. 196.

Use the Breast Cancer Risk Assessment Tool of the National Cancer Institute (http://www.cancer.gov/bcrisktool) or other available clinical models, such as the Gail model, to individualize risk factor assessment for your patients. Ask women beginning in their 20s about any family history of breast or ovarian cancer, or both, on the maternal or paternal side, to help assess risk of BRCA1 or BRCA2 gene mutation. (See http://bcb.dfci.harvard.edu/bayesmendel/software.php.)

Breast Cancer Screening. Mammography combined with the CBE are the most common screening modalities; however, recommendations from professional groups vary about how to screen, when to start screening, and screening intervals, as shown in the table below. Clinicians should be well informed as they counsel individual patients, particularly as more evidence emerges to guide risk-based screening.

Breast Cancer Screening Recommendations

	Mammography	Clinical Breast Examination	Breast Self-Examination
U.S. Preventive Services Task Force—average-risk women (2016)	• 50–74 years—biennially • <50 years—individualize screening based on patient-specific factors • ≥75 years—insufficient evidence to recommend	≥40 years—insufficient evidence to assess additional benefits and harms of CBE beyond screening mammography	Recommends against teaching BSE
American Cancer Society—average-risk women (2015)	• 40–45 years—optional annual screening • 45–54 years—annual screening • ≥55 years—biennial screening with option to continue annual screens • Continue screening if good health and life expectancy ≥10 years	Not recommended due to lack of evidence showing clear benefit	Not recommended due to lack of evidence showing clear benefit
American College of Obstetricians and Gynecologists	≥40 years—annually	• 20–39 years—every 1–3 years • ≥40 years—annually	Encourages breast self-awareness

Sources: U.S. Preventive Services Task Force. Breast Cancer: Screening. January 2016. At http://www.uspreventiveservicestaskforce.org/Page/Document/UpdateSummaryFinal/breast-cancer-screening1?ds=1&s=BREAST CANCER. Accessed 2.11.16; Oeffinger KC, Fontham ETH, Etzioni R, et al. Breast cancer screening for women at average risk 2015 guideline update from the American Cancer Society. *JAMA.* 2015;314:1500. See also http://www.cancer.org/cancer/breastcancer/moreinformation/breastcancerearlydetection/breast-cancer-early-detection-acs-recs. Accessed November 14, 2015.
American College of Obstetricians and Gynecologists. Practice bulletin No. 122: breast cancer screening. *Obstet Gynecol.* 2011;118(2 pt 1):372.

Techniques of Examination

EXAMINATION TECHNIQUES

POSSIBLE FINDINGS

♀ The Female Breast

Inspect the breasts in four positions, identifying the quadrant where changes appear (Figs. 10-1 through 10-5).

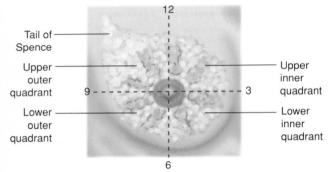

Figure 10-1 Breast quadrants.

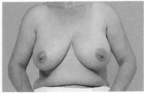

Figure 10-2 Inspect with arms at sides.

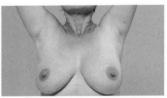

Figure 10-3 Inspect with arms over head.

EXAMINATION TECHNIQUES

POSSIBLE FINDINGS

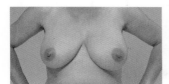

Figure 10-4 Inspect with hands pressed against hips.

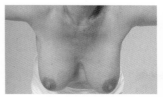

Figure 10-5 Inspect while leaning forward.

Note:

■ Size and symmetry

See Table 10-2, Visible Signs of Breast Cancer, pp. 197–198.

■ Contour

Flattening, dimpling suspicious for malignancy

■ Appearance of the skin

Edema (peau d'orange) in breast cancer

Inspect the nipples.

■ Compare their size, shape, and direction of pointing.

Inversion, retraction, deviation

■ Note any rashes, ulcerations, or discharge.

Paget disease of the nipple, galactorrhea

○— Palpate the breasts, including augmented breasts. Breast tissue should be flattened and the patient supine.

Use a *vertical strip pattern* (currently the best validated technique) or a circular or wedge pattern. Palpate in *small, concentric circles.*

For *the lateral portion of the breast,* ask the patient to roll onto the opposite hip, place her hand on her forehead, but keep shoulders pressed against the bed or examining table (Fig. 10-6).

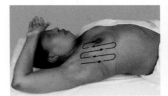

Figure 10-6 Vertical strip pattern— lateral breast.

EXAMINATION TECHNIQUES	POSSIBLE FINDINGS

For *the medial portion of the breast,* ask the patient to lie with her shoulders flat against the bed or examining table, place her hand at her neck, and lift up her elbow until it is even with her shoulder (Fig. 10-7).

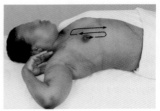

Figure 10-7 Vertical strip pattern— medial breast.

Palpate a rectangular area extending from the clavicle to the inframammary fold, and from the midsternal line to the posterior axillary line and well into the axilla for the tail of Spence.

Note:

- Consistency — **Physiologic nodularity**

- Tenderness — **Infection, premenstrual tenderness**

- Nodules. If present, note *location, size, shape, consistency, delimitation, tenderness,* and *mobility.* — **Cyst, fibroadenoma, cancer**

Palpate each nipple. — **Thickening in cancer**

Compress the areola in a spoke-like pattern around the nipple. Watch for discharge. — **Type and source of discharge may be identified.**

Palpate and inspect along the incision lines of mastectomy. — **Local recurrences of breast cancer**

♀/♂ The Male Breast

Inspect and palpate the nipple and areola. — **Gynecomastia, mass suspicious for cancer, fat**

EXAMINATION TECHNIQUES	POSSIBLE FINDINGS

Axillae

Inspect for rashes, infection, and pigmentation.

Hidradenitis suppurativa, acanthosis nigricans

Palpate the axillary nodes, including the central, pectoral, lateral, and subscapular groups (Figs. 10-8).

Lymphadenopathy

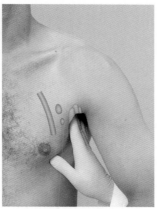

Figure 10-8 Palpate the left axilla.

Special Technique

⚲ Instructions for the Breast Self-Examination. For interested or high-risk patients, instruct the patient about how to perform the BSE.

Patient Instructions for the Breast Self-Examination (BSE)—American Cancer Society

Lying Supine

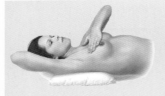
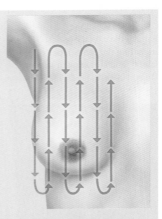

1. Lie down with a pillow under your right shoulder. Place your right arm behind your head.
2. Use the finger pads of the three middle fingers on your left hand to feel for lumps in the right breast. The finger pads are the top third of each finger. Make overlapping, dime-sized circular motions to feel the breast tissue.
3. Apply three levels of pressure in each spot: light, medium, and firm, using firmer pressure for tissue closest to the chest and ribs. A firm ridge in the lower curve of each breast is normal. If you're not sure how hard to press, talk with your health care provider, or try to copy the way the doctor or nurse does it.
4. Examine the breast in an up-and-down or "strip" pattern. Start at an imaginary straight line under the arm, moving up and down across the entire breast, from the ribs to the collarbone, until you reach the middle of the chest bone (the sternum). Remember how your breast feels from month to month.
5. Repeat the examination on your left breast, using the finger pads of the right hand.
6. If you find any masses, lumps, or skin changes, see your clinician right away.

(continued)

Patient Instructions for the Breast Self-Examination (BSE)—American Cancer Society *(Continued)*

Standing

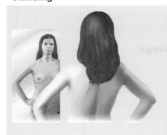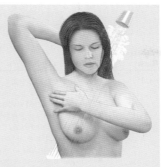

1. While standing in front of a mirror with your hands pressing firmly down on your hips, look at your breasts for any changes of size, shape, contour, or dimpling, or redness or scaliness of the nipple or breast skin. (The pressing down on the hips position contracts the chest wall muscles and enhances any breast changes.)

2. Examine each underarm while sitting up or standing and with your arm only slightly raised so you can easily feel in this area. Raising your arm straight up tightens the tissue in this area and makes it harder to examine.

Adapted from the American Cancer Society. American Cancer Society. Breast awareness and self-exam. Updated April 9, 2015. Available at http://www.cancer.org/cancer/breastcancer/moreinformation/breastcancerearlydetection/breast-cancer-early-detection-acs-recs-bse. Accessed May 7, 2015.

Recording Your Findings

Recording the Breasts and Axillae Examination

"Breasts symmetric and smooth, without masses. Nipples without discharge." (Axillary adenopathy usually included after Neck in section on Lymph Nodes.)
OR
"Breasts pendulous with diffuse fibrocystic changes. Single firm 1 × 1 cm mass, mobile and nontender, with overlying peau d'orange appearance in right breast, upper outer quadrant at 11 o'clock, 2 cm from the nipple." *(These findings suggest possible breast cancer.)*

Aids to Interpretation

Table 10-1 Factors That Increase the Relative Risk for Breast Cancer in Women

Relative Risk	Factor
>4.0	■ Age (65+ vs. <65 years, although risk increases across all ages until age 80) ■ Biopsy-confirmed atypical hyperplasia ■ Certain inherited genetic mutations for breast cancer (*BRCA1* and/or *BRCA2*) ■ Ductal carcinoma in situ ■ Lobular carcinoma in situ ■ Personal history of early-onset (<40 years) breast cancer ■ Two or more first-degree relatives with breast cancer diagnosed at an early age
2.1–4.0	■ High endogenous estrogen or testosterone levels (postmenopausal) ■ High-dose radiation to chest ■ Mammographically extremely dense (>50%) breasts compared to less dense (11%–25%) ■ One first-degree relative with breast cancer
1.1–2.0	■ Alcohol consumption ■ Ashkenazi Jewish heritage ■ Diethylstilbestrol exposure ■ Early menarche (<12 years) ■ Height (>5 feet 3 inches) ■ High socioeconomic status ■ Late age at first full-term pregnancy (>30 years) ■ Late menopause (>55 years) ■ Mammographically dense (26%–50%) breasts compared to less dense (11%–25%) ■ Non-atypical ductal hyperplasia or fibroadenoma ■ Never breastfed a child ■ No full-term pregnancies ■ Obesity (postmenopausal)/adult weight gain ■ Personal history of breast cancer (40+ years) ■ Personal history of endometrium, ovary, or colon cancer ■ Recent and long-term use of menopausal hormone therapy containing estrogen and progestin ■ Recent oral contraceptive use

Source: *American Cancer Society. Facts & Figures 2015–2016*. Atlanta: American Cancer Society Inc, 2015. Available at http://www.cancer.org/acs/groups/content/@research/documents/document/acspc-046381.pdf. Accessed May 1, 2015.

Table 10-2 Visible Signs of Breast Cancer

Retraction Signs

Fibrosis from breast cancer, fat necrosis, and mammary duct ectasia can produce the three retraction signs illustrated here.

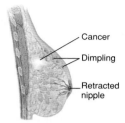

Skin Dimpling

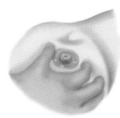

Abnormal Contours

Look for any variation in the normal convexity of each breast, and compare one side with the other.

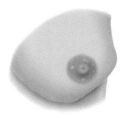

Nipple Retraction and Deviation

A retracted nipple is flattened or pulled inward and may be broadened and thickened. Typically the nipple deviates toward the underlying cancer.

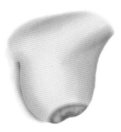

(table continues on page 198)

Table 10-2 Visible Signs of Breast Cancer (*continued*)

Edema of the Skin

From lymphatic blockade, appearing as thickened skin with enlarged pores—the so-called *peau d'orange* (orange peel) *sign*.

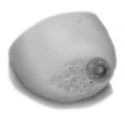

Paget Disease of the Nipple

An uncommon form of breast cancer that usually starts as a scaly, eczema-like lesion that may weep, crust, or erode. A breast mass may be present. Suspect Paget disease in any persisting dermatitis of the nipple and areola.

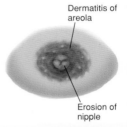

Dermatitis of areola

Erosion of nipple

The Abdomen

The Health History

Common or Concerning Symptoms

Gastrointestinal Disorders

- Abdominal pain, acute and chronic
- Indigestion, nausea, vomiting including blood (*hematemesis*), loss of appetite (*anorexia*), early satiety
- Difficulty swallowing (*dysphagia*) and/or painful swallowing (*odynophagia*)
- Change in bowel function
- Diarrhea, constipation
- Jaundice

Urinary and Renal Disorders

- Suprapubic pain
- Difficulty urinating (*dysuria*), urgency, or frequency
- Hesitancy, decreased stream in males
- Excessive urination (*polyuria*) or excess urination at night (*nocturia*)
- Urinary incontinence
- Blood in the urine (*hematuria*)
- Flank pain and ureteral colic

Mechanisms of Abdominal Pain

Be familiar with three broad categories:

Visceral pain—occurs when hollow abdominal organs such as the intestine or biliary tree contract unusually forcefully or are distended or stretched.

Visceral pain in the right upper quadrant (RUQ) from liver distention against its capsule from the various causes of hepatitis, including alcoholic hepatitis

- May be difficult to localize

- Varies in quality; may be gnawing, burning, cramping, or aching

- When severe, may be associated with sweating, pallor, nausea, vomiting, restlessness.

Parietal pain—from inflammation of the parietal peritoneum.

- Steady, aching

- Usually more severe

- Usually more precisely localized over the involved structure than visceral pain

Referred pain—occurs in more distant sites innervated at approximately the same spinal levels as the disordered structure.

Pain from the chest, spine, or pelvis may be referred to the abdomen.

Visceral periumbilical pain in *early acute appendicitis* from distention of inflamed appendix gradually changes to parietal pain in the right lower quadrant (RLQ) from inflammation of the adjacent parietal peritoneum.

Pain of duodenal or pancreatic origin may be referred to the back; pain from the biliary tree—to the right shoulder or right posterior chest.

Pain from *pleurisy* or *acute myocardial infarction* may be referred to the epigastric area.

The Gastrointestinal Tract

Ask patients to *describe the pain in their own words,* especially timing of the pain (acute or chronic); then ask them to *point to the pain.*

Pursue important details:

"Where does the pain start?"
"Does it radiate or travel?"
"What is the pain like?"
"How severe is it?"
"How about on a scale of 1 to 10?"
"What makes it better or worse?"

Elicit any *symptoms associated with the pain,* such as fever or chills; ask about their sequence.

In emergency rooms, up to 45% of patients have nonspecific pain, but 15% to 30% need surgery, usually for appendicitis, intestinal obstruction, or cholecystitis.

Doubling over with cramping colicky pain signals a renal stone. Sudden knife-like epigastric pain often radiating to the back is typical of pancreatitis.

Epigastric pain occurs with gastroesophageal reflux disease (GERD), pancreatitis, and perforated ulcers. RUQ and upper abdominal pain are common in cholecystitis and cholangitis.

Upper Abdominal Pain, Discomfort, or Heartburn. Ask about chronic or recurrent upper abdominal discomfort, or *dyspepsia.* Related symptoms include bloating, nausea, upper abdominal fullness, and heartburn. Is there:

■ Bloating from excessive gas, especially with frequent belching, abdominal distention, or flatus, the passage of gas by rectum

Bloating may occur with lactose intolerance, inflammatory bowel disease, or ovarian cancer; belching results from aerophagia, or swallowing air.

■ Unpleasant *abdominal fullness* after normal meals or *early satiety,* the inability to eat a full meal

Consider diabetic gastroparesis, anticholinergic drugs, gastric outlet obstruction, gastric cancer. Early satiety may signify *hepatitis.*

■ *Heartburn, dysphagia, or regurgitation?*

Suggests *GERD.* Up to 90% of patients with asthma have GERD-like symptoms. If patient fails empiric therapy, is age >55 years, or has "alarm symptoms" (dysphagia, pain with swallowing or odynophagia, recurrent vomiting, gastrointestinal bleeding, risk factors for gastric cancer, or palpable mass), endoscopy is warranted.

Lower Abdominal Pain or Discomfort—Acute and Chronic. If acute, is the pain sharp and continuous or intermittent and cramping?

RLQ pain, or pain migrating from periumbilical region in *appendicitis;* in women with RLQ pain, possible *pelvic inflammatory disease, ectopic pregnancy, ruptured ovarian follicle*

Left lower quadrant (LLQ) pain in *diverticulitis,* diffuse abdominal pain with abdominal distention, hyperactive bowel sounds, and tenderness on palpation in small or large bowel obstruction; pain with absent bowel sounds, rigidity, percussion tenderness, and guarding in peritonitis

If chronic, is there a change in bowel habits? Alternating diarrhea and constipation?

Colon cancer; irritable bowel syndrome

Abdominal Pain with Associated GI Symptoms

■ Nausea, vomiting, loss of appetite (*anorexia*)

Pregnancy, diabetic ketoacidosis, adrenal insufficiency, hypercalcemia, uremia, liver disease. Induced vomiting without nausea in anorexia/bulimia.

■ Regurgitation	**GERD, esophageal stricture, and esophageal cancer**
■ Coffee ground emesis (hematemesis)	**Esophageal or gastric varices, Mallory–Weiss tears, peptic ulcer disease**

Other GI Symptoms

■ Difficulty swallowing (*dysphagia*)	**If solids and liquids, neuromuscular disorders affecting motility. If only solids, consider structural conditions like *Zenker diverticulum*, *Schatzki ring*, stricture, neoplasm.**
■ Painful swallowing (*odynophagia*)	**Radiation; caustic ingestion, infection from *cytomegalovirus*, herpes simplex, HIV, esophageal ulceration from aspirin or NSAIDs**
■ Diarrhea, acute (<2 weeks) and chronic	**Acute infection (viral, salmonella, shigella, etc.); chronic in *Crohn disease*, ulcerative colitis; oily diarrhea (*steatorrhea*)—in pancreatic insufficiency. See Table 11-1, Diarrhea, pp. 214–215.**
■ Constipation	**Medications, especially anticholinergic agents and opioids; colon cancer, diabetes, hypothyroidism, hypercalcemia, multiple sclerosis, Parkinson disease**
■ Black tarry stools (melena)	**GI bleed**
■ Jaundice from increased levels of bilirubin: Intrahepatic jaundice can be *hepatocellular,* from damage to the hepatocytes, or *cholestatic,* from impaired excretion caused by damaged hepatocytes or intrahepatic bile ducts	**Impaired excretion of conjugated bilirubin in *viral hepatitis, cirrhosis, primary biliary cirrhosis,* drug-induced cholestasis**
Extrahepatic jaundice arises from obstructed extrahepatic bile ducts, commonly the cystic and common bile ducts	**Common bile duct obstruction from gallstones or pancreatic, cholangio-, or duodenal carcinoma**
Ask about the color of *the urine and stool.*	**Dark urine from increased conjugated bilirubin excreted in urine (*hepatitis*); acholic clay-colored stool when bilirubin excretion into intestine is obstructed**

Risk Factors for Liver Disease

- *Hepatitis:* Travel or meals in areas of poor sanitation, ingestion of contaminated water or foodstuffs (*hepatitis A*); parenteral or mucous membrane exposure to infectious body fluids such as blood, serum, semen, and saliva, especially through sexual contact with an infected partner or use of shared needles for injection drug use (*hepatitis B*); illicit injection drug use or blood transfusion (*hepatitis C*)
- *Alcoholic hepatitis* or *alcoholic cirrhosis* (screen patients carefully about alcohol use)
- *Toxic liver damage* from medications, industrial solvents, environmental toxins, or some anesthetic agents
- *Gallbladder disease* or *surgery* that may result in extrahepatic biliary obstruction
- *Hereditary disorders* in the Family History

The Urinary Tract

Ask about *pain on urination,* usually a burning sensation, sometimes termed *dysuria* (also refers to difficulty voiding).

Bladder infection (*cystitis*)

Also seen in *urethritis*, urinary tract infections, bladder stones, tumors, and, in men, *acute prostatitis*. In women, internal burning in *urethritis*, external burning in *vulvovaginitis*

Is there:

- *Urgency,* an unusually intense and immediate desire to void

May lead to urge incontinence

- *Urinary frequency,* or abnormally frequent voiding

Urinary tract infection

- Fever or chills; blood in the urine

Urinary tract infection

- Any pain in the abdomen, flank, or back

Dull, steady pain in *pyelonephritis*; severe colicky pain in ureteral obstruction from renal stone

- In men, *hesitancy* in starting the urine stream, *straining to void, reduced caliber and force of the urine stream,* or *dribbling* as they complete voiding.

Prostatitis, urethritis

Assess any:

◼ *Polyuria,* a significant increase in 24-hour urine volume	Diabetes mellitus, diabetes insipidus
◼ *Nocturia,* urinary frequency at night	Bladder obstruction
◼ *Urinary incontinence,* involuntary loss of urine:	See Table 11-2, Urinary Incontinence, pp. 216–217.
◼ From coughing, sneezing, lifting	*Stress incontinence* (poor urethral sphincter tone)
◼ From urge to void	*Urge incontinence* (detrusor overactivity)
◼ From bladder fullness with leaking but incomplete emptying	*Overflow incontinence* (anatomic obstruction, impaired neural innervation to bladder)

Health Promotion and Counseling: Evidence and Recommendations

Important Topics for Health Promotion and Counseling

- Screening for alcohol abuse
- Viral hepatitis: risk factors, vaccines, and screening
- Screening for colorectal cancer

Screening for Alcohol Abuse. Use the four CAGE questions (see Chapter 3, p. 56) to screen all adults in primary care settings, adolescents, and pregnant women for risky or hazardous alcohol use. Focus on detection, counseling, and, for significant impairment, specific treatment recommendations. Brief counseling interventions have been shown to reduce alcohol consumption by 13% to 34% over 6 to 12 months.

Screening for Problem Drinking

Standard Drink Equivalents: 1 standard drink is equivalent to 12 oz of regular beer or wine cooler, 8 oz of malt liquor, 5 oz of wine, or 1.5 oz of 80-proof spirits

Initial Screening Question: "How many times in the past year have you had 4 or more drinks a day (women), or 5 or more drinks a day (men)?"

(continued)

Screening for Problem Drinking (Continued)

Definitions of Drinking Levels for Adults—National Institute of Alcohol Abuse and Alcoholism

	Women	Men
Moderate drinking	≤1 drink/d	≤2 drinks/d
Unsafe drinking levels (increased risk for developing an alcohol use disorder)[a]	>3 drinks/d and >7 drinks/wk	>4 drinks/d and >14 drinks/wk
Binge drinking[b]	≥4 drinks on one occasion	≥5 drinks on one occasion

[a]Pregnant women and those with health problems that could be worsened by drinking should not drink any alcohol.
[b]Brings blood alcohol level to 0.08 g%, usually within 2 hours.

Viral Hepatitis: Risk Factors, Screening, and Vaccination.

Protective measures against *infectious hepatitis* include counseling about transmission.

■ *Hepatitis A:* Transmission is fecal–oral. Illness occurs approximately 30 days after exposure. Advise hand washing with soap and water after bathroom use or changing diapers and before preparing or eating food. Diluted bleach can be used to clean environmental surfaces.

CDC Recommendations for Hepatitis A Vaccination

- All children at age 1 year
- Individuals with chronic liver disease
- Groups at increased risk of acquiring HAV: travelers to areas with high endemic rates of infection, men who have sex with men, injection and illicit drug users, individuals working with nonhuman primates, and persons who have clotting-factor disorders

  The vaccine alone may be administered at any time before traveling to endemic areas.

■ *Hepatitis B:* Transmission occurs during contact with infected body fluids, such as blood, semen, saliva, and vaginal secretions. Infection increases risk of fulminant hepatitis, chronic infection, and subsequent cirrhosis and hepatocellular carcinoma. Provide counseling and serologic screening for patients at risk.

CDC Recommendations for Hepatitis B Vaccination: High-Risk Groups and Settings

- *Sexual contacts,* including sex partners of hepatitis B surface antigen-positive persons, people with more than one sex partner in the prior 6 months, people seeking evaluation and treatment for sexually transmitted infections, and men who have sex with men
- *People with percutaneous or mucosal exposure to blood,* including injection drug users, household contacts of antigen-positive persons, residents and staff of facilities for the developmentally disabled, health care workers, and people on dialysis
- *Others,* including travelers to endemic areas, people with chronic liver disease and HIV infection, and people seeking protection from hepatitis B infection
- *All adults in high-risk settings,* such as sexually transmitted infection (STI) clinics, HIV testing and treatment programs, drug-abuse treatment programs and programs for injection drug users, correctional facilities, programs for men having sex with men, chronic hemodialysis facilities and end-stage renal disease programs, and facilities for people with developmental disabilities

■ *Hepatitis C:* Hepatitis C, now the most common form of hepatitis, is spread by blood exposure and injection drug use. There is no vaccination for hepatitis C, so prevention targets counseling to avoid risk factors. Serologic screening should be recommended for high-risk groups.

Screening for Colorectal Cancer. Adopt the 2008 recommendations of the U.S. Preventive Services Task Force, listed below.

Screening for Colorectal Cancer

Assess Risk: Begin screening at age 20 years. If high risk, refer for more complex management. If average risk at age 50 (high-risk conditions absent), offer the screening options listed.

- **Common high-risk conditions** (25% of colorectal cancers)
  - Personal history of colorectal cancer or adenoma
  - First-degree relative with colorectal cancer or adenomatous polyps
  - Personal history of breast, ovarian, or endometrial cancer
  - Personal history of ulcerative or Crohn colitis
- **Hereditary high-risk conditions** (6% of colorectal cancers)
  - Familial adenomatous polyposis
  - Hereditary nonpolyposis colorectal cancer

(continued)

Screening for Colorectal Cancer (Continued)

Screening recommendations
- **Adults age 50 to 75 years**—options
  - High-sensitivity fecal occult blood testing (FOBT) annually
  - Sigmoidoscopy every 5 years with FOBT every 3 years
  - Screening colonoscopy every 10 years
- **Adults age 76 to 85 years**—do not screen routinely, as gain in life-years is small compared to colonoscopy risks, and screening benefits not seen for 7 years; use individual decision making if screening for the first time
- **Adults older than age 85**—do not screen, as "competing causes of mortality preclude a mortality benefit that outweighs harms"

Techniques of Examination

EXAMINATION TECHNIQUES | POSSIBLE FINDINGS

The Abdomen

○— Inspect the abdomen, including:

▓ Skin	Scars, striae, veins, ecchymoses (in intra- or retroperitoneal hemorrhages)
▓ Umbilicus	Hernia, inflammation
▓ Contours for shape, symmetry, enlarged organs or masses	Bulging flanks of ascites, suprapubic bulge, large liver or spleen, tumors
▓ Any peristaltic waves	Increased in GI obstruction
▓ Any pulsations	Increased in aortic aneurysm

Auscultate the abdomen for:

▓ Bowel sounds	Increased or decreased motility
▓ Bruits	Bruit of renal artery stenosis
▓ Friction rubs	Liver tumor, splenic infarct

EXAMINATION TECHNIQUES

POSSIBLE FINDINGS

Bowel Sounds and Bruits

Change	Seen with
Increased bowel sounds	Diarrhea Early intestinal obstruction
Decreased, then absent bowel sounds	Adynamic ileus Peritonitis
High-pitched tinkling bowel sounds	Intestinal fluid Air under tension in a dilated bowel
High-pitched rushing bowel sounds with cramping	Intestinal obstruction
Hepatic bruit	Carcinoma of the liver Alcoholic hepatitis
Arterial bruits	Partial obstruction of the aorta or renal, iliac or femoral arteries

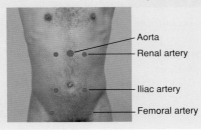

— Aorta
— Renal artery

— Iliac artery

— Femoral artery

Percuss the abdomen for patterns of tympany and dullness.

Ascites, GI obstruction, pregnant uterus, ovarian tumor

Palpate all quadrants of the abdomen:

- Lightly for guarding, rebound, and tenderness (Fig. 11-1)

See Table 11-3, Abdominal Tenderness, p. 217. "Acute abdomen" or peritonitis if:

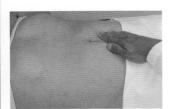

Figure 11-1 Begin with light palpation of the abdomen.

- *Firm, board-like abdominal wall*—suggests peritoneal inflammation.

- *Guarding* if the patient flinches, grimaces, or reports pain during palpation.

- *Rebound tenderness* from peritoneal inflammation; pain is greater when you withdraw your hand than when you press down. Press slowly on a tender area, then quickly "let go."

EXAMINATION TECHNIQUES

POSSIBLE FINDINGS

- Deeply for masses or tenderness (Fig. 11-2)

Tumors, a distended viscus

Abdominal masses may be: physiologic (pregnant uterus), inflammatory (diverticulitis), vascular (an AAA), neoplastic (colon cancer), or obstructive (a distended bladder or dilated loop of bowel).

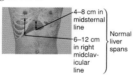

Figure 11-2 Use two hands for deep palpation.

The Liver

● Percuss span of liver dullness in the midclavicular line (MCL), Figure 11-3.

Increased dullness in hepatomegaly from acute hepatitis, heart failure; decreased dullness in cirrhosis

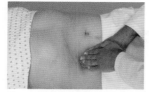

Figure 11-3 Measure the liver span.

Feel the liver edge, if possible, as patient breathes in.

Firm edge of cirrhosis

Starting well below the costal margin, measure distance of the liver edge from the costal margin in the MCL (Fig. 11-4).

Increased distance in hepatomegaly—may be missed (as in Fig. 11-5) by starting palpation too high in the RUQ

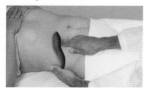

Figure 11-4 Palpate the liver edge.

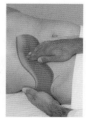

Figure 11-5 Palpating first at the costal margin may miss the liver edge.

Note any tenderness or masses.

Tender liver of hepatitis or heart failure; tumor mass

EXAMINATION TECHNIQUES

POSSIBLE FINDINGS

The Spleen

Percuss across left lower anterior chest (Traube space), noting change from tympany to dullness.

Palpate the spleen with the patient supine then lying on the right side with legs flexed at hips and knees (Fig. 11-6).

Splenomegaly

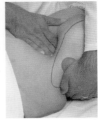

Figure 11-6 Spleen tip (purple) palpable below costal margin.

The Kidneys

Try to palpate each kidney (Fig. 11-7).

Enlargement from cysts, cancer, hydronephrosis

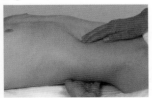

Figure 11-7 Palpate each kidney.

Check for costovertebral angle (CVA) tenderness (Fig. 11-8).

Tender in pyelonephritis

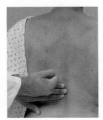

Figure 11-8 Percuss for costovertebral angle tenderness.

| EXAMINATION TECHNIQUES | POSSIBLE FINDINGS |

The Aorta

o— Palpate the aorta's pulsations (Fig. 11-9). In older people, estimate its width.

Periumbilical mass with expansile pulsations ≥3 cm in diameter in abdominal aortic aneurysm. Assess further due to risk of rupture.

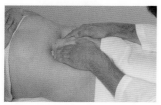

Figure 11-9 Palpate on both sides of the aorta.

Assessing Ascites

o—/o+— Palpate for shifting dullness. Map areas of tympany and dullness with patient supine, then lying on side (Fig. 11-10).

Ascitic fluid usually shifts to dependent side, changing the margin of dullness (Fig. 11-11).

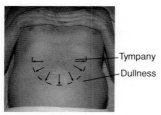

Figure 11-10 Percuss outward to map dullness from ascites.

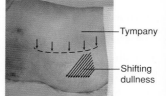

Figure 11-11 Percuss for shifting dullness (here patient turned to right side).

o— Check for a fluid wave (Fig. 11-12). Ask patient or an assistant to press edges of both hands into midline of abdomen. Tap one side and feel for a wave transmitted to the other side.

A palpable wave suggests but does not prove ascites.

EXAMINATION TECHNIQUES | POSSIBLE FINDINGS

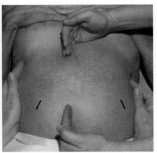

Figure 11-12 Test for a fluid wave.

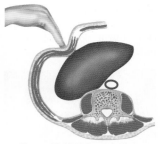

Figure 11-13 Ballotte the liver.

◦— Ballotte an organ or mass in an ascitic abdomen. Place your stiffened and straightened fingers on the abdomen, briefly jab them toward the structure, and try to touch its surface.

Your hand, quickly displacing the fluid, stops abruptly as it touches the solid surface (Fig. 11-13).

Assessing Possible Appendicitis

Ask:

In *classic appendicitis:*

"Where did the pain begin?"

Near the umbilicus

"Where is it now?"

RLQ

Ask patient to cough. "Where does it hurt?"

RLQ at "the McBurney point"

Palpate for local tenderness.

RLQ tenderness

Palpate for muscular rigidity.

RLQ rigidity

Perform a rectal examination and, in women, a pelvic examination (see Chapters 14 and 15).

Local tenderness, especially if appendix is retrocecal

■ *Rovsing sign:* Press deeply and evenly in the *left* lower quadrant. Then quickly withdraw your fingers.

Pain in the *right* lower quadrant during *left*-sided pressure suggests appendicitis (a *positive* Rovsing sign).

EXAMINATION TECHNIQUES

POSSIBLE FINDINGS

■ *Psoas sign:* Place your hand just above the patient's right knee. Ask the patient to raise that thigh against your hand. Or, ask the patient to turn onto the left side. Then extend the patient's right leg at the hip to stretch the psoas muscle.

Pain from irritation of the psoas muscle suggests an inflamed appendix (a *positive* psoas sign).

■ *Obturator sign:* Flex the patient's right thigh at the hip, with the knee bent, and rotate the leg internally at the hip, which stretches the internal obturator muscle.

Right hypogastric pain in a *positive* obturator sign, suggesting irritation of the obturator muscle by an inflamed appendix.

Assessing Possible Acute Cholecystitis

Auscultate, percuss, and palpate the abdomen for tenderness.

Bowel sounds may be active or decreased; tympany may increase with an ileus: Assess any RUQ tenderness.

Assess for the *Murphy sign.* Hook your thumb under the right costal margin at edge of rectus muscle, and ask patient to take a deep breath.

Sharp tenderness and a sudden stop in inspiratory effort constitute a *positive* Murphy sign.

Recording Your Findings

Recording the Abdominal Examination

"Abdomen is protuberant with active bowel sounds. It is soft and nontender; no palpable masses or hepatosplenomegaly. Liver span is 7 cm and in the right MCL; edge is smooth and palpable 1 cm below the right costal margin. Spleen and kidneys not felt. No CVA tenderness."

OR

"Abdomen is flat. No bowel sounds heard. It is firm and board-like, with increased tenderness, guarding, and rebound in the right midquadrant. Liver percusses to 7 cm in the MCL; edge not felt. Spleen and kidneys not felt. No palpable mass. No CVA tenderness." *(These findings suggest peritonitis from possible appendicitis; see pp. 212–213.)*

Aids to Interpretation

Table 11-1   Diarrhea

Problem/Process	Characteristics of Stool
Acute Diarrhea	
Secretory Infection (noninflammatory)	
Infection by viruses; preformed bacterial toxins such as *Staphylococcus aureus, Clostridium perfringens,* toxigenic *Escherichia coli; Vibrio cholerae, Cryptosporidium, Giardia lamblia,* rotavirus	Watery, without blood, pus, or mucus
Inflammatory Infection	
Colonization or invasion of intestinal mucosa as in nontyphoid *Salmonella, Shigella, Yersinia, Campylobacter,* enteropathic *E. coli, Entamoeba histolytica, Clostridium difficile*	Loose to watery, often with blood, pus, or mucus
Drug-Induced Diarrhea	
Action of many drugs, such as magnesium-containing antacids, antibiotics, antineoplastic agents, and laxatives	Loose to watery
Chronic Diarrhea (≥30 days)	
Diarrheal Syndromes	
■ *Irritable bowel syndrome:* A disorder of bowel motility with alternating diarrhea and constipation	Loose; may show mucus but no blood. Small, hard stools with constipation
■ *Cancer of the sigmoid colon:* Partial obstruction by a malignant neoplasm	May be blood-streaked

Table 11-1   Diarrhea (*continued*)

Problem/Process	**Characteristics of Stool**
Inflammatory Bowel Disease	
■ *Ulcerative colitis:* inflammation and ulceration of the mucosa and submucosa of the rectum and colon	Soft to watery, often containing blood
■ *Crohn disease* of the small bowel (regional enteritis) or colon (granulomatous colitis): chronic inflammation of the bowel wall, typically involving the terminal ileum, proximal colon, or both	Small, soft to loose or watery, usually free of gross blood (enteritis) or with less bleeding than ulcerative colitis (colitis)
Voluminous Diarrheas	
■ *Malabsorption syndrome:* Defective absorption of fat, including fat-soluble vitamins, with steatorrhea (excessive excretion of fat) as in pancreatic insufficiency, bile salt deficiency, bacterial overgrowth	Typically bulky, soft, light yellow to gray, mushy, greasy or oily, and sometimes frothy; particularly foul-smelling; usually floats in the toilet
■ *Osmotic Diarrheas*	
■ Lactose intolerance: Deficiency in intestinal lactase	Watery diarrhea of large volume
■ Abuse of osmotic purgatives: Laxative habit, often surreptitious	Watery diarrhea of large volume
■ *Secretory diarrheas* from bacterial infection, secreting villous adenoma, fat or bile salt malabsorption, hormone-mediated conditions (gastrin in Zollinger–Ellison syndrome, vasoactive intestinal peptide): Process is variable.	Watery diarrhea of large volume

Table 11-2   Urinary Incontinence

Problem	Mechanisms
Stress Incontinence: Urethral sphincter weakened. Transient increases in intra-abdominal pressure raise bladder pressure to levels exceeding urethral resistance. Leads to voiding *small amounts* during laughing, coughing, and sneezing.	■ In women, weakness of the pelvic floor with inadequate muscular support of the bladder and proximal urethra and a change in the angle between the bladder and the urethra from childbirth, surgery, and local conditions affecting the internal urethral sphincter, such as postmenopausal atrophy of the mucosa and urethral infection ■ In men, prostatic surgery
Urge Incontinence: Detrusor contractions are stronger than normal and overcome normal urethral resistance. Bladder is typically small. Results in voiding *moderate amounts,* urgency, frequency, and nocturia.	■ Decreased cortical inhibition of detrusor contractions, as in stroke, brain tumor, dementia, and lesions of the spinal cord above the sacral level ■ Hyperexcitability of sensory pathways, as in bladder infection, tumor, and fecal impaction ■ Deconditioning of voiding reflexes, caused by frequent voluntary voiding at low bladder volumes
Overflow Incontinence: Detrusor contractions are insufficient to overcome urethral resistance. Bladder is typically large, even after an effort to void, leading to *continuous dribbling.*	■ Obstruction of the bladder outlet, as by benign prostatic hyperplasia or tumor ■ Weakness of detrusor muscle associated with peripheral nerve disease at the sacral level ■ Impaired bladder sensation that interrupts the reflex arc, as in diabetic neuropathy

Table 11-2   Urinary Incontinence (*continued*)

Problem	Mechanisms
Functional Incontinence: Inability to get to the toilet in time because of impaired health or environmental conditions	■ Problems in mobility from weakness, arthritis, poor vision, other conditions; environmental factors such as unfamiliar setting, distant bathroom facilities, bed rails, physical restraints
Incontinence Secondary to Medications: Drugs may contribute to any type of incontinence listed.	■ Sedatives, tranquilizers, anticholinergics, sympathetic blockers, potent diuretics

Table 11-3   Abdominal Tenderness

Visceral Tenderness

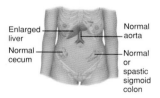

Enlarged liver

Normal cecum

Normal aorta

Normal or spastic sigmoid colon

Peritoneal Tenderness

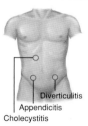

Diverticulitis

Appendicitis

Cholecystitis

Tenderness from Disease in the Chest and Pelvis

Acute Pleurisy

Unilateral or bilateral, upper or lower abdomen

Acute Salpingitis

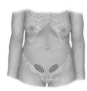

The Peripheral Vascular System

The Health History

Common or Concerning Symptoms

- Abdominal, flank, or back pain
- Pain in the arms or legs
- Exercise-induced pain (intermittent claudication)
- Cold, numbness, pallor in the legs; hair loss
- Swelling in calves, legs, or feet
- Color change in fingertips or toes in cold weather
- Swelling with redness or tenderness

Ask about abdominal, flank, or back pain, especially in older male smokers.

An expanding abdominal aortic aneurysm (AAA) may compress arteries or ureters.

Ask about any pain in the arms and legs.

Cold-induced digital ischemic change with blanching then cyanosis then rubor in Raynaud phenomenon or disease

Is there *intermittent claudication,* exercise-induced pain that is absent at rest, makes the patient stop exertion, and abates within about 10 minutes? Ask "Have you ever had any pain or cramping in your legs when you walk or exercise?" "How far can you walk without stopping to rest?" and "Does pain improve with rest?"

Peripheral arterial disease (PAD) can cause symptomatic limb ischemia with exertion; distinguish this from the neurogenic pain of *spinal stenosis,* which produces leg pain with exertion, often reduced by leaning forward (stretching the spinal cord in the narrowed vertebral canal) and less readily relieved by rest.

Ask also about *coldness, numbness,* or *pallor* in legs or feet or *hair loss* over the anterior tibial surfaces.

Hair loss over the anterior tibiae in PAD. "Dry" or brown–black ulcers from gangrene may ensue.

Because patients have few symptoms, identify risk factors—tobacco abuse, hypertension, diabetes, hyperlipidemia, and coronary artery disease—and PAD warning signs.

Only 10% to 30% of affected patients have the classic symptoms of exertional calf pain relieved by rest.

Peripheral Arterial Disease "Warning Signs"

- Fatigue, aching, numbness, or pain that limits walking or exertion in the legs; if present, identify the location. Ask also about erectile dysfunction.
- Any poorly healing or nonhealing wounds of the legs or feet
- Any pain present when at rest in the lower leg or foot and changes when standing or supine

Symptom location suggests the site of arterial ischemia:
- buttock, hip: *aortoiliac*
- erectile dysfunction: *iliac–pudendal*
- thigh: *common femoral* or *aortoiliac*
- upper calf: *superficial femoral*
- lower calf: *popliteal*
- foot: *tibial* or *peroneal*

- Abdominal pain after meals and associated "food fear" and weight loss

These symptoms suggest intestinal ischemia of the *celiac* or *superior* or *inferior mesenteric arteries.*

- Any first-degree relatives with an AAA

Prevalence of AAAs in first-degree relatives is 15% to 28%.

Ask about *swelling of feet and legs,* or any ulcers on lower legs, often near the ankles from peripheral vascular disease.

Calf swelling in deep venous thrombosis (DVT); hyperpigmentation, edema, and possible cyanosis, especially when legs are dependent, in *venous stasis ulcers;* swelling with redness and tenderness in *cellulitis.*

Health Promotion and Counseling: Evidence and Recommendations

Important Topics for Health Promotion and Counseling

- Screening for peripheral arterial disease
- The ankle–brachial index
- Screening for renal artery disease
- Screening for abdominal aortic aneurysm

Screening for Peripheral Arterial Disease. PAD prevalence increases with age, ranging from around 5% before age 50 years to 15% to 20% in persons aged 80 years and older. Cardiovascular risk factors, particularly smoking and diabetes, increase risk: An estimated 40% to 60% of PAD patients have coexisting coronary artery disease and/or cerebral artery disease, and the presence of PAD significantly increases risk of cardiovascular events. Most patients with PAD have either no symptoms or a range of *nonspecific leg symptoms*, such as *aching, cramping, numbness,* or *fatigue*.

Risk Factors for Lower-Extremity Peripheral Arterial Disease

- Age ≥65 years
- Age ≥50 years with a history of diabetes or smoking
- Leg symptoms with exertion
- Nonhealing wounds

The Ankle–Brachial Index. To diagnose PAD, use the ankle–brachial index (ABI), which is reliable, reproducible, noninvasive, easy to perform in the office, and highly specific. The ABI is the ratio of blood pressure measurements in the foot and arm; values <0.9 are considered abnormal.

A wide range of interventions reduces both onset and progression of PAD, including: supervised exercise programs; tobacco cessation; treatment of hyperlipidemia; optimal control of diabetes and hypertension; use of antiplatelet agents; meticulous foot care and well-fitting shoes, particularly for diabetic patients; and revascularization.

Screening for Renal Artery Disease. The American College of Cardiology and the American Heart Association recommend renal artery disease (RAS) screening with duplex ultrasonography, magnetic resonance angiography, or computed tomographic angiography in patients with the conditions listed in the box below.

Conditions Suspicious for Renal Artery Disease

- Onset of hypertension at age ≤30 years
- Onset of severe hypertension at age ≥55 years
- Accelerated (sudden and persistent worsening of previously controlled hypertension), resistant (not controlled with three drugs), or malignant hypertension (evidence of acute end-organ damage)

(continued)

Conditions Suspicious for Renal Artery Disease *(Continued)*

- New worsening of renal function or worsening function after use of an angiotensin-converting enzyme inhibitor or an angiotensin-receptor blocking agent
- An unexplained small kidney or size discrepancy of >1.5 cm between the two kidneys
- Sudden unexplained pulmonary edema, especially in the setting of worsening renal function

---

Screening for Abdominal Aortic Aneurysm. An AAA is present when the infrarenal aortic diameter exceeds 3 cm. Rupture and mortality rates dramatically increase for AAAs exceeding 5.5 cm in diameter. Additional risk factors are smoking, age older than 65 years, family history, coronary artery disease, PAD, hypertension, and elevated cholesterol level. Because symptoms are rare, and screening is now shown to reduce mortality by 50% over 13 to 15 years, the U.S. Preventive Services Task Force recommends one-time screening by ultrasound in men between 65 and 75 years of age with a history of "ever smoking," defined as more than 100 cigarettes in a lifetime.

Techniques of Examination

EXAMINATION TECHNIQUES	POSSIBLE FINDINGS

⚕ Arms

Inspect for:

▪ Size and symmetry, any swelling	**Lymphedema, venous obstruction**
▪ Venous pattern	**Visible venous collaterals, swelling, edema, and discoloration signal upper-extremity DVT.**
▪ Color and texture of skin and nails	**Sharply demarcated pallor of the fingers in Raynaud disease**

Palpate and grade the pulses:

Grading Arterial Pulses

3+	Bounding
2+	**Brisk, expected (normal)**
1+	Diminished, weaker than expected
0	Absent, unable to palpate

EXAMINATION TECHNIQUES	**POSSIBLE FINDINGS**

▦ Radial (Fig. 12-1)

Bounding radial, carotid, and femoral pulses in *aortic regurgitation*

Lost in thromboangiitis obliterans or acute arterial occlusion

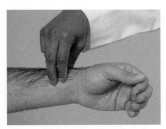

Figure 12-1 Palpate the radial pulse.

▦ Brachial (Fig. 12-2)

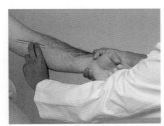

Figure 12-2 Palpate the brachial pulse.

Feel for the epitrochlear nodes.

Lymphadenopathy from local or distal infection, lymphoma, or human immunodeficiency virus (HIV)

॰— Abdomen

Auscultate for aortic, renal, and femoral bruits.

Palpate and estimate the width of the abdominal aorta between your two fingers (see p. 211).

Pulsatile mass, AAA if width ≥4 cm.

Palpate the superficial inguinal nodes (Fig. 12-3). Note size, consistency, discreteness, and any tenderness.

Lymphadenopathy in genital infections, lymphoma, AIDS

▦ Horizontal group

▦ Vertical group

<table>
<tr><td>**EXAMINATION TECHNIQUES**</td><td>POSSIBLE FINDINGS</td></tr>
</table>

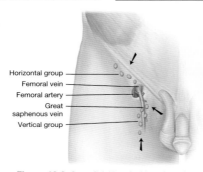

Horizontal group
Femoral vein
Femoral artery
Great saphenous vein
Vertical group

Figure 12-3 Superficial inguinal lymph nodes.

ᗧ Legs

Inspect for:

See Table 12-1, Chronic Insufficiency of Arteries and Veins, p. 228, and Table 12-2, Common Ulcers of the Feet and Ankles, p. 229.

■ Size and symmetry, any swelling in thigh or calf

Venous insufficiency, lymphedema; DVT. Calf asymmetry >3 cm (measure 10 cm below tibial tuberosity) doubles the risk of DVT.

■ Venous pattern

Varicose veins

■ Color and texture of skin

Pallor, rubor, cyanosis; erythema, warmth in *cellulitis, thrombophlebitis;* pigmentation, ulcers of the feet in PAD

■ Hair distribution, temperature

Atrophic hairless cool skin in PAD

Palpate and grade the pulses:

Loss of pulses in acute arterial occlusion and arteriosclerosis obliterans

■ Femoral

■ Popliteal (Fig. 12-4)

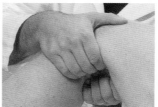

Figure 12-4 Palpate the popliteal pulse.

EXAMINATION TECHNIQUES

■ Dorsalis pedis and posterior tibial (Figs. 12-5 and 12-6)

Absent pedal pulses with normal femoral and popliteal pulses make PAD highly likely. Confirm with the ABI (see Table 12-3, Using the Ankle–Brachial Index, pp. 230–231).

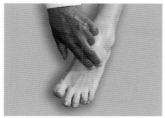

Figure 12-5 Palpate the dorsalis pedis pulse.

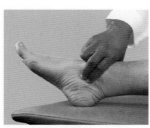

Figure 12-6 Palpate the posterior tibial pulse.

Palpate for pitting edema.

Dependent edema, heart failure, hypoalbuminemia, nephrotic syndrome

Palpate the calves.

Possible cord and tenderness in DVT (not always present)

Ask patient to stand, and reinspect the venous pattern.

Varicose veins

Special Techniques

⚲ Evaluating Arterial Supply to the Hand. Feel ulnar pulse, if possible. Perform an *Allen test*.

EXAMINATION TECHNIQUES	POSSIBLE FINDINGS

1. Ask the patient to make a tight fist, palm up. Occlude both radial and ulnar arteries with your thumb (Fig. 12-7).

2. Ask the patient to open hand into a relaxed, slightly flexed position (Fig. 12-8).

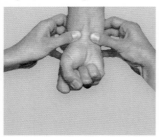

Figure 12-7 Compress the radial and ulnar arteries.

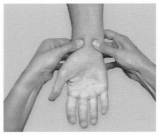

Figure 12-8 Pallor when hand relaxed.

3. Release your pressure over one artery. Palm should flush within 3 to 5 seconds (Fig. 12-9).

4. Repeat, releasing other artery. Persisting pallor of palm indicates occlusion of the released artery or its distal branches (Fig. 12-10).

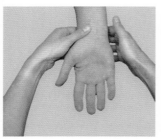

Figure 12-9 Palmar flushing—Allen test negative.

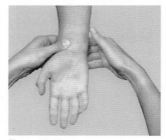

Figure 12-10 Palmar pallor—Allen test positive.

⚲/⚲ Postural Color Changes of Chronic Arterial Insufficiency.

Raise both legs to 60 degrees for about 1 minute. Then ask patient to sit up with legs dangling down. Note time required for (1) return of pinkness (normally 10 seconds) and (2) filling of veins on feet and ankles (normally about 15 seconds).

Marked pallor of feet on elevation, delayed color return and venous filling, and rubor of dependent feet suggest arterial insufficiency.

Recording Your Findings

Recording the Peripheral Vascular System Examination

"Extremities are warm and without edema. No varicosities or stasis changes. Calves are supple and nontender. No femoral or abdominal bruits. Brachial, radial, femoral, popliteal, dorsalis pedis (DP), and posterior tibial (PT) pulses are 2+ and symmetric."

OR

"Extremities are pale below the midcalf, with notable hair loss. Rubor noted when legs dependent but no edema or ulceration. Bilateral femoral bruits; no abdominal bruits heard. Brachial and radial pulses 2+; femoral, popliteal, DP, and PT pulses 1+." Alternatively, pulses can be recorded as below. *(These findings suggest atherosclerotic PAD.)*

	Radial	Brachial	Femoral	Popliteal	Dorsalis Pedis	Posterior Tibial
RT	2+	2+	1+	1+	1+	1+
LT	2+	2+	1+	1+	1+	1+

Aids to Interpretation

Table 12-1   Chronic Insufficiency of Arteries and Veins

Condition	Characteristics
Chronic Arterial Insufficiency 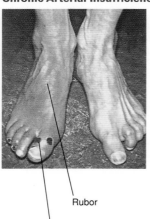 Rubor Ischemic ulcer	Intermittent claudication progressing to pain at rest. Decreased or absent pulses. Pale, especially on elevation; dusky red on dependency. Cool. Absent or mild edema, which may develop on lowering the leg to relieve pain. Thin, shiny, atrophic skin; hair loss over foot and toes; thickened, ridged nails. Possible ulceration on toes or points of trauma on feet. Potential for gangrene.
Chronic Venous Insufficiency 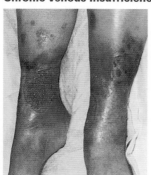	No pain to aching pain on dependency. Normal pulses, though may be hard to feel because of edema. Color normal or cyanotic on dependency; petechiae or brown pigment may develop. Often marked edema. Stasis dermatitis, possible thickening of skin, and narrowing of leg as scarring develops. Potential ulceration at sides of ankles. No gangrene.

Table 12-2   Common Ulcers of the Feet and Ankles

Ulcer	Characteristics
Arterial Insufficiency 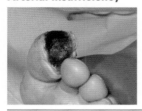	Located on toes, feet, or possible areas of trauma. No callus or excess pigment. May be atrophic. Pain often severe, unless masked by neuropathy. Possible gangrene. Decreased pulses, trophic changes, pallor of foot on elevation, dusky rubor on dependency.
Chronic Venous Insufficiency 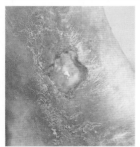	Located on inner or outer ankle. Pigmented, sometimes fibrotic. Pain not severe. No gangrene. Edema, pigmentation, stasis dermatitis, and possibly cyanosis of feet on dependency.
Neuropathic Ulcer 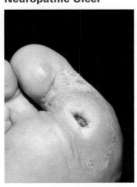	Located on pressure points in areas with diminished sensation, as in diabetic neuropathy. Skin calloused. No pain (which may cause ulcer to go unnoticed). Usually no gangrene. Decreased sensation, absent ankle jerks.

Table 12-3 Using the Ankle–Brachial Index

Instructions for Measuring the Ankle–Brachial Index (ABI)

1. Patient should rest supine in a warm room for at least 10 min before testing.

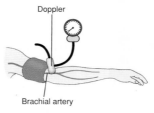

Doppler

Brachial artery

2. Place blood pressure cuffs on both arms and ankles as illustrated, then apply ultrasound gel over brachial, dorsalis pedis, and posterior tibial arteries.
3. Measure systolic pressures in the arms
   - Use vascular Doppler to locate brachial pulse
   - Inflate cuff 20 mm Hg above last audible pulse
   - Deflate cuff slowly and record pressure at which pulse becomes audible
   - Obtain 2 measures in each arm and record the average as the brachial pressure in that arm

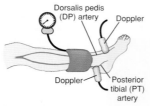

Dorsalis pedis (DP) artery   Doppler

Doppler   Posterior tibial (PT) artery

4. Measure systolic pressures in ankles
   - Use vascular Doppler to locate dorsalis pedis pulse
   - Inflate cuff 20 mm Hg above last audible pulse
   - Deflate cuff slowly and record pressure at which pulse becomes audible
   - Obtain 2 measures in each ankle and record the average as the dorsalis pedis pressure in that leg
   - Repeat above steps for posterior tibial arteries

Table 12-3 Using the Ankle–Brachial Index (*continued*)

5. Calculate ABI

$$\text{Right ABI} = \frac{\text{highest right average ankle pressure (DP or PT)}}{\text{highest average arm pressure (right or left)}}$$

$$\text{Left ABI} = \frac{\text{highest left average ankle pressure (DP or PT)}}{\text{highest average arm pressure (right or left)}}$$

Interpretation of Ankle–Brachial Index

Ankle–Brachial Index Result	Clinical Interpretation
>0.90 (with a range of 0.90 to 1.30)	Normal lower-extremity blood flow
<0.89 to >0.60	Mild PAD
<0.59 to >0.40	Moderate PAD
<0.39	Severe PAD

Source: Wilson JF, Laine C, Goldman D. In the clinic: peripheral arterial disease. *Ann Int Med.* 2007;146(5):ITC3.

Male Genitalia and Hernias

The Health History

Common or Concerning Symptoms

- Sexual health
- Penile discharge or lesions
- Scrotal pain, swelling, or lesions
- Sexually transmitted infections (STIs)

Sexual Health. Explain your concern for the patient's sexual health. Pose questions in a neutral and nonjudgmental way.

▪ "Are you currently dating, sexually active, or in a relationship?" "How would you identify your sexual orientation?" Continue with "How would you describe your gender identity?"

▪ "How is your current relationship?" "Are you satisfied with your relationship and your sexual activity?" "What about your ability to perform sexually?"

To assess *libido*, or desire: "How is your desire for sex?"

Decreased libido from depression, endocrine dysfunction, or side effects of medications.

For the *arousal* phase: "Can you achieve and maintain an erection?"

Erectile dysfunction from psychogenic causes, especially if early morning erection is preserved; also from decreased testosterone, decreased blood flow in hypogastric arterial system, impaired neural innervation, diabetes.

If *ejaculation* is premature or early: "About how long does intercourse last?" "Do you climax too soon?" For reduced or absent ejaculation: "Do you find that you cannot have orgasm even though you can have an erection?" "Does the problem involve the pleasurable sensation of *orgasm*, the ejaculation of seminal fluid, or both?"

Premature ejaculation is common, especially in young men. Less common is reduced or absent ejaculation affecting middle-aged or older men. Consider medications, surgery, neurologic deficits, or lack of androgen. Lack of orgasm with intact ejaculation is usually psychogenic.

Penile Discharge or Lesions, Scrotal Swelling or Pain, STIs and HIV. To assess possible infection from STIs, ask about any *discharge from the penis*.

Penile discharge in *gonococcal* (usually yellow) and *nongonococcal* (clear or white) *urethritis*.

Inquire about sores or growths on the penis and any pain or swelling in the scrotum.

See Table 13-1, Abnormalities of the Penis and Scrotum, p. 241, and Table 13-2, Sexually Transmitted Infections of Male Genitalia, pp. 242–243.

STIs may involve other parts of the body. Ask about practices of oral and anal sex and any related sore throat, oral itching or pain, diarrhea, or rectal bleeding.

Rash in disseminated gonococcal infection.

Ask "Do you have any concerns about HIV infection?" and discuss the need for *universal testing for HIV.*

Health Promotion and Counseling: Evidence and Recommendations

Important Topics for Health Promotion and Counseling

- Screening for STIs and HPV
- Screening for HIV infection and AIDS; counseling about sexual practices
- Screening for testicular cancer; testicular self-examination

Screening for STIs and HPV. Focus on patient education about STIs and HPV, early detection of infection during history taking and physical examination, and identification and treatment of infected partners. Identify the patient's sexual orientation, the number of sexual partners in the past month, and any history of STIs. Also query use of alcohol and drugs, particularly injection drugs. Counsel patients at risk about limiting the number of partners, using condoms, and establishing regular medical care for treatment. *Correct use of male condoms* is highly effective in preventing the transmission of STIs, HPV, and HIV.

Routine HPV vaccination is recommended in males age 11 or 12 years and through age 21 years if not vaccinated previously (age 26 years if immunocompromised or having sex with other men). The vaccine can prevent HPV-related diseases in males (genital warts, anal cancer, and penile cancer) and possibly reduce HPV transmission to female sex partners and lower the risk of oropharyngeal cancers.

Screening for HIV Infection and AIDS. The USPSTF recommends HIV screening for all adolescents and adults from age 15 to 65 years and all pregnant women. At least annual testing is recommended for high-risk groups (including adolescents younger than 15 years and older adults), defined as men with male sex partners, individuals with multiple sexual partners, past or present injection-drug users, persons who exchange sex for money or drugs, and sex partners of persons who are HIV-infected, bisexual, or injection-drug users. The presence of any STI, or requests for STI testing, warrants testing for coinfection with HIV.

Patient counseling should be interactive and combine information about general risk reduction with personalized messages based on the patient's personal risk behaviors.

Screening for Testicular Cancer; Testicular Self-Examination. Testicular cancer is rare but highly treatable when detected early. It is the most commonly diagnosed cancer in white men ages 20 to 34 years. Risk factors are white ethnicity, family history, HIV infection, and a history of cryptorchidism. The American Cancer Society encourages men, especially those between 15 and 35 years of age, to perform monthly testicular self-examinations.

Techniques of Examination

EXAMINATION TECHNIQUES | POSSIBLE FINDINGS

Male Genitalia

Wear gloves to examine the male genitalia (Fig. 13-1). The patient may be standing or supine.

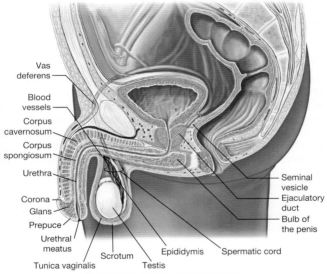

Vas deferens
Blood vessels
Corpus cavernosum
Corpus spongiosum
Urethra
Corona
Glans
Prepuce
Urethral meatus
Tunica vaginalis
Scrotum
Testis
Epididymis
Spermatic cord
Seminal vesicle
Ejaculatory duct
Bulb of the penis

Figure 13-1 Anatomy of male genitalia.

⚬⎯/ The Penis

Inspect the:

■ Development of the penis and the skin and hair at its base — Sexual maturation, lice

■ Prepuce (if present, retract the foreskin) — Phimosis, cancer

■ Glans — *Balanitis, chancre, herpes, warts, cancer*

EXAMINATION TECHNIQUES	POSSIBLE FINDINGS

■ Urethral meatus (compress the glans to inspect the meatus for discharge)

Hypospadias, discharge of *urethritis*

Palpate:

■ Any visible lesions

Chancre, cancer

■ The shaft

Urethral stricture or cancer

The Scrotum and Its Contents

Inspect:

■ Skin of scrotum

Rashes

■ Contours of scrotum

Hernia, *hydrocele, cryptorchidism*

■ Inguinal areas

Fungal infection

Palpate each:

■ Testis (Fig. 13-2), noting any:

See Table 13-3, Abnormalities of the Testis, p. 244.

   ■ Lumps

Testicular carcinoma

   ■ Tenderness

Acute epididymitis, acute orchitis, torsion of the spermatic cord, strangulated inguinal hernia.

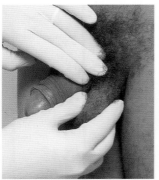

Figure 13-2 Palpate the testis and epididymis.

EXAMINATION TECHNIQUES	POSSIBLE FINDINGS

- Epididymis

Epididymitis, cyst

- Spermatic cord and adjacent areas (Fig. 13-3)

Varicocele if multiple tortuous veins; cystic structure may be a hydrocele

See Table 13-4, Abnormalities of the Epididymis and Spermatic Cord, p. 245.

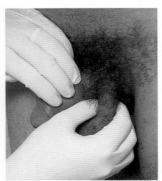

Figure 13-3 Palpate the spermatic cord.

Hernias

Patient is usually standing.

See Table 13-5, Hernias in the Groin, p. 246.

Inspect inguinal and femoral areas as patient strains down.

Inguinal and femoral hernias

Palpate external inguinal ring through scrotal skin and ask patient to strain down (Fig. 13-4).

Indirect and direct inguinal hernias

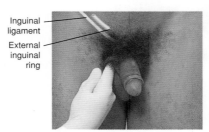

Inguinal ligament

External inguinal ring

Figure 13-4 Invaginate the scrotum.

Special Technique

Patient Instructions for the Testicular Self-Examination

This examination is best performed after a warm bath or shower. This way the scrotal skin is warm and relaxed. It is best to do the test while standing.

- Standing in front of a mirror, check for any swelling on the skin of the scrotum.
- With the penis out of the way, gently feel your scrotal sac to locate a testicle. Examine each testicle separately.

  As noted by the American Cancer Society, "It's normal for one testicle to be slightly larger than the other, and for one to hang lower than the other. You should also know that each normal testicle has a small, coiled tube (epididymis) that can feel like a small bump on the upper or middle outer side of the testicle. Normal testicles also have blood vessels, supporting tissues, and tubes that carry sperm. Some men may confuse these with abnormal lumps at first. If you have any concerns, ask your doctor or clinician."

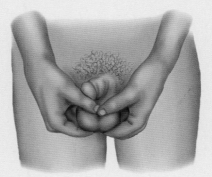

- Use one hand to stabilize the testicle. Using the fingers and thumb of your other hand, firmly but gently feel or roll the testicle between your fingers. Feel the entire surface. Find the epididymis. This is a soft, tube-like structure at the back of the testicle that collects and carries sperm, and is not an abnormal lump. Check the other testicle and epididymis the same way.
- If you find a hard lump, an absent or enlarged testicle, a painful swollen scrotum, or any other differences that do not seem normal, do not wait. See your health care provider right away.

Sources: American Cancer Society. Testicular self-exam. Updated January 21, 2015. Available at http://www.cancer.org/cancer/testicularcancer/moreinformation/doihavetesticularcancer/do-i-have-testicular-cancer-self-exam. Accessed May 13, 2015; U.S. National Library of Medicine, National Institutes of Health. MedlinePlus—Testicular self-exam. Updated December 27, 2013. Available at http://www.nlm.nih.gov/medlineplus/ency/article/003909.htm. Accessed May 13, 2015.

Recording Your Findings

Recording the Male Genitalia and Hernia Examination

"Circumcised male. No penile discharge or lesions. No scrotal swelling or discoloration. Testes descended bilaterally, smooth, without masses. Epididymis nontender. No inguinal or femoral hernias."

OR

"Uncircumcised male; prepuce easily retractible. No penile discharge or lesions. No scrotal swelling or discoloration. Testes descended bilaterally; right testicle smooth; 1×1 cm firm nodule on left lateral testicle. It is fixed and nontender. Epididymis nontender. No inguinal or femoral hernias." *(These findings are suspicious for testicular carcinoma, the most common form of cancer in men between ages 15 and 35 years).*

Aids to Interpretation

Table 13-1 Abnormalities of the Penis and Scrotum

Hypospadias

A congenital displacement of the urethral meatus to the inferior surface of the penis. A groove extends from the actual urethral meatus to its normal location on the tip of the glans.

Scrotal Edema

Pitting edema may make the scrotal skin taut; seen in heart failure or nephrotic syndrome.

Peyronie Disease

Palpable, nontender, hard plaques are found just beneath the skin, usually along the dorsum of the penis. The patient complains of crooked, painful erections.

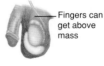
Fingers can get above mass

Hydrocele

A nontender, fluid-filled mass within the tunica vaginalis. It transilluminates, and the examining fingers can get above the mass within the scrotum.

Carcinoma of the Penis

An indurated nodule or ulcer that is usually nontender. Limited almost completely to men who are not circumcised, it may be masked by the prepuce. Any persistent penile sore is suspicious.

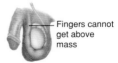
Fingers cannot get above mass

Scrotal Hernia

Usually an *indirect inguinal hernia* that comes through the external inguinal ring, so the examining fingers cannot get above it within the scrotum.

Table 13-2 Sexually Transmitted Infections of Male Genitalia

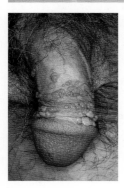

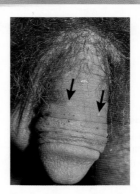

Genital Warts (Condylomata Acuminata)

- *Appearance:* Single or multiple papules or plaques of variable shapes; may be round, acuminate (or pointed), or thin and slender. May be raised, flat, or cauliflower-like (verrucous).
- *Causative organism: Human papillomavirus (HPV),* usually from subtypes 6, 11; carcinogenic subtypes rare, approximately 5%–10% of all anogenital warts.
- *Incubation:* Weeks to months; infected contact may have no visible warts.
- Can arise on penis, scrotum, groin, thighs, anus; usually asymptomatic, occasionally cause itching and pain.
- May disappear without treatment.

Genital Herpes Simplex

- *Appearance:* Small scattered or grouped vesicles, 1–3 mm in size, on glans or shaft of penis. Appear as erosions if vesicular membrane breaks.
- *Causative organism:* Usually *Herpes simplex virus 2* (90%), a double-stranded DNA virus. *Incubation:* 2–7 days after exposure.
- Primary episode may be asymptomatic; recurrence usually less painful, of shorter duration.
- Associated with fever, malaise, headache, arthralgias; local pain and edema, lymphadenopathy.
- Need to distinguish from genital herpes zoster (usually in older patients with dermatomal distribution); candidiasis.

Table 13-2   Sexually Transmitted Infections of Male Genitalia (*continued*)

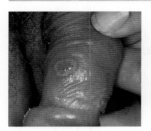

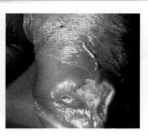

Primary Syphilis

- *Appearance:* Small red papule that becomes a chancre, or painless erosion up to 2 cm in diameter. Base of chancre is clean, red, smooth, and glistening; borders are raised and indurated. Chancre heals within 3–8 weeks.
- *Causative organism: Treponema pallidum,* a spirochete.
- *Incubation:* 9–90 days after exposure.
- May develop inguinal lymphadenopathy within 7 days; lymph nodes are rubbery, nontender, mobile.
- 20%–30% of patients develop secondary syphilis while chancre still present (suggests coinfection with HIV).
- Distinguish from: genital herpes simplex, chancroid, granuloma inguinale from *Klebsiella granulomatis* (rare in the United States; four variants, so difficult to identify).

Chancroid

- *Appearance:* Red papule or pustule initially, then forms a painful deep ulcer with ragged nonindurated margins; contains necrotic exudate, has a friable base.
- *Causative organism: Haemophilus ducreyi,* an anaerobic bacillus.
- *Incubation:* 3–7 days after exposure.
- Painful inguinal adenopathy; suppurative bobos in 25% of patients.
- Need to distinguish from: primary syphilis; genital herpes simplex; lymphogranuloma venereum, granuloma inguinale from *Klebsiella granulomatis* (both rare in the United States).

Table 13-3 Abnormalities of the Testis

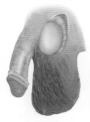 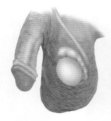 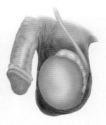

Cryptorchidism
Testis is atrophied and may lie in the inguinal canal or the abdomen, resulting in an unfilled scrotum. As above, there is no palpable left testis or epididymis. Cryptorchidism markedly raises the risk for testicular cancer.

Small Testis
In adults, testicular length is usually ≤3.5 cm. Small, firm testes seen in *Klinefelter syndrome,* usually ≤2 cm. Small, soft testes suggesting atrophy seen in cirrhosis, myotonic dystrophy, use of estrogens, and hypopituitarism; may also follow orchitis.

Acute Orchitis
The testis is acutely inflamed, painful, tender, and swollen. It may be difficult to distinguish from the epididymis. The scrotum may be reddened. Seen in mumps and other viral infections; usually unilateral.

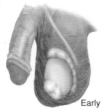

Early

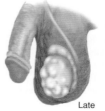

Late

Tumor of the Testis
Usually appears as a painless nodule. Any nodule within the testis warrants investigation for malignancy.

As a testicular neoplasm grows and spreads, it may seem to replace the entire organ. The testicle characteristically feels heavier than normal.

Table 13-4   Abnormalities of the Epididymis and Spermatic Cord

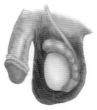

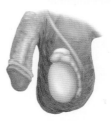

Acute Epididymitis

An acutely inflamed epididymis is tender and swollen and may be difficult to distinguish from the testis. The scrotum may be reddened and the vas deferens inflamed. It occurs chiefly in adults. Coexisting urinary tract infection or prostatitis supports the diagnosis.

Spermatocele and Cyst of the Epididymis

A painless, movable cystic mass just above the testis suggests a spermatocele or an epididymal cyst. Both transilluminate. The former contains sperm, and the latter does not, but they are clinically indistinguishable.

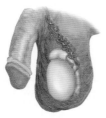

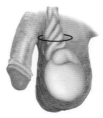

Varicocele of the Spermatic Cord

Varicocele refers to varicose veins of the spermatic cord, usually found on the left. It feels like a soft "bag of worms" separate from the testis, and slowly collapses when the scrotum is elevated in the supine patient.

Torsion of the Spermatic Cord

Twisting of the testicle on its spermatic cord produces an acutely painful and swollen organ that is retracted upward in the scrotum, which becomes red and edematous. There is no associated urinary infection. It is a surgical emergency because of obstructed circulation.

Table 13-5 Hernias in the Groin

Indirect Inguinal

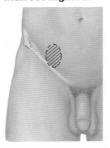

Most common hernia at all ages, both sexes. Originates above inguinal ligament and often passes into scrotum. *May touch examiner's fingertip in inguinal canal.*

Direct Inguinal

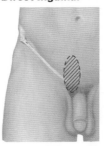

Less common than indirect hernia, usually occurs in men older than 40 years. Originates above inguinal ligament near external inguinal ring and *rarely enters scrotum. May bulge anteriorly, touching side of examiner's finger.*

Femoral

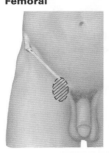

Least common hernia, more common in women than in men. Originates below inguinal ligament, more lateral than inguinal hernia. *Never enters scrotum.*

Female Genitalia

The Health History

Common Concerns

- Menarche, menstruation, menopause, postmenopausal bleeding
- Pregnancy
- Vulvovaginal symptoms
- Sexual health
- Pelvic pain—acute and chronic
- Sexually transmitted infections (STIs)

Menarche, Menstruation, Menopause, Postmeno-pausal Bleeding; Pregnancy.
For the *menstrual history*, ask when menstrual periods began (age at menarche).

When did her last menstrual period (LMP) start, and the one prior menstrual period (PMP)? What is the interval between periods, from the first day of one to the first day of the next? Are menses regular or irregular? How long do they last? How heavy is the flow?

Changes in the interval between periods can signal possible pregnancy or menstrual irregularities.

Amenorrhea is the absence of periods. Failure to begin periods is *primary amenorrhea*, whereas cessation of established periods is *secondary amenorrhea*.

Secondary amenorrhea from pregnancy, lactation, menopause; low body weight from conditions of malnutrition, *anorexia nervosa*, stress, chronic illness, and hypothalamic–pituitary–ovarian dysfunction

In amenorrhea from *pregnancy,* common early symptoms are tenderness, tingling, or increased size of breasts; urinary frequency; nausea and vomiting; easy fatigability; and feelings that the baby is moving (usually noted at about 20 weeks).

Amenorrhea followed by heavy bleeding in threatened abortion or dysfunctional uterine bleeding

Dysmenorrhea, or painful menses, is common.

Primary dysmenorrhea from increased prostaglandin production; secondary dysmenorrhea from *endometriosis, adenomyosis, pelvic inflammatory disease,* and endometrial polyps

Menopause, the absence of menses for 12 consecutive months, usually occurs between 48 and 55 years. Associated symptoms include hot flashes, flushing, sweating, and sleep disturbances.

Postmenopausal bleeding, or bleeding occurring 6 months after cessation of menses, from endometrial cancer, hormone replacement therapy (HRT), or uterine or cervical polyps

Vulvovaginal Symptoms. For *vaginal discharge* and local *itching,* inquire about amount, color, consistency, and odor of discharge.

See Table 14-1, Lesions of the Vulva, pp. 258–259; and Table 14-2, Vaginal Discharge, p. 260.

Sexual Health. Ask neutral questions about sexual orientation and gender identity: "Are you currently dating, sexually active, or in a relationship?" "How would you identify your sexual orientation?" Then, "How would you describe your gender identity?" and "Do you use protection such as birth control or condoms? . . . Has anyone ever tried to touch or have sex with you without your consent?"

To assess sexual health, be nonjudgmental. Ask "How is sex for you?" "Are you having any problems with sex? This includes sexual intercourse and anal and oral sex." Or, "Are you satisfied with your sex life as it is now?"

Direct questions help you assess desire, arousal, and orgasm.

"Do you have an interest in (appetite for) sex?" "Do you get sexually aroused?" "Are you able to reach climax?"

Ask also about *dyspareunia*, or discomfort or pain during intercourse.

Superficial pain suggests local inflammation, atrophic vaginitis, or inadequate lubrication; deeper pain may result from pelvic disorders or pressure on a normal ovary.

Pelvic Pain. Assess acute and chronic (>6 months) pelvic pain.

Acute pelvic pain in PID, ruptured ovarian cyst, appendicitis; ectopic pregnancy; also mittelschmerz, ruptured ovarian cyst, tubo-ovarian abscess. Chronic pelvic pain in endometriosis, PID, adenosis and fibroids, history of sexual abuse; pelvic floor spasm.

Sexually Transmitted Infection. Identify sexual preference (male, female, or both) and the number of sexual partners in the previous month. Ask if the patient has concerns about HIV infection, desires HIV testing, or has current or past partners at risk.

In women, some STIs do not produce symptoms, but do increase the risk of infertility.

Health Promotion and Counseling: Evidence and Recommendations

Important Topics for Health Promotion and Counseling

- Cervical cancer screening
- Ovarian cancer
- STIs and HIV infection
- Options for family planning
- Menopause and hormone replacement therapy

Cervical Cancer Screening. In 2012, five major societies released common guidelines for cervical cancer screening.

Current Cervical Cancer Screening Guidelines for Average-Risk Women[a]: USPSTF, ACS/ASCCP/ASCP, and ACOG

Variable	Recommendation
Age at which to begin screening	21 years
Screening method and interval	Ages 21–65 years: cytology every 3 years OR
	Ages 21–29 years: cytology every 3 years
	Ages 30–65 years: cytology plus HPV testing (for high-risk or oncogenic HPV types) every 5 years
Age at which to end screening	Age >65 years, assuming three consecutive negative results on cytology or two consecutive negative results on cytology plus HPV testing within 10 years before cessation of screening, with the most recent test performed within 5 years
Screening after hysterectomy with removal of the cervix	Not recommended

USPSTF, U.S. Preventive Services Task Force; ACS/ASCCP/ASCP, American Cancer Society/American Society for Colposcopy and Cervical Pathology/American Society for Clinical Pathology; ACOG, American College of Obstetricians and Gynecologists; HPV, human papillomavirus.
[a]**Definition of Average Risk:** No history of high-grade, precancerous cervical lesion (cervical intraepithelial neoplasia grade 2 or a more severe lesion) or cervical cancer; not immunocompromised (including being HIV-infected); and no in utero exposure to diethylstilbestrol.
Source: Sawaya GF, Kulasingam S, Denberg T, et al. Cervical cancer screening in average-risk women: best practice advice from the Clinical Guidelines Committee of the American College of Physicians. *Ann Intern Med.* 2015;162:851.

The most important risk factor for cervical cancer is HPV infection from HPV strains 16, 18, 6, or 11. The three-dose HPV vaccination series prevents HPV infection from the strains when given *before* sexual exposure at age 11 years. The vaccine is also recommended for unvaccinated and immunocompromised girls and women up to age 26 years.

Ovarian Cancer. There are no effective screening tests to date. Risk factors include family history of breast or ovarian cancer and BRCA1 or BRCA2 mutation. Watch for the nonspecific symptoms of new abdominal distention, abdominal bloating, and urinary frequency.

STIs and HIV Infection. Assess risk factors by taking a careful sexual history and counseling patients about spread of disease and ways to reduce high-risk practices. *Chlamydia trachomatis* is the most commonly reported STI in the United States and the most common STI in women. The CDC and the USPSTF strongly recommend screening for STIs as summarized in the box below.

CDC STD and HIV Screening Recommendations 2014

- Chlamydia and gonorrhea screening annually for all sexually active women ages <25 years and older women with risk factors such as new or multiple sex partners, or a sex partner infected with an STD.
- Chlamydia, syphilis, hepatitis B, and HIV screening for all pregnant women and gonorrhea screening for at-risk pregnant women starting early in pregnancy, with repeat testing as needed to protect the health of mothers and their infants.
- Chlamydia, gonorrhea, and syphilis screening at least once a year for all sexually active gay, bisexual, and other MSM. MSM who have multiple or anonymous partners should be screened more frequently for STDs (i.e., at 3- to 6-month intervals).
- HIV testing at least once for all adults and adolescents from ages 13–64 years.
- HIV testing at least once a year for anyone having unsafe sex or using injection drug equipment. Sexually active gay and bisexual men may benefit from testing every 3–6 months.

Source: Centers for Disease Control and Prevention. Sexually transmitted diseases. STD and HIV screening recommendations. Updated December 16, 2014. Available at http://www.cdc.gov/std/prevention/screeningreccs.htm. Accessed May 20, 2015.

Options for Family Planning. More than half of U.S. pregnancies are unintended. Counsel women, particularly adolescents, about the *timing of ovulation,* midway in the regular menstrual cycle. Discuss methods for contraception and their effectiveness.

Options for Family Planning

Methods	Types of Contraception
Natural	Fertility awareness/periodic abstinence, withdrawal, lactation
Barrier	Male condom, female condom, diaphragm, cervical cap, sponge
Implantable	Intrauterine device, subdermal implant of levonorgestrel
Pharmacologic/hormonal	Spermicide, oral contraceptives (estrogen and progesterone; progestin only), estrogen/progesterone injectables and patch, hormonal vaginal contraceptive ring, emergency contraception
Surgery (permanent)	Tubal ligation; transcervical sterilization; vasectomy

Menopause and Hormone Replacement Therapy. Be familiar with the psychological and physiologic changes of *menopause*. Help the patient to weigh the risks of HRT, including increased risk of stroke, pulmonary embolism, and breast cancer.

Techniques of Examination

Tips for the Successful Pelvic Examination

The Patient	**The Examiner**
• Avoids intercourse, douching, or use of vaginal suppositories for 24–48 hours before examination	• Obtains permission; selects chaperone
	• Explains each step of the examination in advance
• Empties bladder before examination	• Drapes patient from midabdomen to knees; depresses drape between knees to provide eye contact with patient
• Lies supine, with head and shoulders elevated, arms at sides or folded across chest to enhance eye contact and reduce tightening of abdominal muscles	• Avoids unexpected or sudden movements
	• Chooses a speculum that is the correct size
	• Warms speculum with tap water
	• Monitors comfort of the examination by watching the patient's face
	• Uses excellent but gentle technique, especially when inserting the speculum

Male examiners should be accompanied by female chaperones. Female examiners should be assisted whenever possible.

EXAMINATION TECHNIQUES	POSSIBLE FINDINGS

External Genitalia

⚬— Observe pubic hair to assess sexual maturity.

Normal or *delayed puberty*

⋀⋀ Examine the external genitalia (Fig. 14-1).

See Table 14-1, Lesions of the Vulva, pp. 258–259.

▪ Labia minora

Ulceration in herpes simplex, syphilitic chancre; inflammation in Bartholin cyst

▪ Clitoris

Enlarged in masculinization

▪ Urethral orifice

Urethral caruncle or prolapse; tenderness in interstitial cystitis

EXAMINATION TECHNIQUES   POSSIBLE FINDINGS

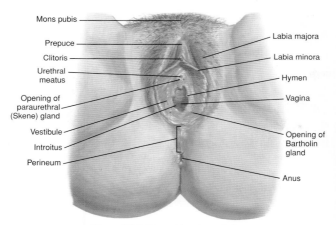

Mons pubis
Prepuce
Clitoris
Urethral meatus
Opening of paraurethral (Skene) gland
Vestibule
Introitus
Perineum

Labia majora
Labia minora
Hymen
Vagina
Opening of Bartholin gland
Anus

Figure 14-1 External female genitalia.

■ Introitus   Imperforate hymen

Milk the urethra for discharge if   Discharge of urethritis
indicated.

Internal Genitalia and Pap Smear
Locate the cervix with a gloved and
water-lubricated index finger.

Assess support of vaginal outlet by   Cystocele, cystourethrocele, rectocele
asking patient to strain down.

Enlarge the introitus by pressing its
posterior margin downward.

Insert a water-lubricated speculum
of suitable size. Start with speculum held obliquely (Fig. 14-2),
then rotate to horizontal position
for full insertion (Fig. 14-3).

EXAMINATION TECHNIQUES

POSSIBLE FINDINGS

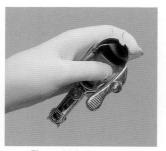

Figure 14-2 Entry angle.

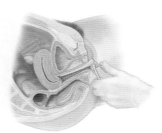

Figure 14-3 Carefully insert the speculum to full length.

Open the speculum gently and inspect cervix:

■ Position

Cervix faces forward if uterus is retroverted.

■ Color

Purplish in pregnancy

■ Shape of the cervical os (Fig. 14-4); epithelial surface (squamous–columnar epithelial junction)

Oval (normal) or slit-like or transverse os from delivery; raised, friable, or lobed wart-like lesions in condylomata or cervical cancer (see Table 14-3, Abnormalities of the Cervix, p. 261)

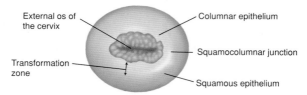

Figure 14-4 Cervical epithelial surface.

■ Any discharge or bleeding

Discharge from os in mucopurulent cervicitis from *Chlamydia* or *gonorrhea* (see Table 14-2, Vaginal Discharge, p. 260)

■ Any ulcers, nodules, or masses

Herpes, polyp, cancer

EXAMINATION TECHNIQUES

POSSIBLE FINDINGS

Obtain specimens for cytology (Pap smears) with:

Early cancer before it is clinically evident

- An endocervical broom (Fig. 14-5) or brush with scraper (except in pregnant women), to collect both squamous and columnar cells

- Or, if the woman is pregnant, use a cotton-tipped applicator moistened with water

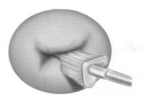

Figure 14-5 Endocervical broom.

Inspect the vaginal mucosa as you withdraw the speculum.

Bluish color and deep rugae in pregnancy; vaginal cancer (rare); vaginal discharge from infection from *Candida*, *Trichomonas vaginalis*, bacterial vaginosis (see Table 14-2, Vaginal Discharge, p. 260)

Palpate, by means of a bimanual examination (Fig. 14-6):

- The cervix and fornices

Pain on moving cervix in PID

- The uterus

Pregnancy, myomas; soft isthmus in early pregnancy (see Table 14-4, Positions of the Uterus and Uterine Myomas, p. 262)

- Right and left adnexa (ovaries)

Ovarian cysts or masses, salpingitis, PID, tubal pregnancy

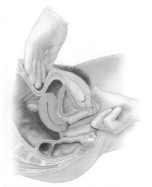

Figure 14-6 Palpate the cervix, uterus, and adnexa.

EXAMINATION TECHNIQUES	POSSIBLE FINDINGS

Assess strength of pelvic muscles. With your vaginal fingers clear of the cervix, ask patient to tighten her muscles around your fingers as hard and long as she can.

A firm squeeze that compresses your fingers, moves them up and inward, and lasts more than 3 seconds is full strength (see Table 14-5, Relaxations of the Pelvic Floor, p. 263).

⚬⃫/⋀⋀ When indicated, perform a rectovaginal examination as shown in Figure 14-7 to palpate a retroverted uterus, uterosacral ligaments, cul-de-sac, and adnexa or screen for colorectal cancer in women 50 years or older (see p. 269).

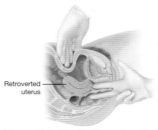

Retroverted — uterus

Figure 14-7 Examine the rectovaginal area.

Hernias

Ask the woman to strain down, as you palpate for a bulge in:

- The femoral canal

Femoral hernia

- The labia majora up to just lateral to the pubic tubercle

Indirect inguinal hernia

Special Technique

Assessing Urethritis. Insert your index finger into the vagina and milk the urethra gently outward from the inside (Fig. 14-8). Note any discharge.

Discharge in *C. trachomatis* and *Neisseria gonorrhoeae* infection

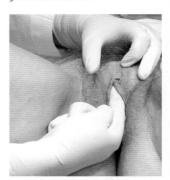

Figure 14-8 Milk the urethra if indicated.

Recording Your Findings

Recording the Female Genitalia Examination

"No inguinal adenopathy. External genitalia without erythema, lesions, or masses. Vaginal mucosa pink. Cervix parous, pink, and without discharge. Uterus anterior, midline, smooth, and not enlarged. No adnexal tenderness. Pap smear obtained. Rectovaginal wall intact. Rectal vault without masses. Stool brown and Hemoccult negative."

OR

"Bilateral shotty inguinal adenopathy. External genitalia without erythema or lesions. Vaginal mucosa and cervix coated with thin, white homogeneous discharge with mild fishy odor. After swabbing cervix, no discharge visible in cervical os. Uterus midline; no adnexal masses. Rectal vault without masses. Stool brown and Hemoccult negative." *(These findings suggest bacterial vaginosis.)*

Aids to Interpretation

Table 14-1 Lesions of the Vulva

Epidermoid Cyst

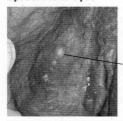

Cystic nodule in skin

A small, firm, round cystic nodule in the labia suggests an *epidermoid cyst.* They are yellowish in color. Look for the dark punctum marking the blocked opening of the gland.

Venereal Wart (*Condyloma Acuminatum*)

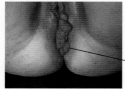

Warts

Warty lesions on the labia and within the vestibule suggest *condyloma acuminata* from infection with human papillomavirus.

Genital Herpes

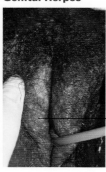

Shallow ulcers on red bases

Shallow, small, painful ulcers on red bases suggest a herpes infection. Initial infection may be extensive, as illustrated here. Recurrent infections are usually confined to a small local patch.

Table 14-1 Lesions of the Vulva (*continued*)

Syphilitic Chancre

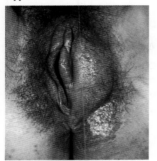

A firm, painless ulcer suggests the chancre of *primary syphilis*. Because most chancres in women develop internally, they often go undetected.

Secondary Syphilis (*Condyloma Latum*)

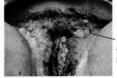

Flat, gray papules

Slightly raised, round or oval flat-topped papules covered by a gray exudate suggest *condylomata lata*, a manifestation of *secondary syphilis*. They are contagious.

Carcinoma of the Vulva

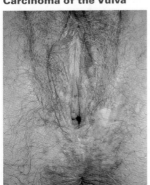

An ulcerated or raised red vulvar lesion in an elderly woman may indicate vulvar carcinoma.

Table 14-2 Vaginal Discharge

Note: Accurate diagnosis depends on laboratory assessment and cultures.

Trichomonas vaginitis

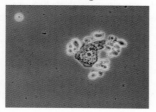

Discharge: Yellowish green, often profuse, may be malodorous

Other Symptoms: Itching, vaginal soreness, dyspareunia

Vulva: May be red

Vagina: May be normal or red, with red spots, petechiae

Laboratory Assessment: Saline wet mount for trichomonads

Candida vaginitis

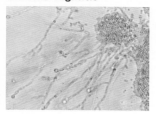

Discharge: White, curdy, often thick, not malodorous

Other Symptoms: Itching, vaginal soreness, external dysuria, dyspareunia

Vulva: Often red and swollen

Vagina: Often red with white patches of discharge

Laboratory Assessment: KOH preparation for branching hyphae

Bacterial vaginosis

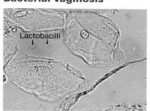

Lactobacilli

Discharge: Gray or white, thin, homogeneous, scant, malodorous

Other Symptoms: Fishy genital odor

Vulva: Usually normal

Vagina: Usually normal

Laboratory Assessment: Saline wet mount for "clue cells," "whiff test" with KOH for fishy odor

Table 14-3 Abnormalities of the Cervix

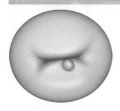

Endocervical polyp. A bright red, smooth mass that protrudes from the os suggests a polyp. It bleeds easily.

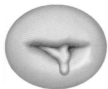

Mucopurulent cervicitis. A yellowish exudate emerging from the cervical os suggests infection from *Chlamydia, gonorrhea* (often asymptomatic), or herpes.

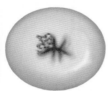

Carcinoma of the cervix. An irregular hard mass suggests carcinoma from HPV infection. Early lesions are best detected by pap smear and HPV screening, followed by colposcopy.

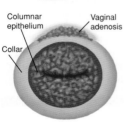

Columnar epithelium

Vaginal adenosis

Collar

Fetal exposure to diethylstilbestrol (DES). Several changes may occur: a collar of tissue around the cervix, columnar epithelium that covers the cervix or extends to the vaginal wall (then termed *vaginal adenosis*), and, rarely, carcinoma of the vagina.

Table 14-4 Positions of the Uterus and Uterine Myomas

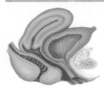

An anteverted uterus lies in a forward position at roughly a right angle to the vagina. This is the most common position. *Anteflexion*—a forward flexion of the uterine body in relation to the cervix—often coexists.

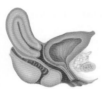

A retroverted uterus is tilted posteriorly with its cervix facing anteriorly.

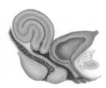

A retroflexed uterus has a posterior tilt that involves the uterine body but not the cervix. A uterus that is retroflexed or retroverted may be felt only through the rectal wall; some cannot be felt at all.

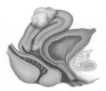

A myoma of the uterus is a very common benign tumor that feels firm and often irregular. There may be more than one. A myoma on the posterior surface of the uterus may be mistaken for a retrodisplaced uterus; one on the anterior surface may be mistaken for an anteverted uterus.

Table 14-5   Relaxations of the Pelvic Floor

When the pelvic floor is weakened, various structures may become displaced. These displacements are seen best when the patient strains down.

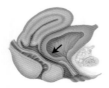 **A cystocele** is a bulge of the anterior wall of the upper part of the vagina, together with the urinary bladder above it.

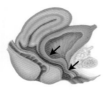 **A cystourethrocele** involves both the bladder and the urethra as they bulge into the anterior vaginal wall throughout most of its extent.

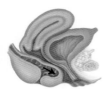 **A rectocele** is a bulge of the posterior vaginal wall, together with a portion of the rectum.

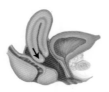 **A prolapsed uterus** has descended down the vaginal canal. There are three degrees of severity: first, still within the vagina (as illustrated); second, with the cervix at the introitus; and third, with the cervix outside the introitus.

The Anus, Rectum, and Prostate

The Health History

Common or Concerning Symptoms

- Change in bowel habits
- Blood in the stool
- Pain with defecation; rectal bleeding or tenderness
- Anal warts or fissures
- Weak stream of urine
- Burning with urination
- Blood in urine

Ask about any change in bowel habits or stool size or caliber, and any diarrhea or constipation. Is there any blood in the stool, or dark tarry stools? Any mucus in the stool?

Pencil-like stool or blood in stool in *colon cancer;* dark tarry stools if polyps, carcinoma, gastrointestinal bleeding; mucus in villous adenoma, inflammatory bowel disease (IBD), or irritable bowel syndrome (IBS)

Any pain with defecation, or rectal bleeding or tenderness?

Hemorrhoids; proctitis from sexually transmitted infections (STIs)

Any anal warts, fissures, or ulcerations?

Human papillomavirus (HPV), *condylomata lata* in secondary syphilis; fissures in Crohn disease, proctitis from receptive anal intercourse, ulcerations of herpes simplex, or chancres of primary syphilis

In men, is there difficulty starting the urine stream or holding back urine? Is the flow weak? What about frequent urination, especially at night? Or pain or burning when passing urine? Any blood in the urine or semen or pain with ejaculation? Is there frequent pain or stiffness in the lower back, hips, or upper thighs?

These symptoms suggest urethral obstruction from *benign prostatic hyperplasia (BPH)* or *prostate cancer,* especially in men age ≥70 years. The American Urological Association (AUA) Symptom Index helps quantify BPH severity (see Table 15-1, BPH Symptom Score Index: American Urological Association (AUA), p. 271).

Health Promotion and Counseling: Evidence and Recommendations

Important Topics for Health Promotion and Counseling

- Prostate cancer screening
- Colorectal cancer screening
- Counseling for sexually transmitted infections

Prostate Cancer Screening. Prostate cancer is the leading nonskin cancer diagnosed in the United States and the second leading cause of death in men. Risk factors are age, family history of prostate cancer, and African American ethnicity.

Screening methods such as prostate-specific antigen (PSA) test and the digital rectal examination (DRE) are not highly accurate, which complicates decisions about screening men *without symptoms*.

The PSA. PSA screening remains controversial, so warrants shared decision making about risks and benefits and patient preferences. About 12% of men have a PSA screening test above 4 ng/mL, but only 30% of these men have prostate cancer on biopsy. At 4 ng/mL, PSA sensitivity is 21% and specificity is 91%. See recommendations of major societies below.

Prostate Cancer Screening Guidelines

	American Urological Association	American Cancer Society	United States Preventive Services Task Force
Shared decision making	Yes	Yes (consider using decision aid)	Yes (when patient requests screening)
Age to begin offering screening			No recommendation
Average-risk	40 years	50 years	
High-risk	40 years	40–45 years	
Age to stop offering screening	Life expectancy <10 years	Life expectancy <10 years	No recommendation
Screening tests	PSA DRE (optional)	PSA DRE (optional)	No recommendation

(*continued*)

Prostate Cancer Screening Guidelines (Continued)

	American Urological Association	American Cancer Society	United States Preventive Services Task Force
Frequency of screening	Annual	Annual (biennial when PSA <2.5 ng/mL)	No recommendation
Biopsy referral criteria		PSA ≥4 ng/mL Abnormal DRE Individualized risk assessment for PSA levels 2.5–4 ng/mL	No recommendation

Abbreviations: PSA, prostate-specific antigen; DRE, digital rectal examination.

The DRE. reaches only the posterior and lateral surfaces of the prostate, missing findings in the anterior and central areas. DRE sensitivity for prostate cancers is only 59%.

Encourage men with symptomatic disorders such as incomplete emptying of the bladder, urinary frequency or urgency, weak or intermittent stream or straining to initiate flow, hematuria, nocturia, or even bony pains in the pelvis to seek evaluation and treatment early.

Colorectal Cancer Screening. In 2008, screening recommendations were revised to promote more aggressive surveillance:

■ Clinicians should first identify whether patients are at average or increased risk, ideally by age 20 years. High-risk factors include a personal history of colorectal neoplasia or long-standing IBD—or a family history of colorectal neoplasia, including hereditary syndromes. People at increased risk should undergo colonoscopy at intervals ranging from 3 to 5 years.

■ Average-risk patients 50 years or older should be offered a range of screening options to increase compliance: annual screening with high-sensitivity fecal occult blood tests (including guaiac-based Hemoccult tests and fecal immunochemical tests), colonoscopy every 10 years, or sigmoidoscopy every 5 years (which can be combined with high-sensitivity fecal occult blood testing performed every 3 years).

Counseling for STIs. Anal intercourse increases risk for HIV and STIs. Promote abstinence from high-risk behaviors, use of condoms, vaccination for hepatitis B and HPV, and good hygiene.

Techniques of Examination

EXAMINATION TECHNIQUES

POSSIBLE FINDINGS

⊶ Wear gloves to examine the anus, rectum, and prostate (Fig. 15-1).

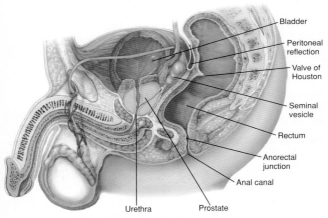

Bladder

Peritoneal reflection

Valve of Houston

Seminal vesicle

Rectum

Anorectal junction

Anal canal

Urethra   Prostate

Figure 15-1 Anus and rectum—sagittal view.

Male

Position the patient on his side, or standing leaning forward over the examining table and hips flexed (Fig. 15-2).

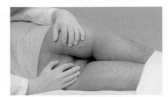

Figure 15-2 Position the patient on the left side.

Inspect the:

▪ Sacrococcygeal area

Pilonidal cyst or sinus

▪ Perianal area

Hemorrhoids, warts, herpes, chancre, cancer, fissures from proctitis, STIs, or Crohn disease, fistula from anorectal abscess

EXAMINATION TECHNIQUES	POSSIBLE FINDINGS

Palpate the anal canal and rectum with a lubricated and gloved finger. Palpate the:

Lax sphincter tone in some neurologic disorders; tightness in proctitis

■ Walls of the rectum

Cancer of the rectum, polyps

■ Prostate gland, as shown in Figure 15-3, including median sulcus

Prostate nodule or cancer (Fig. 15-4); BPH; tenderness in prostatitis

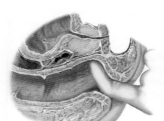

Figure 15-3 Palpate the prostate gland.

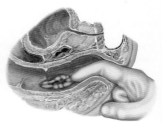

Figure 15-4 Rectal cancer.

Try to palpate above the prostate for irregularities or tenderness, if indicated.

See Table 15-2, Abnormalities on Rectal Examination, pp. 272–273.

♂—/♀♀ Female

The patient is usually in the lithotomy position or lying on her side.

Rectal shelf of peritoneal metastases; tenderness of inflammation

Inspect the anus.

Hemorrhoids

Palpate the anal canal and rectum.

Rectal cancer, normal uterine cervix or tampon (felt through the rectal wall)

Recording Your Findings

Recording the Anus, Rectum, and Prostate Examination

"No perirectal lesions or fissures. External sphincter tone intact. Rectal vault without masses. Prostate smooth and nontender with palpable median sulcus. (Or in a female, uterine cervix nontender.) Stool brown and Hemoccult negative."

OR

"Perirectal area inflamed; no ulcerations, warts, or discharge. Cannot examine external sphincter, rectal vault, or prostate because of spasm of external sphincter and marked inflammation and tenderness of anal canal." *(These findings suggest proctitis from infectious cause.)*

OR

"No perirectal lesions or fissures. External sphincter tone intact. Rectal vault without masses. Left lateral prostate lobe with 1 × 1 cm firm hard nodule; right lateral lobe smooth; medial sulcus is obscured. Stool brown and Hemoccult negative." *(These findings are suspicious for prostate cancer.)*

Aids to Interpretation

Table 15-1   BPH Symptom Score Index: American Urological Association (AUA)

Score or ask the patient to score each of the questions below on a scale of 1 to 5, with 0 = not at all, 1 = less than 1 time in 5, 2 = less than half the time, 3 = about half the time, 4 = more than half the time, and 5 = almost always.

Higher scores (maximum 35) indicate more severe symptoms; scores ≤7 are considered mild and generally do not warrant treatment.

PART A	**Score**
1. **Incomplete emptying:** Over the past month, how often have you had a sensation of not emptying your bladder completely after you finished urinating?	_____
2. **Frequency:** Over the past month, how often have you had to urinate again <2 hours after you finished urinating?	_____
3. **Intermittency:** Over the past month, how often have you stopped and started again several times when you urinated?	_____
4. **Urgency:** Over the past month, how often have you found it difficult to postpone urination?	_____
5. **Weak stream:** Over the past month, how often have you had a weak urinary stream?	_____
6. **Straining:** Over the past month, how often have you had to push or strain to begin urination?	_____
PART A TOTAL SCORE	_____

For Part B, 0 = none, 1 = 1 time, 2 = 2 times, 3 = 3 times, 4 = 4 times, 5 = 5 times.

PART B	**Score**
7. **Nocturia:** Over the past month, how many times did you most typically get up to urinate from the time you went to bed at night until the time you got up in the morning? (Score 0 to 5 times on night)	_____
TOTAL PARTS A and B (maximum 35)	_____

Adapted from: Madsen FA, Burskewitz RC. Clinical manifestations of benign prostatic hyperplasia. *Urol Clin North Am.* 1995;22:291.

Table 15-2 Abnormalities on Rectal Examination

External Hemorrhoids (Thrombosed). Dilated hemorrhoidal veins that originate below the pectinate line, covered with skin; a tender, swollen, bluish ovoid mass is visible at the anal margin.

Anal Fissure. Painful longitudinal oval ulceration usually in posterior midline with swollen sentinel tag just below it.

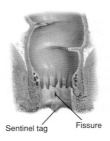

Sentinel tag   Fissure

Anorectal Fistula. An inflammatory tract or tube opening inside the anus or rectum and also onto the perianal area or into another viscus.

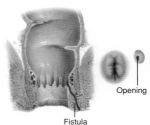

Opening

Fistula

Polyps of the Rectum. A soft mass that may or may not be on a stalk; may not be palpable.

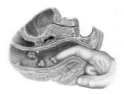

Table 15-2 Abnormalities on Rectal Examination (*continued*)

Benign Prostatic Hyperplasia.
An enlarged, nontender, smooth, firm but slightly elastic prostate gland; can cause symptoms without palpable enlargement.

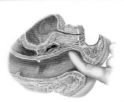

Acute Prostatitis. A prostate that is very tender, swollen, and firm because of acute infection.

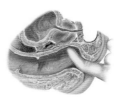

Cancer of the Prostate. A hard area in the prostate that may or may not feel nodular.

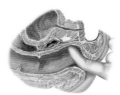

Cancer of the Rectum. Firm, nodular, rolled edge of an ulcerated cancer.

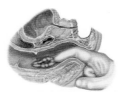

Benign Prostatic Hyperplasia

Acute Prostatitis

Cancer of the Prostate

Cancer of the Rectum

The Musculoskeletal System

Fundamentals for Assessing Joints

Musculoskeletal disorders are the leading primary diagnosis during office visits in the United States. Your first goal is to assess four key features of the patient's complaint. Is the joint problem:

- Articular or extra-articular;

- Acute (usually <6 weeks) or chronic (usually >12 weeks);

- Inflammatory or noninflammatory; and

- Localized (monoarticular) or diffuse (polyarticular)?

Assessing joints requires knowledge of each joint's structure and function. Learn the surface landmarks and underlying anatomy of each of the major joints. Use the descriptive terms below.

Joint Anatomy—Important Terms

- *Articular structures* include the *joint capsule* and *articular cartilage*, the *synovium* and *synovial fluid*, *intra-articular ligaments*, and *juxta-articular bone*. Articular cartilage is composed of a collagen matrix containing charged ions and water, allowing the cartilage to change shape in response to pressure or load, acting as a cushion for underlying bone. Synovial fluid provides nutrition to the adjacent relatively avascular articular cartilage.
- *Extra-articular structures* include periarticular ligaments, tendons, bursae, muscle, fascia, bone, nerve, and overlying skin.
  - *Ligaments* are rope-like bundles of collagen fibrils that connect bone to bone.
  - *Tendons* are collagen fibers connecting muscle to bone.
  - *Bursae* are pouches of synovial fluid that cushion the movement of tendons and muscles over bone or other joint structures.

Age also provides clues to causes of joint pain.

Common Causes of Joint Pain by Age

Age <60 Years	Age >60 Years
• Repetitive strain or overuse syndromes (tendinitis, bursitis)	• Osteoarthritis (OA)
	• Osteoporotic fracture
• Crystalline arthritis (gout; crystalline pyrophosphate deposition disease [CPPD])	• Gout and pseudogout
• Rheumatoid arthritis (RA), psoriatic arthritis and reactive (Reiter) arthritis (in inflammatory bowel disease [IBD])	• Polymyalgia rheumatica (PMR)
• Infectious arthritis from gonorrhea, Lyme disease, or viral or bacterial infections	• Septic bacterial arthritis

Review the three primary types of joint articulation—synovial, cartilaginous, and fibrous—and the varying degrees of movement each type allows. Note that joint anatomy determines its function and range of motion.

Types of Joints

Synovial Joints
- Freely movable within limits of surrounding ligaments
- Separated by **articular cartilage** and a **synovial cavity**
- Lubricated by synovial fluid
- Surrounded by a joint capsule
- *Example:* knee, shoulder

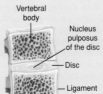

Bone
Ligament
Synovial membrane
Joint space
Joint capsule
Synovial cavity
Articular cartilage

Cartilaginous Joints
- Slightly movable
- Contain fibrocartilaginous discs that separate the bony surfaces
- Have a central *nucleus pulposus* of discs that cushions bony contact
- *Example:* vertebral bodies

Vertebral body

Nucleus pulposus of the disc

Disc

Ligament

Fibrous Joints
- No appreciable movement
- Consist of fibrous tissue or cartilage
- Lack a joint cavity
- *Example:* skull sutures

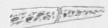

Review the types of synovial joints and their associated features as well.

Types of Synovial Joints

Spheroidal (ball and socket)
Articular shape: Convex surface in concave
   cavity
Movement: Wide-ranging flexion, extension,
   abduction, adduction, rotation,
   circumduction
Example: Shoulder, hip

Hinge
Articular shape: Flat, planar
Movement: Motion in one plane; flexion,
   extension
Example: Interphalangeal joints of hand and
   foot; elbow

Condylar
Articular shape: Convex or concave
Movement: Movement of two articulating
   surfaces, not dissociable
Example: Knee; temporomandibular joint

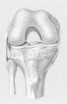

The Health History

Common or Concerning Symptoms

- Joint pain: articular or extra-articular, acute or chronic, inflammatory or
  noninflammatory, localized or diffuse
- Joint pain: associated constitutional symptoms and systemic manifestations
  from other organ systems
- Neck pain
- Low back pain

Assess the seven features of any joint pain (see p. 47).

Tips for Assessing Joint Pain

- Ask the patient to "point to the pain." This may save considerable time because many patients have trouble pinpointing pain location in words.
- Clarify and record when the pain started and the mechanism of injury, particularly if there is a history of trauma.
- Determine whether the pain is articular or extra-articular, acute or chronic, inflammatory or noninflammatory, and localized (monoarticular) or diffuse (polyarticular).

Joint Pain

Articular or Extra-articular. Ask "Do you have any pains in your joints?" Ask the patient to *point to the pain.* If *localized* and involving only one joint, it is *monoarticular.*

See Table 16-1, Patterns of Pain in and Around the Joints, p. 304.

Consider trauma, monoarticular arthritis, tendinitis, or bursitis. Hip pain near the greater trochanter suggests trochanteric bursitis.

If *polyarticular,* does it migrate from joint to joint, or steadily spread from one joint to multiple joint involvement? Is the involvement symmetric?

Migratory pattern in *rheumatic fever* or *gonococcal arthritis;* progressive and symmetric pattern in *rheumatoid arthritis*

If pain is extra-articular, are there generalized "aches and pains" (*myalgia* if in muscles, *arthralgia* if in joints with no evidence of arthritis)?

Bursitis if inflammation of bursae; *tendinitis* if in tendons, and tenosynovitis if in tendon sheaths; also *sprains* from stretching or tearing of ligaments

Ask if there is decreased joint movement or stiffness.

In articular pain, decreased active and passive range of motion and morning stiffness ("gelling"); in nonarticular joint pain, periarticular tenderness and only passive range of motion intact

Acute or Chronic. Acute joint pain typically lasts up to 6 weeks; *chronic pain* lasts >12 weeks. Assess the timing, quality, and severity of joint symptoms.

Severe pain of rapid onset in red swollen joint in acute septic arthritis or crystalline arthritis (gout; CPPD). In children, osteomyelitis in bone contiguous to a joint.

If from trauma, what was the *mechanism of injury* or series of events that caused the joint pain? Furthermore, what aggravates or relieves the pain? What are the effects of exercise, rest, and treatment?

See Table 16-1, Patterns of Pain in and Around the Joints, p. 304.

Inflammatory or Noninflammatory. Is the problem inflammatory or noninflammatory? Is there fever, chills, tenderness, warmth, or redness?

If inflammatory, consider infectious causes (*Neisseria gonorrhoeae* or *Mycobacterium tuberculosis*), crystal-induced (gout, pseudogout), immune-related (RA, SLE), reactive (rheumatic fever, reactive arthritis), or idiopathic arthritis. If noninflammatory, consider trauma (rotator cuff tear), repetitive use (bursitis, tendinitis), OA, fibromyalgia.

Assess any stiffness or *limitations of motion*.

Morning stiffness that gradually improves with activity in inflammatory disorders like RA and PMR; intermittent stiffness and gelling in OA

Localized or Diffuse. Ask the patient to point to the joints that are painful to determine if joint pain is be monoarticular, oligoarticular involving two to four joints, or polyarticular.

Monoarticular arthritis in traumatic, crystalline, or septic arthritis; oligoarticular arthritis gonorrhea or rheumatic fever, connective tissue disease, and OA; polyarthritis if may be viral or inflammatory from RA, SLE, or psoriasis

Joint Pain: Associated Constitutional Symptoms and Systemic Manifestations from Other Organ Systems. Assess *constitutional symptoms* such as fever, chills, rash, fatigue, anorexia, weight loss, and weakness.

Common in RA, SLE, PMR, and other inflammatory arthritides. High fever and chills suggest an infectious cause.

Neck Pain. Ask about location, radiation into the shoulders or arms, arm or leg weakness, bladder or bowel dysfunction.

C7 or C6 spinal nerve compression from foraminal impingement more common than disc herniation. See Table 16-2, Pains in the Neck, p. 305.

If the patient reports neck trauma, common in motor vehicle accidents, ask about neck tenderness and consider clinical decision rules that identify risk of cervical cord injury (NEXUS criteria and Canadian C-Spine Rule).

Low Back Pain. There are numerous clinical guidelines, but most categorize low back pain into three groups: nonspecific (>90%), nerve root entrapment with radiculopathy or spinal stenosis (~5%), and pain from a specific underlying disease (1% to 2%). Ask, "Do you have any pains in your back?" and "Is the pain in the midline over the vertebrae, or off midline?"

See Table 16-3, Low Back Pain, pp. 306–307. *Midline back pain* in vertebral collapse, disc herniation, epidural abscess, spinal cord compression, or spinal cord metastases. *Pain off the midline* in muscle strain, sacroiliitis, trochanteric bursitis, sciatica, hip arthritis, renal conditions such as pyelonephritis or renal stones

If the pain radiates into the legs, ask about any associated numbness, tingling, or weakness. Ask about history of trauma.

Sciatica if radicular gluteal and posterior leg pain in the S1 distribution that increases with cough or Valsalva

Check for bladder or bowel dysfunction.

Present in *cauda equina syndrome* from S2–S4 tumor or disc herniation, especially if "saddle anesthesia" from perianal numbness

Elicit any "red flags" for serious underlying systemic disease.

Red Flags for Low Back Pain from Underlying Systemic Disease

- Age <20 years or >50 years
- History of cancer
- Unexplained weight loss, fever, or decline in general health
- Pain lasting more than 1 month or not responding to treatment
- Pain at night or present at rest
- History of intravenous drug use, addiction, or immunosuppression
- Presence of active infection or human immunodeficiency virus (HIV) infection
- Long-term steroid therapy
- Saddle anesthesia, bladder or bowel incontinence
- Neurologic symptoms or progressive neurologic deficit

Health Promotion and Counseling: Evidence and Recommendations

Important Topics for Health Promotion and Counseling

- Nutrition, weight, and physical activity
- Low back pain
- Osteoporosis: risk factors, screening, and assessing fracture risk
- Treating osteoporosis and preventing falls

Nutrition, Weight, and Physical Activity. Good nutrition supplies the calcium and vitamin D needed for bone mineralization and bone density, with supplements advised in selected age groups. Optimal weight reduces excess mechanical stress on weight-bearing joints like the hips and knees. Exercise helps maintain bone mass and improves outlook and stress management.

Physical Activity Guidelines for Americans

- At least 2 hours and 30 minutes a week of moderate-intensity, or 1 hour and 15 minutes a week of vigorous-intensity, *aerobic physical activity*, or an equivalent combination
- Moderate- or high-intensity *muscle-strengthening activity* that involves all major muscle groups on 2 or more days a week

Low Back Pain. The estimated lifetime prevalence of low back pain in the U.S. population is over 80%. Most patients with acute low back pain get better within 6 weeks; for patients with nonspecific symptoms, clinical guidelines emphasize reassurance, staying active, analgesics, muscle relaxants, and spinal manipulation therapy. About 10% to 15% of these patients develop chronic symptoms, often associated with long-term disability. Poor outcomes are linked to inappropriate beliefs about low back pain as a serious clinical condition, maladaptive pain-coping behaviors (avoiding work, movement, or other activities for fear of causing back damage), multiple nonorganic physical examination findings, psychiatric disorders, poor general health, high levels of baseline functional impairment, and low work satisfaction.

Osteoporosis: Risk Factors, Screening, and Assessing Fracture Risk. Osteoporosis is a major public health threat and a common U.S. health problem—9% of adults over age 50 years have osteoporosis at the femoral neck or lumbar spine, including 16% of women and 4% of men. Half of all postmenopausal women sustain an osteoporosis-related fracture during their lifetime; 25% develop vertebral deformities, and 15% suffer hip fractures that increase risk of chronic pain, disability, loss of independence, and increased mortality.

The U.S. Preventive Services Task Force (USPSTF) gives a grade B recommendation supporting osteoporosis screening for women age ≥65 years and for younger women whose 10-year fracture risk equals or exceeds that of an average-risk 65-year-old white woman.

Risk Factors for Osteoporosis

- Postmenopausal status in women
- Age ≥50 years
- Prior fragility fracture
- Low body mass index
- Low dietary calcium
- Vitamin D deficiency
- Tobacco and excessive alcohol use
- Family history of fracture in a first-degree relative, particularly with history of fragility fracture

- Clinical conditions such as thyrotoxicosis, celiac sprue, IBD, cirrhosis, chronic renal disease, organ transplantation, diabetes, HIV, hypogonadism, multiple myeloma, anorexia nervosa, and rheumatologic and autoimmune disorders
- Medications such as oral and high-dose inhaled corticosteroids, anticoagulants (long-term use), aromatase inhibitors for breast cancer, methotrexate, selected antiseizure medications, immunosuppressive agents, proton-pump inhibitors (long-term use), and antigonadal therapy for prostate cancer

■ Use the country-specific FRAX calculator to assess fracture risk. If risk is >9.3% for any fracture and >3% for hip fracture, bone density screening is warranted. The website for the FRAX Calculator for Assessing Fracture Risk for the United States is http://www.shef.ac.uk/FRAX/tool.jsp?country=9.

■ Use the World Health Organization scoring criteria to determine bone density.

World Health Organization Bone Density Criteria

Osteoporosis: T score <−2.5 (>2.5 standard deviations below the mean for young adult white women)

Osteopenia: T score between −1.0 and −2.5 (1.0 to 2.5 SDs below the young adult mean)

Treating Osteoporosis and Preventing Falls. Learn the therapeutic uses of agents that inhibit bone resorption: calcium and vitamin D; antiresorptive agents such as bisphosphonates, selective estrogen-receptor modulators (SERMs), calcitonin, and postmenopausal estrogen; and anabolic agents such as PTH.

More than one in three adults over age 65 years falls each year. Risk factors for falls include increasing age, impaired gait and balance, postural hypotension, loss of strength, medication use, comorbid illness, depression, cognitive impairment, and visual deficits.

The USPSTF gives a grade B recommendation for providing exercise or physical therapy and/or vitamin D supplementation to prevent falls among at-risk community-dwelling adults age ≥65 years. Effective exercise interventions target balance, gait, and strength training. Urge patients to correct poor lighting, dark or steep stairs, chairs at awkward heights, slippery or irregular surfaces, and ill-fitting shoes. Scrutinize any medications affecting balance, especially benzodiazepines, vasodilators, and diuretics.

Techniques of Examination

Steps for Examining the Joints

1. Inspect for joint symmetry, alignment, bony deformities, and swelling
2. Inspect and palpate surrounding tissues for skin changes, nodules, muscle atrophy, tenderness
3. Assess range of motion and maneuvers to test joint function and stability and the integrity of ligaments, tendons, bursae, especially if pain or trauma
4. Assess any areas of inflammation, especially tenderness, swelling, warmth, redness

Inspect and palpate any joints with signs of inflammation.

The Four Signs of Inflammation

- *Swelling.* Palpable swelling may involve: (1) the synovial membrane, which can feel boggy or doughy; (2) effusion from excess synovial fluid within the joint space; or (3) soft tissue structures, such as bursae, tendons, and tendon sheaths.
- *Warmth.* Use the backs of your fingers to compare the involved joint with its unaffected contralateral joint, or with nearby tissues if both joints are involved.

(continued)

The Four Signs of Inflammation *(Continued)*

- *Redness.* Redness of the overlying skin is the least common sign of inflammation near the joints and is usually seen in more superficial joints like fingers, toes, and knees.
- *Pain or tenderness.* Try to identify the specific anatomic structure that is tender.

EXAMINATION TECHNIQUES

POSSIBLE FINDINGS

Temporomandibular Joint

Inspect the temporomandibular joint (TMJ) for swelling or redness.

Palpate the TMJ as the patient opens and closes the mouth (Fig. 16-1).

Palpate the muscles of mastication: the *masseters, temporal muscles,* and *pterygoid muscles.*

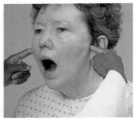

Figure 16-1 Palpate the TMJ.

Shoulders

Inspect the contour of the shoulders and shoulder girdles from front and back.

Muscle atrophy; anterior or posterior dislocation of humeral head; scoliosis if shoulder heights asymmetric

See Table 16-4, Painful Shoulders, p. 308.

Palpate:

■ The clavicle from the sternoclavicular joint to the acromioclavicular joint (Fig. 16-2)

■ The bicipital tendon

"Step-offs" if fracture from trauma

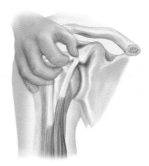

Figure 16-2 Palpate the bicipital groove and tendon.

EXAMINATION TECHNIQUES

POSSIBLE FINDINGS

- The subacromial and subdeltoid bursae after lifting arm posteriorly (Fig. 16-3)

Subacromial or subdeltoid bursitis; tenderness over the SITS (**S**upraspinatus, **I**nfraspinatus, **T**eres minor, and **S**ubscapularis) muscle insertions and difficulty abducting the arm above shoulder level occurs in sprains, tears, tendon rupture of rotator cuff.

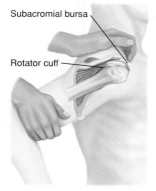

Subacromial bursa

Rotator cuff

Figure 16-3 Palpate the subacromial bursa.

Assess range of motion.

- Flexion—"Raise your arm in front of you and overhead."

Intact glenohumeral motion if patient raises arms to shoulder level, palms facing *down*

- Extension—"Move your arms behind you."

Intact scapulothoracic motion if patient raises arms an additional 60 degrees, palms facing *up*

- Abduction—"Raise your arms out to the side and overhead."

- Adduction—"Cross your arm in front of your body, keeping the arm straight."

Acromioclavicular joint arthritis

EXAMINATION TECHNIQUES	POSSIBLE FINDINGS

- External and internal rotation (Figs. 16-4 and 16-5)

Shoulder arthritis

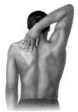

Figure 16-4 Test abduction and external rotation.

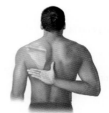

Figure 16-5 Test adduction and internal rotation.

Perform five maneuvers to assess the "SITS" muscles of the *rotator cuff* and the bicipital tendon.

Pain or inability to perform these maneuvers in rotator cuff sprains, tendinitis, rupture

Five Maneuvers for SITS Muscle Assessment

Pain Provocation Test
Painful arc test (Fig. 16-6). Fully adduct the patient's arm from o to 180 degrees.

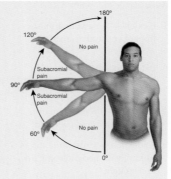

Figure 16-6 Painful arc test.

(continued)

EXAMINATION TECHNIQUES | POSSIBLE FINDINGS

Five Maneuvers for SITS Muscle Assessment (Continued)

Strength Tests

- *External rotation lag test (Fig. 16-7).* With the patient's arm flexed to 90 degrees with palm up, rotate the arm into full external rotation.

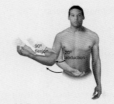

Figure 16-7 Internal rotation lag test.

- *Internal rotation lag test (Fig. 16-8).* Ask the patient to place the dorsum of the hand on the low back with the elbow flexed to 90 degrees. Then you lift the hand off the back, which further internally rotates the shoulder. Ask the patient to keep the hand in this position.

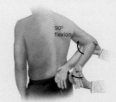

Figure 16-8 External rotation lag test.

- *Drop-arm test (Fig. 16-9).* Ask the patient to fully abduct the arm to shoulder level, up to 90 degrees, and lower it slowly. Note that abduction above shoulder level, from 90 to 120 degrees, reflects action of the deltoid muscle.

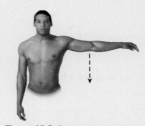

Figure 16-9 Drop arm test.

Composite Test

External rotation resistance test (Fig. 16-10). Ask the patient to adduct and flex the arm to 90 degrees, with the thumbs turned up. Stabilize the elbow with one hand and apply pressure proximal to the patient's wrist as the patient presses the wrist outward in external rotation.

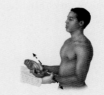

Figure 16-10 External rotation resistance test.

EXAMINATION TECHNIQUES | POSSIBLE FINDINGS

Elbows

Inspect and palpate:

- Olecranon process

  Olecranon bursitis; posterior dislocation from direct trauma or supracondylar fracture

- Medial and lateral epicondyles

  Tenderness distal to epicondyle in epicondylitis (medial → "tennis elbow"; lateral → "pitcher's elbow")

- Extensor surface of the ulna

  Rheumatoid nodules

- Grooves between the epicondyles and the olecranon

  Tender in arthritis

Ask patient to:

- Flex and extend elbows

- Turn forearms and palms up and down (supination and pronation), as shown in Figure 16-11

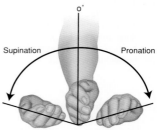

Figure 16-11 Elbow supination and pronation.

Wrists and Hands

Inspect:

- Movement of the wrist (flexion, extension, ulnar and medial deviation), hands, and fingers

  Guarded movement in injury

- Contours of wrists, hands, and fingers

  Asymmetric DIP, PIP deformities in OA; symmetric deformities in PIP, MCP, wrist joints in RA; swelling in arthritis, ganglia; impaired alignment of fingers in flexor tendon damage; flexion contractures in Dupuytren contractures

- Contours of palms

  Thenar atrophy in median nerve compression (*carpal tunnel syndrome*); hypothenar atrophy in ulnar nerve compression

| EXAMINATION TECHNIQUES | POSSIBLE FINDINGS |

Palpate:

■ Wrist joints (Fig. 16-12)

Swelling and tenderness in *rheumatoid arthritis, gonococcal infection* of joint or extensor tendon sheaths

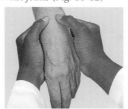

Figure 16-12 Palpate the wrist joint.

■ Distal radius and ulna

Tenderness over ulnar styloid in *Colles fracture*

■ "Anatomic snuffbox," the hollow space distal to the radial styloid bone; thumb extensor and abductor tendons (Fig. 16-13).

Tenderness suggests *scaphoid fracture*. Tenderness over extensor and abductor tendons in de Quervain tenosynovitis.

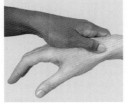

Figure 16-13 Palpate the anatomic snuffbox.

■ Metacarpophalangeal joints (Fig. 16-14)

Swelling in *rheumatoid arthritis*

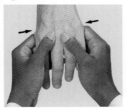

Figure 16-14 Palpate the MCP joints.

EXAMINATION TECHNIQUES	POSSIBLE FINDINGS
▪ Proximal and distal interphalangeal joint	Proximal nodules in RA; Bouchard (PIP) and Heberden (DIP) nodes in OA
Assess range of motion:	
▪ Wrists: Flexion, extension, adduction (radial deviation), abduction (lateral deviation)	*Arthritis, tenosynovitis*
▪ Fingers: Flexions, extension, abduction/adduction (spread fingers apart and back)	**Trigger finger, Dupuytren contracture**
▪ Thumbs (Figs. 16-15 to 16-18)	

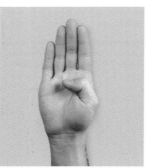

Figure 16-15 Flexion.

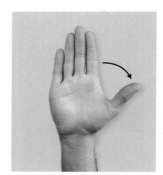

Figure 16-16 Extension.

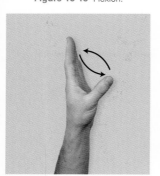

Figure 16-17 Abduction and adduction.

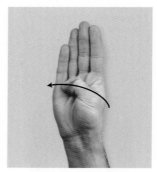

Figure 16-18 Opposition.

EXAMINATION TECHNIQUES

POSSIBLE FINDINGS

Perform selected maneuvers.

■ Hand grip strength (Fig. 16-19)

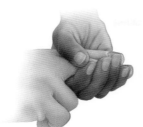

Figure 16-19 Test grip strength.

Decreased grip strength if weakness of finger flexors or intrinsic hand muscles

■ Thumb movement (Fig. 16-20)

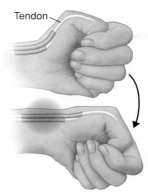

Tendon

Figure 16-20 Test thumb function.

Pain if de Quervain tenosynovitis

■ Carpal tunnel testing

■ *Thumb adduction* (Fig. 16-21)

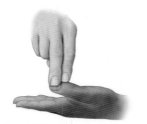

Figure 16-21 Test thumb abduction.

Weakness of abductor pollicis longus is specific to the median nerve.

■ Tinel sign: Tap lightly over median nerve at volar wrist (Fig. 16-22)

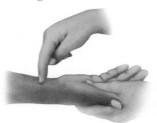

Figure 16-22 Test Tinel sign.

Aching, tingling, and numbness in second, third, and fourth fingers is a positive Tinel sign.

EXAMINATION TECHNIQUES	POSSIBLE FINDINGS

■ Phalen sign: Patient flexes wrists for 60 seconds (Fig. 16-23)

Aching, tingling, and numbness in second, third, and fourth volar fingers is a positive Phalen sign.

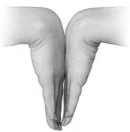

Figure 16-23 Test Phalen sign.

Spine

Inspect spine from the side and back, noting any abnormal curvatures.

Kyphosis, scoliosis, lordosis, gibbus, list curvatures

Look for asymmetric heights of shoulders, iliac crests, or buttocks.

Scoliosis, pelvic tilt, unequal leg length

Identify and palpate (Fig. 16-24):

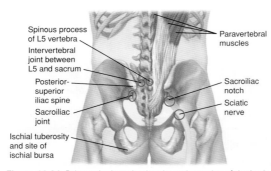

Spinous process of L5 vertebra

Intervertebral joint between L5 and sacrum

Posterior-superior iliac spine

Sacroiliac joint

Ischial tuberosity and site of ischial bursa

Paravertebral muscles

Sacroiliac notch

Sciatic nerve

Figure 16-24 Palpate the bony landmarks and muscles of the back.

■ Spinous processes of each vertebra

Tender if trauma, infection; "step-offs" in spondylolisthesis, fracture

EXAMINATION TECHNIQUES

- Sacroiliac joints

Sacroiliitis, ankylosing spondylitis

- Paravertebral muscles, if painful

Paravertebral muscle spasm in abnormal posture, degenerative and inflammatory muscle disorders, overuse

- Sciatic nerve (midway between greater trochanter and ischial tuberosity), Figure 16-25

Herniated disc or nerve root compression

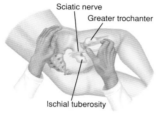

Sciatic nerve
Greater trochanter

Ischial tuberosity

Figure 16-25 Palpate the sciatic nerve.

Test the range of motion in the neck and spine in: flexion, extension, rotation, and lateral bending.

Decreased mobility in arthritis

Hips

Inspect gait (Fig. 16-26) for:

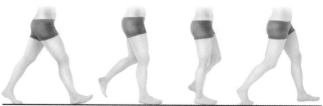

Heelstrike   Foot flat   Midstance   Push-off
Figure 16-26 The stance phase of gait.

EXAMINATION TECHNIQUES	POSSIBLE FINDINGS

■ *Stance* (see Fig. 16-26) and *swing* (foot moves forward, does not bear weight)

Most problems arise during the weight-bearing stance phase.

■ *Width of base* (usually 2 to 4 inches from heel to heel), shift of pelvis, flexion of knee

Cerebellar disease or foot problems if wide base; impaired shift of pelvis in arthritis, hip dislocation, abductor weakness; disrupted gait if poor knee flexion

Palpate:

■ Bony landmarks: anterior—iliac crest and tubercle, anterior-superior iliac spine, greater trochanter, pubic tubercle; posterior—posterior-superior iliac spine, greater trochanter, ischial tuberosity, sacroiliac joint

■ Along the inguinal ligament. Identify the **N**erve–**A**rtery–**V**ein–**E**mpty space–**L**ymph node (NAVEL).

Bulges in inguinal hernia, aneurysm

■ The *trochanteric bursa,* on the greater trochanter of the femur (Fig. 16-27)

Focal tenderness in *trochanteric bursitis,* often described by patients as "low back pain"

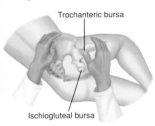

Trochanteric bursa

Ischiogluteal bursa

Figure 16-27 Trochanteric and ischio-gluteal bursae.

■ The *ischiogluteal bursa,* superficial to the ischial tuberosity

Tender in bursitis ("weaver's bottom") from prolonged sitting

EXAMINATION TECHNIQUES

POSSIBLE FINDINGS

Check range of motion, including:

- Flexion—"Bend your knee and pull it against your abdomen." (Fig. 16-28)

Flexion of opposite leg suggests deformity of that hip.

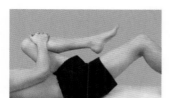

Figure 16-28 Hip flexion and flattening of lumbar lordosis.

- Extension (Fig. 16-29)

Painful in iliopsoas abscess

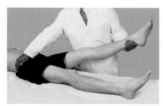

Figure 16-29 Abduct the leg.

- Abduction and adduction

Restricted in hip arthritis

- Internal and external rotation (Fig. 16-30)

Restricted in hip arthritis

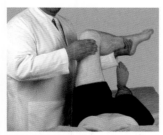

Figure 16-30 Test internal and external rotation of the hip.

<table>
<tr><td>EXAMINATION TECHNIQUES</td><td>POSSIBLE FINDINGS</td></tr>
</table>

Knees

Identify the medial (Fig. 16-31)
and lateral structures of the knee.

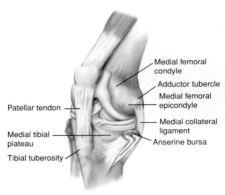

Figure 16-31 Medial compartment of the knee.

Inspect:

■ Gait for knee extension at heel strike, flexion during all other phases of swing and stance	Stumbling or "giving way" during heel strike in *quadriceps weakness* or abnormal patellar tracking
■ Alignment of knees	Bowlegs, knock-knees; flexion contractures in limb paralysis or hamstring tightness.
■ Contours of knees, including any atrophy of the quadriceps muscles	Quadriceps atrophy with patellofemoral disorder; swelling over the patella in prepatellar bursitis (housemaid's knee), over the tibial tubercle in infrapatellar or if more medial anserine bursitis

Inspect and palpate:

See Table 16-5, Painful Knees, pp. 309–310.

■ The tibiofemoral joint—with knees flexed, including:	
■ Joint line—place thumbs on either side of the patellar tendon.	Irregular, bony ridges in osteoarthritis.

EXAMINATION TECHNIQUES

| | POSSIBLE FINDINGS |

- ▣ Medial and lateral meniscus

  Tenderness if meniscus tear

- ▣ Medial and lateral collateral ligaments

  Tenderness if MCL tear (LCL injuries less common)

- ▣ The patellofemoral compartment:

  - ▣ Patella

    Swelling over the patella in prepatellar bursitis ("housemaid's knee")

  - ▣ Palpate the patellar tendon and ask patient to extend the leg.

    Tenderness or inability to extend the leg in partial or complete tear of the patellar tendon

  - ▣ Press the patella against the underlying femur.

    Pain, crepitus, and a history of knee pain in *patellofemoral disorder*

  - ▣ Push patella distally and ask patient to tighten knee against table.

    Pain during contraction of quadriceps in *chondromalacia*

- ▣ Also:

  - ▣ Suprapatellar pouch

    Swelling in synovitis and arthritis

  - ▣ Infrapatellar spaces (hollow areas adjacent to patella)

    Swelling in arthritis

  - ▣ Medial tibial condyle

    Swelling in *pes anserine* bursitis

  - ▣ Popliteal surface

    Popliteal or Baker cyst

Assess any effusions.

- ▣ *Bulge sign* (minor effusions): Compress the suprapatellar pouch, stroke downward on medial surface (Fig. 16-32), apply pressure to force fluid to lateral surface (Fig. 16-33), and then tap knee behind lateral margin of patella (Fig. 16-34).

  A fluid wave returning to the medial surface after a lateral tap confirms an effusion—a positive "bulge sign."

EXAMINATION TECHNIQUES

POSSIBLE FINDINGS

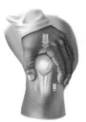

Figure 16-32 Milk downward.

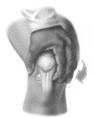

Figure 16-33 Apply medial pressure.

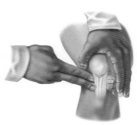

Figure 16-34 Tap and watch for fluid wave.

■ *Balloon sign* (major effusions): Compress suprapatellar pouch with one hand; with thumb and finger of other hand, feel for fluid entering the spaces next to the patella (Fig. 16-35).

A palpable fluid wave is a positive sign.

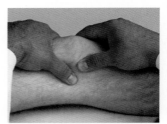

Figure 16-35 Test for the balloon sign.

■ *Ballotte the patella* (major effusion): Push the patella sharply against the femur; watch for fluid returning to the suprapatellar space.

Visible wave is a positive sign.

EXAMINATION TECHNIQUES

POSSIBLE FINDINGS

Assess range of motion: flexion, extension, internal and external rotation.

Use maneuvers to assess menisci and ligaments.

■ *Medial meniscus and lateral meniscus—McMurray test* (*Fig. 16-36*): With the patient supine, grasp the heel and flex the knee. Cup your other hand over the knee joint with fingers and thumb along the medial joint line. From the heel, externally rotate the lower leg, then push on the lateral side to apply a valgus stress on the medial side of the joint. Slowly extend the lower leg in external rotation.

Click or pop along the medial joint with valgus stress, external rotation, and leg extension in tear of posterior medial meniscus.

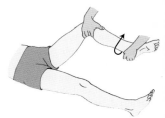

Figure 16-36 McMurray test.

The same maneuver with internal rotation stresses the lateral meniscus.

■ *Medial collateral ligament* (*Fig. 16-37*): With knee slightly flexed, push medially against lateral surface of knee with one hand and pull laterally at the ankle with the other hand (*abduction* or *valgus stress*).

Pain or a gap in the medial joint line points to a partial or complete MCL tear.

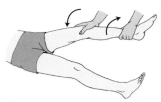

Figure 16-37 Medial collateral ligament test.

EXAMINATION TECHNIQUES

POSSIBLE FINDINGS

■ *Lateral collateral ligament (LCL)* *(Fig. 16-38):* With knee slightly flexed, push laterally along medial surface of knee with one hand and pull medially at the ankle with the other hand (an *adduction* or *varus stress*).

Pain or a gap in the lateral joint line points to a partial or complete LCL tear.

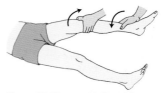

Figure 16-38 Lateral collateral ligament test.

■ *Anterior cruciate ligament (ACL)* *(Fig. 16-39):* (1) With knee flexed, place thumbs on medial and lateral joint line and place fingers on hamstring insertions. Pull tibia forward, observe if tibia slides forward "like a drawer." Compare to opposite knee.

Forward slide of proximal tibia is a positive *anterior drawer sign* in ACL laxity or tear.

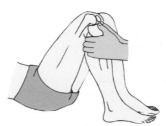

Figure 16-39 Anterior cruciate ligament test.

(2) *Lachman test (Fig. 16-40):* Grasp the distal femur with one hand and the proximal tibia with the other (place the thumb on the joint line). Move the femur forward and the tibia back.

Significant forward excursion of tibia in ACL tear

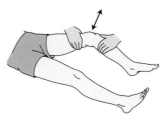

Figure 16-40 Lachman test.

EXAMINATION TECHNIQUES

POSSIBLE FINDINGS

■ *Posterior cruciate ligament (PCL): Posterior drawer sign (Fig. 16-41): Position patient and hands as in the ACL test. Push the tibia posteriorly and observe for posterior movement, like a drawer sliding posteriorly.*

Isolated PCL tears are rare.

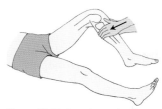

Figure 16-41 Posterior cruciate ligament test (posterior drawer sign).

Ankles and Feet

Inspect ankles and feet.

Hallux valgus, corns, calluses

Palpate:

■ Ankle joint

Tender joint in arthritis

■ Ankle ligaments: medial-deltoid; lateral-anterior and posterior talofibular, calcaneofibular

Tenderness in sprain: lateral ligaments weaker, making inversion injuries (ankle bows outward, heel bows inward) more common

■ Achilles tendon

Rheumatoid nodules, tenderness in tendinitis

■ Compress the metatarsophalangeal joints; then palpate each joint between the thumb and forefinger (Figs. 16-42 and 16-43).

Tenderness in arthritis, Morton neuroma third and fourth MTP joints; inflammation of first MTP joint in gout

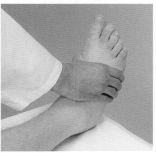

Figure 16-42 Palpate the MTP joints.

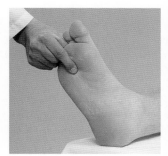

Figure 16-43 Palpate the metatarsal heads.

EXAMINATION TECHNIQUES

POSSIBLE FINDINGS

Assess range of motion.

- Dorsiflex and plantar flex the ankle (*tibiotalar joint*).

Arthritic joint often painful when moved in any direction; sprain, when injured ligament is stretched.

- Stabilize the ankle and invert (Fig. 16-44) and evert (Fig. 16-45) the heel (*subtalar* or *talocalcaneal joint*).

Ankle sprain

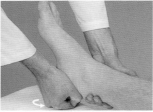

Figure 16-44 Invert the heel.

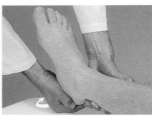

Figure 16-45 Evert the heel.

- Stabilize the heel and invert (Fig. 16-46) and evert (Fig. 16-47) the forefoot (*transverse tarsal joints*).

Trauma, arthritis

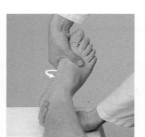

Figure 16-46 Invert the forefoot.

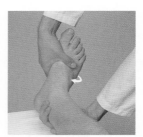

Figure 16-47 Evert the forefoot.

- Move proximal phalanx of each toe up and down (metatarsophalangeal joints).

EXAMINATION TECHNIQUES

POSSIBLE FINDINGS

Special Techniques

o— Measuring Leg Length.
Patient's legs should be aligned
symmetrically. With a tape, measure distance from anterior-superior iliac spine to medial malleolus.
Tape should cross knee medially.

Unequal leg length may be the cause of
scoliosis.

**♀/o— Measuring Range of
Motion.** To measure range of
motion precisely, a simple pocket
goniometer is needed. Estimates
may be made visually. Movement
in the elbow at the right is limited
to range indicated by red lines
(Fig. 16-48).

A flexion deformity of 45 degrees
and further flexion to 90 degrees
(45 degrees → 90 degrees)

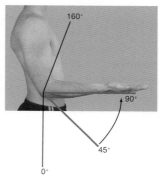

Figure 16-48 Degrees of elbow flexion.

Recording Your Findings

Recording the Musculoskeletal System Examination

"Full range of motion in all joints. No evidence of swelling or deformity."
OR
"Full range of motion in all joints. Hand with degenerative changes of Heberden
nodes at the distal interphalangeal joints, Bouchard nodes at proximal interphalangeal joints. Mild pain with flexion, extension, and rotation of both hips. Full
range of motion in the knees, with moderate crepitus; no effusion but boggy
synovium and osteophytes along the tibiofemoral joint line bilaterally. Both feet
with hallux valgus at the first metatarsophalangeal joints." *(These findings suggest osteoarthritis.)*

Aids to Interpretation

Table 16-1 Patterns of Pain in and Around the Joints

	Rheumatoid Arthritis	**Osteoarthritis (Degenerative Joint Disease, or DJD)**
Process	Chronic inflammation of *synovial membranes* with secondary erosion of adjacent cartilage and bone, damage to ligaments and tendons	Degeneration and progressive loss of *cartilage* within joints, damage to underlying bone, formation of new bone at margins of cartilage
Common Locations	Hands (proximal interphalangeal and metacarpophalangeal joints), feet (metatarsophalangeal joints), wrists, knees, elbows, ankles	Knees, hips, hands (distal, sometimes proximal interphalangeal joints), cervical and lumbar spine, and wrists (first carpometacarpal joint); also joints previously injured or diseased
Pattern of Spread	Symmetrically additive: progresses to other joints; persists in initial ones	Additive; however, sometimes only one joint affected
Onset	Usually insidious	Usually insidious
Progression and Duration	Often chronic, with remissions and exacerbations	Slowly progressive, with exacerbations after overuse
Associated Symptoms	Frequent swelling of synovial tissue in joints or tendon sheaths; also subcutaneous nodules	Small joint effusions may be present, especially in knees; also bony enlargement
	Tender, often warm but seldom red	Tender, seldom warm or red
	Prominent stiffness, often for >1 hour in mornings	Frequent but brief stiffness in the morning

Table 16-2 Pains in the Neck

Patterns	**Physical Signs**
Mechanical Neck Pain	
Aching pain in the cervical paraspinal muscles and ligaments with associated muscle spasm, stiffness, and tightness in the upper back and shoulder, lasting up to 6 weeks. No associated radiation, paresthesias, or weakness. Headache may be present.	Local muscle tenderness, pain on movement. No neurologic deficits. Possible trigger points in *fibromyalgia. Torticollis* if prolonged abnormal neck posture and muscle spasm.
Mechanical Neck Pain— Whiplash	
Also mechanical neck pain with aching paracervical pain and stiffness, often beginning the day after injury. Occipital headache, dizziness, malaise, and fatigue may be present. Chronic whiplash syndrome if symptoms last more than 6 months, present in 20–40% of injuries.	Localized paracervical tenderness, decreased neck range of motion, perceived weakness of the upper extremities. Causes of cervical cord compression such as fracture, herniation, head injury, or altered consciousness are excluded.
Cervical Radiculopathy— from nerve root compression	
Sharp burning or tingling pain in the neck and one arm, with associated paresthesias and weakness. Sensory symptoms often in myotomal pattern, deep in muscle, rather than dermatomal pattern.	C7 nerve root affected most often (45–60%), with weakness in triceps and finger flexors and extensors. C6 nerve root involvement also common, with weakness in biceps, brachioradialis, wrist extensors.
Cervical Myelopathy—from cervical cord compression	
Neck pain with bilateral weakness and paresthesias in both upper and lower extremities, often with urinary frequency. Hand clumsiness, palmar paresthesias, and gait changes may be subtle. Neck flexion often exacerbates symptoms.	Hyperreflexia; clonus at the wrist, knee, or ankle; extensor plantar reflexes (positive Babinski signs); and gait disturbances. May also see *Lhermitte sign:* neck flexion with resulting sensation of electrical shock radiating down the spine. Confirmation of cervical myelopathy warrants neck immobilization and neurosurgical evaluation.

Table 16-3   Low Back Pain

Patterns	Physical Signs
Mechanical Low Back Pain Aching pain in lumbosacral area; may radiate into lower leg, along L5 or S1 dermatomes. Usually acute, work related, in age group 30 to 50 years; no underlying pathology	Paraspinal muscle or facet tenderness, muscle spasm or pain with back movement, loss of normal lumbar lordosis but no motor or sensory loss or reflex abnormalities. In osteoporosis, check for thoracic kyphosis, percussion tenderness over a spinous process, or fractures in the thoracic spine or hip.
Sciatica (Radicular Low Back Pain) Usually from disc herniation; more rarely from nerve root compression, primary or metastatic tumor	Disc herniation most likely if calf wasting, weak ankle dorsiflexion, absent ankle jerk, positive *crossed straight-leg raise* (pain in affected leg when healthy leg tested); negative straight-leg raise makes diagnosis highly unlikely.
Lumbar Spinal Stenosis Pseudoclaudication pain in the back or legs that improves with rest, forward lumbar flexion. Pain vague but usually bilateral, with paresthesias in one or both legs; usually from arthritic narrowing of spinal canal	Posture may be flexed forward with lower extremity weakness and hyporeflexia; straight-leg raise usually negative

Table 16-3   Low Back Pain (*continued*)

Patterns	Physical Signs
Chronic Back Stiffness	
Consider ankylosing spondylitis in inflammatory polyarthritis, most common in men younger than 40 years. Diffuse idiopathic skeletal hyperostosis (DISH) affects men more than women, usually age older than 50 years.	Loss of the normal lumbar lordosis, muscle spasm, limited anterior and lateral flexion; improves with exercise. Lateral immobility of the spine, especially thoracic segment
Nocturnal Back Pain, Unrelieved by Rest	
Consider metastasis to spine from cancer of the prostate, breast, lung, thyroid, and kidney, and multiple myeloma.	Findings vary with the source. Local vertebral tenderness may be present.
Pain Referred from the Abdomen or Pelvis	
Usually a deep, aching pain, the level of which varies with the source (~2% of low back pain)	Spinal movements are not painful and range of motion is not affected. Look for signs of the primary disorder, such as peptic ulcer, pancreatitis, dissecting aortic aneurysm.

Table 16-4   Painful Shoulders

Acromioclavicular Arthritis

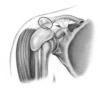

Tenderness over the acromioclavicular joint, especially with adduction of the arm across the chest. Pain often increases with shrugging the shoulders, due to movement of scapula.

Subacromial and Subdeltoid Bursitis

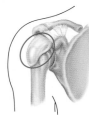

Pain over anterior-superior aspect of shoulder, particularly when raising the arm overhead. Tenderness common anterolateral to the acromion, in hollow recess formed by the acromiohumeral sulcus. Often seen in overuse syndromes.

Rotator Cuff Tendinitis

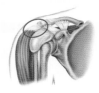

Tenderness over the rotator cuff, when elbow passively lifted posteriorly or with five maneuvers (pp. 286–287).

Bicipital Tendinitis

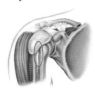

Tenderness over the long head of the biceps when rolled in the bicipital groove or when flexed arm is supinated against resistance suggests *bicipital tendinitis*.

Table 16-5   Painful Knees

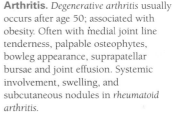

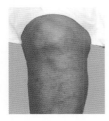

Arthritis. *Degenerative arthritis* usually occurs after age 50; associated with obesity. Often with medial joint line tenderness, palpable osteophytes, bowleg appearance, suprapatellar bursae and joint effusion. Systemic involvement, swelling, and subcutaneous nodules in *rheumatoid arthritis*.

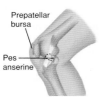

Prepatellar bursa

Pes anserine

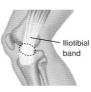

Iliotibial band

Bursitis. Inflammation and thickening of bursa seen in repetitive motion and overuse syndromes. Can involve *prepatellar bursa* ("housemaid's knee"), *pes anserine* bursa medially (runners, osteoarthritis), *iliotibial band* laterally (over lateral femoral condyle), especially in runners.

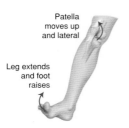

Patella moves up and lateral

Leg extends and foot raises

Patellofemoral instability. During flexion and extension of knee, due to subluxation and/or malalignment, patella tracks laterally instead of centrally in trochlear groove of femoral condyle. Inspect or palpate for lateral motion with leg extension. May lead to chondromalacia, osteoarthritis.

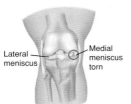

Lateral meniscus

Medial meniscus torn

Meniscal tear. Commonly arises from twisting injury of knee; in older patients may be degenerative, often with clicking, popping, or locking sensation. Check for tenderness along joint line over medial or lateral meniscus and for effusion. May have associated tears of medial collateral of anterior cruciate ligaments.

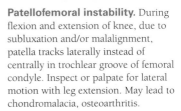

(table continues on page 310)

Table 16-5 Painful Knees (*continued*)

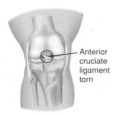

Anterior cruciate tear or sprain.
In twisting injuries of the knee, often with popping sensation, immediate swelling, pain with flexion/extension, difficulty walking, and sensation of knee "giving way." Check for anterior drawer sign, swelling of hemarthrosis, injuries to medial meniscus or medial collateral ligament. Consider evaluation by an orthopedic surgeon.

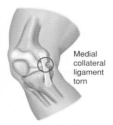

Collateral ligament sprain or tear.
From force applied to medial or lateral surface of knee (valgus or varus stress), producing localized swelling, pain, stiffness. Patients able to walk but may develop an effusion. Check for tenderness over affected ligament and ligamentous laxity during valgus or varus stress.

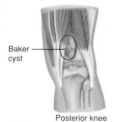

Posterior knee

Baker cyst. Cystic swelling palpable on the medial surface of the popliteal fossa, prompting complaints of aching or fullness behind the knee. Inspect, palpate for swelling adjacent to medial hamstring tendons. If present, suggests involvement of posterior horn of medial meniscus. In rheumatoid arthritis, cyst may expand into calf or ankle.

The Nervous System

Fundamentals for Assessing the Nervous System

Approach to Assessment

The history and neurologic examination respond to four guiding questions. These questions are not answered separately, but iteratively as you learn about the patient during the interview and establish your neurologic findings. To acquire the skills of nervous system examination, it is important to test your physical findings against those of your teachers and neurologists to refine your clinical expertise.

Guiding Questions for Examination of the Nervous System

- Does the patient have neurologic disease?
- If so, what is the localization of the lesion or lesions? Are your findings symmetric?
- What is the pathophysiology of abnormal findings?
- What is the preliminary differential diagnosis?

Central and Peripheral Nervous Systems

Central Nervous System. The *central nervous system* (CNS) consists of the brain and spinal cord.

The Brain. The brain has four regions: the *cerebrum*, the *diencephalon*, the *brainstem*, and the *cerebellum* (Fig. 17-1). Each cerebral hemisphere is subdivided into frontal, parietal, temporal, and occipital lobes. The brain consists of gray matter and myelinated neuronal axons, or white matter. Important structures include the *basal ganglia*, the *thalamus*, the *hypothalamus*, the *brainstem* (*midbrain*, *pons*, and *medulla*), which connects the cortex with the spinal cord, the *reticular activating (arousal) system* linked to consciousness, and the *cerebellum*.

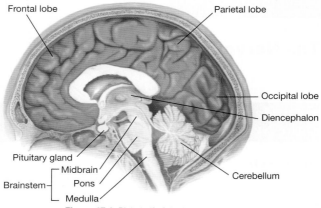

Frontal lobe
Parietal lobe
Occipital lobe
Diencephalon
Pituitary gland
Midbrain
Brainstem — Pons
Medulla
Cerebellum

Figure 17-1 Right half of the brain, medial view.

Spinal Cord. The spinal cord extends from the medulla to the first or second lumbar vertebrae. The spinal cord:

■ is divided into five segments: cervical (C1–C8), thoracic (T1–T12), lumbar (L1–L5), sacral (S1–S5), and coccygeal. Its roots fan out like a horse's tail at L1–L2, the *cauda equina.*

■ contains important motor and sensory nerve pathways that exit and enter the cord via anterior and posterior nerve roots and spinal and peripheral nerves.

■ mediates the monosynaptic muscle stretch reflexes.

Peripheral Nervous System. The peripheral nervous system consists of the 12 pairs of cranial nerves and the spinal and peripheral nerves. Most peripheral nerves contain both motor and sensory fibers.

Cranial Nerves. The twelve pairs of cranial nerves (CNs) emerge from the cranial vault through skull foramina and canals to structures in the head and neck. Some are limited to general motor and/or sensory functions, whereas others are specialized, serving smell, vision, or hearing (I, II, VIII).

Peripheral Nerves. Thirty-one pairs of nerves carry impulses to and from the cord: 8 cervical, 12 thoracic, 5 lumbar, 5 sacral, and 1 coccygeal. Each nerve has an anterior (ventral) root containing motor fibers, and a posterior (dorsal) root containing sensory fibers. These merge to form a short (<5 mm) *spinal nerve.* Spinal nerve fibers commingle with similar fibers in plexuses outside the cord—from these emerge *peripheral nerves.*

The Health History

Common or Concerning Symptoms

- Headache
- Dizziness or vertigo
- Weakness (generalized, proximal, or distal)
- Numbness, abnormal or lost sensations
- Fainting or blacking out (near-syncope and syncope)
- Seizures
- Tremors or involuntary movements

Headache. Ask about location, severity, duration, and any associated symptoms, such as visual changes, weakness, or loss of sensation. Always elicit unusual headache warning signs, such as sudden onset "like a thunderclap," onset after age 50 years, and associated symptoms such as fever and stiff neck, which warrant examination for papilledema and focal neurologic signs.

See Table 7-1, Primary Headaches, p. 128, and Table 7-2, Secondary Headaches, pp. 129–131. *Subarachnoid hemorrhage* may evoke "the worst headache of my life." Dull headache especially on awakening and in the same location, especially when affected by examination maneuvers, may arise from mass lesions like a brain tumor or abscess.

Dizziness or Vertigo. Dizziness or vertigo can have many meanings. Is the patient lightheaded or feeling faint (*presyncope*)? Is there unsteady gait from disequilibrium or ataxia, or true *vertigo*, a perception that the room is spinning or rotating?

Lightheadedness in palpitations; near-syncope from vasovagal stimulation, low blood pressure, febrile illness, and others; vertigo in benign positional vertigo, Ménière disease, brainstem tumor

Are any medications contributing to dizziness?

Are associated symptoms present, such as double vision (*diplopia*), difficulty forming words (*dysarthria*), or difficulty with gait or balance (*ataxia*)? Is there any weakness?

Diplopia, dysarthria, ataxia in vertebrobasilar *transient ischemic attack* (*TIA*) or *stroke*

See Table 17-1, Types of Stroke, pp. 335–336, and Table 17-2, Disorders of Speech, pp. 347–348.

Weakness or paralysis in *TIA* or *stroke*

Weakness. Distinguish *proximal* from *distal* weakness. For *proximal weakness,* ask about combing hair, reaching for things on a high shelf, difficulty getting out of a chair or taking a high step up.

Bilateral proximal limb weakness with intact sensation in myopathies from alcohol, drugs like glucocorticoids, and inflammatory muscle disorders like polymyositis and dermatomyositis

In myasthenia gravis, weakness is asymmetric and gets worse with effort (fatigability), and often has bulbar symptoms such as diplopia, ptosis, dysarthria, and dysphagia.

For *distal weakness,* ask about hand movements such as opening a jar or can or using hand tools (e.g., scissors, pliers, screwdriver). Ask about frequent tripping.

Bilateral predominantly distal weakness, often with sensory loss, in polyneuropathy, as in diabetes

Sensory Loss. Is there any loss of sensation or altered sensation such as tingling or pins and needles without an obvious stimulus (*paresthesias*)? *Dysesthesias,* or disordered sensations in response to a stimulus, may last longer than the stimulus itself.

Consider: paresthesias in hands and around the mouth in hyperventilation; local nerve compression or "entrapment," seen in hand numbness from median, ulnar, or radial nerve disorders; nerve root compression with dermatomal sensory loss from vertebral bone spurs or herniated discs; or central lesions from stroke or multiple sclerosis.

Syncope. "Have you ever fainted or passed out?" leads to discussion of any *loss of consciousness (syncope).*

Syncope is complete but temporary loss of consciousness from decreased cerebral blood flow, commonly called *fainting.*

Get a complete description of the event including setting and triggers, any warning signs, position (standing, sitting, lying down), and duration. What brought on the episode? Could voices be heard while passing out and coming to? How rapid was recovery? Were onset and offset slow or fast?

Young people with emotional stress and warning symptoms of flushing, warmth, or nausea may have *vasodepressor (or vasovagal) syncope* of slow onset, slow offset.

Consider:
- seizures
- "neurocardiogenic" conditions such as vasovagal syncope, postural tachycardia syndrome, carotid sinus syndrome, and orthostatic hypotension
- arrhythmias, especially ventricular tachycardia and bradyarrhythmias, often with syncope of sudden onset and offset

Also ask if anyone observed the episode. What did the patient look like before, during, and after the episode? Was there any seizure-like movement of the arms or legs? Any incontinence of the bladder or bowel?

Tonic–clonic motor activity, incontinence, and *postictal state* in generalized *seizures*. Unlike in syncope, tongue biting or bruising of limbs may occur.

Depending on the type of seizure, there may be loss of consciousness or abnormal feelings, thought processes, and sensations, including smells, as well as abnormal movements.

Seizure. A seizure is a sudden excessive electrical discharge from cortical neurons, and may be symptomatic, with an identifiable cause, or idiopathic. Elicit a careful history.

If acute symptomatic seizures, consider head trauma; alcohol, cocaine, and other drugs; withdrawal from alcohol, benzodiazepines, and barbiturates; metabolic insults from low or high glucose or low calcium or sodium; acute stroke; and meningitis or encephalitis.

Tremors or Involuntary Movements. Ask about any tremor, shaking, or body movements that the patient is unable to control. Does the tremor occur at rest? Get worse with voluntary intentional movement or with sustained postures?

Low-frequency unilateral resting tremor, rigidity, and bradykinesia in Parkinson disease.

Essential tremors if high-frequency, bilateral, upper extremity tremors that occur with both limb movement and sustained posture and subside when the limb is relaxed.

Health Promotion and Counseling: Evidence and Recommendations

Important Topics for Health Promotion and Counseling

- Preventing stroke and transient ischemic attack (TIA)
- Carotid artery screening
- Reducing risk of peripheral neuropathy
- Herpes zoster vaccination
- Detecting the "three Ds": delirium, dementia, and depression

Preventing Stroke or TIA. Cerebrovascular disease is the fourth leading cause of death in the United States. *Stroke* is a sudden neurologic deficit caused by cerebrovascular ischemia (87%) or hemorrhage (13%).

Hemorrhagic strokes may be intracerebral (10% of all strokes) or subarachnoid (3% of all strokes). Decreased vascular perfusion results in sudden focal but transient brain dysfunction in *TIA,* or in permanent neurologic deficits in *stroke,* as determined by neurodiagnostic imaging. Detecting TIAs is important—in the first 3 months after a TIA, subsequent stroke occurs in approximately 15% of patients.

AHA/ASA Stroke Warning Signs and Symptoms

F	**Face Drooping**—Does one side of the face droop or is it numb? Ask the person to smile. Is the person's smile uneven?
A	**Arm Weakness**—Is one arm weak or numb? Ask the person to raise both arms. Does one arm drift downward?
S	**Speech Difficulty**—Is speech slurred? Is the person unable to speak or hard to understand? Ask the person to repeat a simple sentence, like "The sky is blue." Is the sentence repeated correctly?
T	**Time to call 9-1-1**—If someone shows any of these symptoms, even if the symptoms go away, call 9-1-1 and get the person to the hospital immediately. Check the time so you'll know when the first symptoms appeared.

Beyond FAST: Other important symptoms

- Sudden numbness or weakness of the leg, arm, or face
- Sudden confusion or trouble understanding
- Sudden trouble seeing in one or both eyes
- Sudden trouble walking, dizziness, loss of balance or coordination
- Sudden severe headache with no known cause

AHA, American Heart Association; ASA, American Stroke Association.

Primary prevention of stroke requires aggressive management of risk factors and patient education.

■ Target modifiable risk factors: hypertension, smoking, dyslipidemia, excess weight, diabetes, poor diet and nutrition, physical inactivity, and alcohol use.

■ Address disease-specific risk factors: atrial fibrillation, carotid artery disease, and sleep apnea.

Carotid Artery Screening. Screen symptomatic patients with duplex ultrasound. The U.S. Preventive Services Task Force recommends against screening asymptomatic patients in the general population.

Reducing Risk of Peripheral Neuropathy. In diabetics, promote optimal glucose control to reduce risk of sensorimotor polyneuropathy, autonomic dysfunction, mononeuritis multiplex, or diabetic neuropathy.

Examine diabetics regularly for neuropathy, including testing pinprick sensation, ankle reflexes, vibration perception (with a 128-Hz tuning fork) and plantar light touch sensation (with a Semmes-Weinstein monofilament), as well as checking for skin breakdown, poor circulation, and musculoskeletal abnormalities.

Herpes Zoster Vaccination. The herpes zoster vaccine reduces the short-term risks for zoster and postherpetic neuralgia in adults ≥50 years. The Advisory Committee on Immunization Practices (ACIP) currently recommends routinely offering onetime vaccination for adults ≥60 years; the vaccine is FDA-approved for adults ≥50 years.

Detecting the "Three Ds": Delirium, Dementia, and Depression. *Delirium* is an acute confusional state marked by sudden onset, fluctuating course, inattention and changes in the level of consciousness; it is often undetected. Learn to use the Confusional Assessment Method (CAM) algorithm.

The Confusion Assessment Method (CAM) Diagnostic Algorithm

1. Acute change in mental status and fluctuating course
   - Is there evidence of an acute change in cognition from baseline?
   - Does the abnormal behavior fluctuate during the day?
2. Inattention
   - Does the patient have difficulty focusing attention?
3. Disorganized thinking
   - Does the patient have rambling or irrelevant conversations, unclear or illogical flow of ideas, or unpredictable switching from subject to subject?
4. Abnormal level of consciousness
   - Is the patient anything besides alert—hyperalert, lethargic, stuporous, or comatose?

Diagnosing delirium requires features 1 and 2 and either 3 or 4.

Dementia is best assessed by the Mini-Mental State examination and the Mini-Cog (see Chapter 20, Table 20-3, p. 420), but may be difficult to distinguish from *benign forgetfulness* and *mild cognitive impairment*.

Depression is common in individuals with significant medical conditions. Ask the well-validated screening questions: "Have you been feeling down, depressed, or hopeless (depressed mood)?" and, "Have you felt little interest or pleasure in doing things (anhedonia)?"

See also Chapter 20, The Older Adult, pp. 405–406, and Table 20-2, Delirium and Dementia, pp. 418–419.

Techniques of Examination

Cranial Nerves and Function

No.	Cranial Nerve	Function
I	Olfactory	Sense of smell
II	Optic	Vision
III	Oculomotor	Pupillary constriction, opening the eye (lid elevation), most extraocular movements
IV	Trochlear	Downward, internal rotation of the eye
V	Trigeminal	*Motor*—temporal and masseter muscles (jaw clenching), lateral pterygoids (lateral jaw movement) *Sensory*—facial; the nerve has three divisions: (1) ophthalmic, (2) maxillary, and (3) mandibular
VI	Abducens	Lateral deviation of the eye
VII	Facial	*Motor*—facial movements, including those of facial expression, closing the eye, closing the mouth *Sensory*—taste for salty, sweet, sour, and bitter substances on anterior two thirds of tongue; sensation from the ear
VIII	Acoustic	Hearing (cochlear division) and balance (vestibular division)
IX	Glossopharyngeal	*Motor*—pharynx *Sensory*—posterior portions of the eardrum and ear canal, the pharynx, and the posterior tongue, including taste (salty, sweet, sour, bitter)
X	Vagus	*Motor*—palate, pharynx, and larynx *Sensory*—pharynx and larynx
XI	Spinal accessory	*Motor*—sternocleidomastoid; upper portion of the trapezius
XII	Hypoglossal	*Motor*—tongue

EXAMINATION TECHNIQUES	POSSIBLE FINDINGS

Cranial Nerves

CN I (Olfactory). Test sense of smell on each side.

Loss of smell in sinus conditions, head trauma, smoking, aging, cocaine use, Parkinson disease

CN II (Optic). Assess visual acuity.

Blindness

Check visual fields.

Hemianopsia

Inspect optic discs.

Papilledema, optic atrophy, glaucoma

EXAMINATION TECHNIQUES

POSSIBLE FINDINGS

CN II, III (Optic and Oculomotor). Test pupillary reactions to light. If abnormal, test reactions to near effort.

Blindness, CN III paralysis, tonic pupils; Horner syndrome may affect light reactions

CN III, IV, VI (Oculomotor, Trochlear, and Abducens). Assess extraocular movements.

Strabismus and binocular diplopia in CN III, IV, and VI neuropathy; diplopia in eye muscle disorders from myasthenia gravis, trauma, thyroid ophthalmopathy, and internuclear ophthalmoplegia; nystagmus

CN V (Trigeminal). Palpate the contractions of temporal and masseter muscles. Test pain and light touch sensations on face in (1) ophthalmic, (2) maxillary, and (3) mandibular zones (Fig. 17-2).

Motor or sensory loss from lesions of CN V or its higher motor pathways.

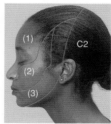

Figure 17-2 Test for facial sensory loss.

Test corneal reflexes (Fig. 17-3).

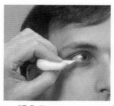

Figure 17-3 Test the corneal reflex.

CN VII (Facial). Ask patient to raise both eyebrows, frown, close eyes tightly, show teeth, smile, and puff out cheeks.

Weakness from lesion of peripheral nerve, as in Bell palsy, or of CNS, as in a stroke. See Table 17-3, Types of Facial Paralysis, p. 339.

EXAMINATION TECHNIQUES	POSSIBLE FINDINGS

CN VIII (Acoustic). Test hearing of whispered voice. If decreased:

- Test for lateralization if unilateral hearing loss (*Weber test*).

In unilateral sensorineural loss, sound is heard in the good ear where AC > BC. In conductive loss lateralization is to the affected ear where BC > AC. See p. 125.

- Compare air and bone conduction (*Rinne test*).

In sensorineural hearing loss, sound is heard longer through air than bone (AC > BC). In conductive loss sound is heard through bone longer than air (BC = AC or BC > AC). See p. 125.

CN IX, X (Glossopharyngeal and Vagus). Observe any difficulty swallowing.

A weakened palate or pharynx impairs swallowing.

Listen to the voice.

Hoarseness in vocal cord paralysis; nasal voice in paralysis of palate

Watch soft palate rise with "ah."

Deviated uvula, palatal paralysis in CVA

Test gag reflex on each side.

Absent reflex is often normal.

CN XI (Spinal Accessory). *Trapezius muscles.* Assess muscles for bulk, involuntary movements, and strength of shoulder shrug (Fig. 17-4).

Atrophy, fasciculations, weakness

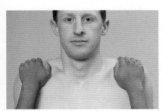

Figure 17-4 Test trapezius strength.

Sternocleidomastoid muscles. Assess strength as head turns against your hand.

Weakness of sternocleidomastoid muscle when head turns to *opposite* side

EXAMINATION TECHNIQUES	POSSIBLE FINDINGS

CN XII (Hypoglossal). Listen to patient's articulation.

Dysarthria from damage to CN X or CN XII

Inspect the resting tongue.

Atrophy, fasciculations in ALS, polio

Inspect the protruded tongue.

In a unilateral cortical lesion, the protruded tongue deviates away from the side of cortical lesion; in CN XII lesion, tongue deviates to the weak side.

℞ The Motor System

See Table 17-4, Motor Disorders, p. 340.

Body Position. Observe the patient's body position during movement and at rest.

Hemiplegia in stroke

Involuntary Movements. If present, observe location, quality, rate, rhythm, amplitude, and setting.

Tremors, fasciculations, tics, chorea, athetosis, oral–facial dyskinesias. See Table 17-5, Involuntary Movements, p. 341.

Muscle Bulk and Tone. Inspect muscle contours.

Atrophy of bulk. See Table 17-6, Disorders of Muscle Tone, p. 342.

Assess resistance to passive stretch of arms and legs.

Spasticity, rigidity, flaccidity of tone

Muscle Strength. Test and grade the major muscle groups, with the examiner trying to overcome the strength of the *patient's resistance.*

Is the pattern *focal,* from a lower motor neuron lesion in peripheral nerve or nerve root? Is there unilateral paralysis from an upper motor neuron cortical or subcortical lesion? Is there a symmetric distal weakness from *polyneuropathy,* or proximal weakness from *myopathy*?

Grading Muscle Strength

Grade	Description
0	No muscular contraction detected
1	A barely detectable trace of contraction
2	Active movement with gravity eliminated
3	Active movement against gravity
4	Active movement against gravity and some resistance
5	**Active movement against full resistance (normal)**

EXAMINATION TECHNIQUES

POSSIBLE FINDINGS

- *Flexion* (C5, C6)—biceps and brachioradialis and *extension* (C6, C7, C8)—triceps *at the elbow*

- Wrist *extension* (C6, C7, C8, radial nerve)—extensor carpi radialis longus and brevis

  Peripheral radial nerve damage; central *stroke* or *multiple sclerosis* if hemiplegia

- Grip (C7, C8, T1)

  Weak grip in cervical radiculopathy, de Quervain tenosynovitis, carpal tunnel syndrome

- Finger abduction (C8, T1, ulnar nerve) (Fig. 17-5)

  Weak in ulnar nerve disorders

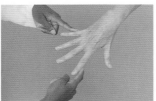

Figure 17-5 Test finger abduction.

- Thumb opposition (C8, T1)— median nerve (Fig. 17-6)

  Weak in carpal tunnel syndrome

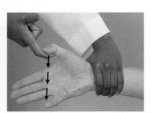

Figure 17-6 Test opposition of the thumb.

- ⓘ Trunk—flexion extension, lateral bending

EXAMINATION TECHNIQUES

- ⚲ Hip flexion (L2, L3, L4)—iliopsoas (Fig. 17-7)

- Hip extension (S1)—gluteus maximus

- Hip adduction (L2, L3, L4)—adductors

- Hip abduction (L4, L5, S1)—gluteus medius and minimus

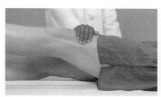

Figure 17-7 Test hip flexion.

- Knee extension (L2, L3, L4)—quadriceps

- Knee flexion (L4, L5, S1, S2)—hamstrings

- Ankle dorsiflexion (L4, L5)—tibialis anterior

- Ankle plantar flexion (S1)—gastrocnemius, soleus

Coordination. Test *rapid alternating movements* in hands (tap fingers), arms, and legs (tap foot) (Fig. 17-8)

Clumsy, slow movements in cerebellar disease

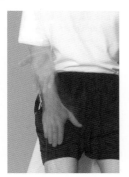

Figure 17-8 Test rapid alternating arm movement.

EXAMINATION TECHNIQUES	POSSIBLE FINDINGS

Point-to-point movements in arms and legs—finger-to-nose, heel-to-shin

Clumsy, unsteady movements in cerebellar disease

Gait. Ask patient to:

■ Walk away, turn, and come back

CVA, cerebellar ataxia, parkinsonism, or loss of position sense may affect performance.

■ Walk heel-to-toe

Ataxia

■ Walk on toes, then on heels

Corticospinal tract injury

■ Hop in place on each foot; do one-leg shallow knee bends. Substitute rising from a chair and climbing on a stool for hops and bends as indicated.

Proximal hip girdle weakness increases risk of falls.

Stance

■ Do a *Romberg test* (a sensory test of stance). Ask patient to stand with feet together and eyes open, then closed for 20 to 30 seconds. Mild swaying may occur. Stand close by to prevent falls.

Loss of balance when eyes are closed is a *positive* Romberg test, suggesting poor position sense.

■ Inspect for a *pronator drift* as patient holds arms forward, with eyes closed, for 20 to 30 seconds (Fig. 17-9).

Flexion and pronation at elbow and downward drift of arm from *contralateral corticospinal tract lesion* (Fig. 17-10)

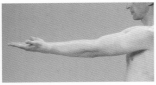

Figure 17-9 Test for pronator drift.

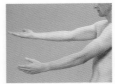

Figure 17-10 Positive test for pronator drift.

Ask patient to keep arms up and tap them downward. A smooth return to position is normal.

Weakness, incoordination, poor position sense

EXAMINATION TECHNIQUES

POSSIBLE FINDINGS

♀/♂ The Sensory System

Use an object like a sharp pin or stick portion of a broken cotton swab to test sharp and dull sensation; *compare symmetric areas on the two sides of the body.* Do not reuse the object on another patient.

A hemisensory loss pattern suggests a contralateral cortical lesion.

Compare proximal and distal areas of arms and legs for *pain, temperature,* and *touch sensation.* Scatter stimuli to sample most dermatomes and major peripheral nerves.

"Glove-and-stocking" loss of peripheral neuropathy, often seen in alcoholism and diabetes

See Table 17-7, Dermatomes, pp. 343–344.

Map any area of abnormal response, including dermatomes, if present.

Dermatomal sensory loss in herpes zoster, nerve root compression.

Assess response to the following stimuli, with the patient's eyes closed.

- *Pain.* Use the sharp end of a pin or other suitable tool. The dull end serves as a control.

Analgesia, hypalgesia, hyperalgesia

- *Temperature* (if indicated). Use test tubes with hot and cold water, or other objects of suitable temperature.

Temperature and pain sensation usually correlate.

- *Light touch.* Use a fine wisp of cotton.

Anesthesia, hyperesthesia

Test for *vibration* and *proprioception* (*joint position sense*). If responses are abnormal, test more proximally. Vibration and position senses, both carried in the posterior columns, often correlate.

Loss of vibration and position senses in peripheral neuropathy from diabetes or alcoholism and in posterior column disease from tertiary syphilis or vitamin B_{12} deficiency

EXAMINATION TECHNIQUES

POSSIBLE FINDINGS

- *Vibration.* Use a 128-Hz tuning fork, held on a *bony* prominence at the ankle and wrist (Fig. 7-11).

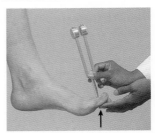

Figure 17-11 Test vibration sense.

- *Proprioception (joint position sense).* Holding patient's finger or big toe by its sides, move it up or down (Fig. 17-12).

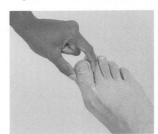

Figure 17-12 Test proprioception.

Assess *discriminative* sensations:

- *Stereognosis.* Ask for identification of a common object placed in patient's hand.

Lesions in the posterior columns or sensory cortex impair stereognosis, number identification, and two-point discrimination.

- *Number identification* (graphesthesia). Draw a number on patient's palm with blunt end of a pen and ask the patient to identify the number.

- *Two-point discrimination* (Fig. 17-13). Use two pins of the sides of a paper clip to find minimal distance on pad of patient's finger at which two points can be distinguished (normally <5 mm).

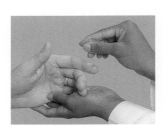

Figure 17-13 Test two-point discrimination.

EXAMINATION TECHNIQUES

■ *Point localization.* Touch skin briefly, and ask patient to open both eyes and identify the place touched.

■ *Extinction.* Simultaneously touch opposite, corresponding areas of the body; ask whether the patient feels one touch or two.

Reflexes

Hold the reflex hammer loosely between your thumb and index finger so that it swings freely in an arc within the limits set by your palm and other fingers. Use the common grading system below.

POSSIBLE FINDINGS

A lesion in the sensory cortex may impair point localization on the contralateral side and cause contralateral extinction of the touch sensation.

Hyperactive deep tendon reflexes, absent abdominal reflexes, and a positive Babinski response in *upper motor neuron lesions.*

Grading Reflexes

Grade	Description
4+	Hyperactive (clonus must be present)
3+	Brisker than average, not necessarily abnormal
2+	**Average, normal**
1+	Diminished, low normal
0	No response

 Biceps (C5, C6) (Fig. 17-14)

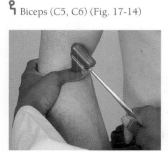

Figure 17-14 Biceps reflex—patient sitting.

 Triceps (C6, C7) (Fig. 17-15)

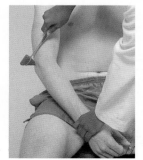

Figure 17-15 Triceps reflex—patient sitting.

EXAMINATION TECHNIQUES	POSSIBLE FINDINGS

Brachioradialis (C5, C6) (Fig. 17-16)

Quadriceps (patellar) (L2, L3, L4) (Fig. 17-17)

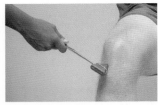

Figure 17-17 Quadriceps (patellar) reflex.

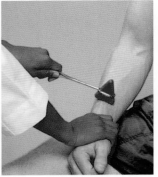

Figure 17-16 Brachioradialis reflex.

Achilles (ankle) (S1) (Fig. 17-18)

Check for clonus if reflexes seem hyperactive (Fig. 17-19).

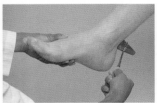

Figure 17-18 Achilles reflex—patient sitting.

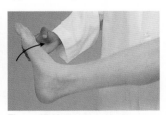

Figure 17-19 Test for ankle clonus.

Ankle jerks symmetrically, decreased or absent in peripheral polyneuropathy; slowed ankle jerk in hypothyroidism.

EXAMINATION TECHNIQUES

POSSIBLE FINDINGS

∿ Cutaneous or Superficial Stimulation Reflexes

Abdominal reflexes (upper T8, T9, T10; lower T10, T11, T12) (Fig. 17-20)

May be absent in both central and peripheral nerve disorders

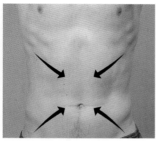

Figure 17-20 Test the abdominal reflexes.

Plantar response (L5, S1), normally flexor (Fig. 17-21)

Babinski extensor response (big toe fans up) from corticospinal tract lesion (Fig. 17-22)

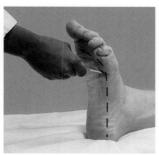

Figure 17-21 Test the plantar response.

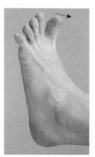

Figure 17-22 Babinski response (abnormal).

∿ *Anal reflex.* With a dull object, stroke outward from anus in four quadrants. Watch for anal contraction.

Loss of reflex suggests cauda equina lesion at the S2, S3, S4 level.

EXAMINATION TECHNIQUES	POSSIBLE FINDINGS

Special Techniques

o— Meningeal Signs. *Make sure there is no injury or fracture to the cervical vertebrae or cervical cord. This often requires radiologic evaluation.* With patient supine, flex head and neck toward chest. Note resistance or pain, and watch for flexion of hips and knees (*Brudzinski sign*).

Inflammation in the subarachnoid space causes resistance to movement that stretches the spinal nerves (neck flexion), the femoral nerve (Brudzinski sign), and the sciatic nerve (Kernig sign).

Flex one of patient's legs at hip and knee, then straighten knee (Fig. 17-23). Note resistance or pain (*Kernig sign*).

A compressed lumbosacral nerve root also causes pain on straightening the knee of the raised leg.

The frequency of Brudzinski and Kernig signs in meningitis ranges from 5% to 60%.

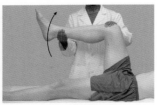
Figure 17-23 Test for Kernig sign.

o— Lumbosacral Radiculopathy: Straight-Leg Raise. With patient supine, raise relaxed and straightened leg, flexing the leg at the hip. Then dorsiflex the foot (Fig. 17-24).

Pain radiating into the ipsilateral leg is a positive straight-leg test for lumbosacral radiculopathy. Foot dorsiflexion can further increase leg pain in lumbosacral radiculopathy, sciatic neuropathy, or both. Increased pain when the contralateral healthy leg is raised is a positive crossed straight-leg raise sign.

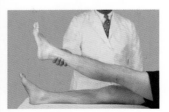
Figure 17-24 Test the straight-leg raise.

EXAMINATION TECHNIQUES

POSSIBLE FINDINGS

ᶜⳆAsterixis. Ask patient to hold both arms forward, with hands cocked up and fingers spread, like "stopping traffic." Watch for 1 to 2 minutes.

Sudden brief flexions in liver disease, uremia and hypercapnia.

ᵀⳆWinging of the Scapula. Ask patient to push against the wall of your hand with a partially straightened arm (Fig. 17-25). Inspect scapula. It should stay close to the chest wall.

Winging of scapula away from chest wall suggests weakness of the serratus anterior muscle, seen in muscular dystrophy or injury to long thoracic nerve (Fig. 17-26).

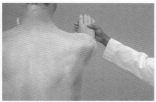

Figure 17-25 Test for scapular winging.

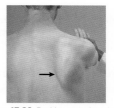

Figure 17-26 Positive scapular winging.

The Stuporous or Comatose Patient

⟋ Assess ABCs (airway, breathing, and circulation).

See Table 17-8, Metabolic and Structural Coma, p. 345, Table 17-9, Glasgow Coma Scale, p. 346, and Table 17-10, Pupils in Comatose Patients, p. 347.

■ Take pulse, blood pressure, and rectal temperature.

■ Establish level of consciousness with escalating stimuli.

Lethargy, obtundation, stupor, coma

However, do not dilate pupils, and *do not flex patient's neck* if any suspicion of cervical cord injury.

EXAMINATION TECHNIQUES | POSSIBLE FINDINGS

Levels of Consciousness

Alertness	Patient is awake and aware of self and environment. When spoken to in a normal voice, patient looks at you and responds fully and appropriately to stimuli.
Lethargy	When spoken to in a loud voice, patient appears drowsy but opens eyes and looks at you, responds to questions, and then falls asleep.
Obtundation	When shaken gently, patient opens eyes and looks at you but responds slowly and is somewhat confused. Alertness and interest in environment are decreased.
Stupor	Patient arouses from sleep only after painful stimuli. Verbal responses are slow or absent. Patient lapses into unresponsiveness when stimulus stops. Patient has minimal awareness of self or environment.
Coma	Despite repeated painful stimuli, patient remains unarousable with eyes closed. No evident response to inner need or external stimuli is shown.

Neurologic Examination

Conduct neurologic examination, looking for asymmetric findings. Observe:

- Breathing pattern

  Cheyne–Stokes, ataxic breathing

- Pupils

  Asymmetrical pupils and loss of the light reaction in structural lesions from stroke, abscess, or tumor

- Ocular movements

  Deviation to affected side in hemispheric stroke

Check for the *oculocephalic reflex* (*doll's eye movements*), as shown in Figure 17-27. Holding upper eyelids open, turn head quickly to each side, and then flex and extend patient's neck. This patient's head will be turned to her right.

In a comatose patient with an **intact brainstem,** the eyes move in the opposite direction, in this case to her left (doll's eye movements) as in Figure 17-28.

Very deep coma or a lesion in the midbrain or pons abolishes this reflex, so eyes do not move.

EXAMINATION TECHNIQUES

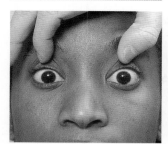

Figure 17-27 Test the oculocephalic reflex.

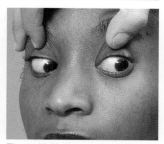

Figure 17-28 Oculocephalic reflex intact.

Note posture of body.

Decorticate rigidity, decerebrate rigidity, flaccid hemiplegia

Test for flaccid paralysis.

- Hold forearms vertically; note wrist positions.

A flaccid hand droops to the horizontal.

- From 12 to 18 inches above bed, drop each arm.

A flaccid arm drops more rapidly.

- Support both knees in a somewhat flexed position, and then extend each knee and let leg drop to the bed.

The flaccid leg drops more rapidly.

- From a similar starting position, release both legs.

A flaccid leg falls into extension and external rotation.

Complete the neurologic and general physical examination.

Recording Your Findings

Recording the Nervous System Examination

"**Mental Status:** Alert, relaxed, and cooperative. Thought process coherent. Oriented to person, place, and time. Detailed cognitive testing deferred. **Cranial Nerves:** I—not tested; II through XII intact. **Motor:** Good muscle bulk and tone.

(continued)

Recording the Nervous System Examination *(Continued)*

Strength 5/5 throughout. *Cerebellar:* Rapid alternating movements (RAMs), finger-to-nose (F→N), heel-to-shin (H→S) intact. Gait with normal base. Romberg—maintains balance with eyes closed. No pronator drift. *Sensory:* Pinprick, light touch, position, and vibration intact. *Reflexes:* 2+ and symmetric with plantar reflexes downgoing."

OR

"*Mental Status:* The patient is alert and tries to answer questions but has difficulty finding words. *Cranial Nerves:* I—not tested; II—visual acuity intact; visual fields full; III, IV, VI—extraocular movements intact; V motor—temporal and masseter strength intact, sensory corneal reflexes present; VII motor—prominent right facial droop and flattening of right nasolabial fold, left facial movements intact, sensory—taste not tested; VIII—hearing intact bilaterally to whispered voice; IX, X—gag intact; XI—strength of sternocleidomastoid and trapezius muscles 5/5; XII—tongue midline. *Motor:* strength in right biceps, triceps, iliopsoas, gluteals, quadriceps, hamstring, and ankle flexor and extensor muscles 3/5 with good bulk but increased tone and spasticity; strength in comparable muscle groups on the left 5/5 with good bulk and tone. Gait—unable to test. Cerebellar—unable to test on right due to right arm and leg weakness; RAMs, F→N, H→S intact on left. Romberg—unable to test due to right leg weakness. Right pronator drift present. *Sensory:* decreased sensation to pinprick over right face, arm, and leg; intact on the left. Stereognosis and two-point discrimination not tested. *Reflexes* (can record in two ways):

(These findings suggest left hemispheric CVA in distribution of the left middle cerebral artery, with right-sided hemiparesis.)

	Biceps	Triceps	Brach	Knee	Ankle	Pl
RT	4+	4+	4+	4+	4+	↑
LT	2+	2+	2+	2+	1+	↓

OR

Aids to Interpretation

Table 17-1   Types of Stroke

Clinical Features and Vascular Territories of Stroke

Assessment of stroke requires careful history taking and a detailed physical examination. Focus on three fundamental questions: *What brain area and related vascular territory explain the patient's findings? Is the stroke ischemic or hemorrhagic? If ischemic, is the mechanism thrombosis or embolus?* This brief overview is intended to prompt further study and practice.

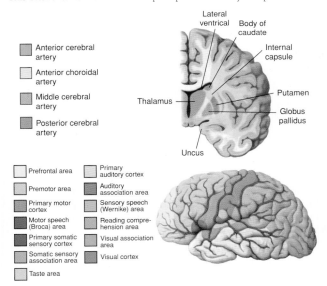

Major Clinical Features	Vascular Territory
Contralateral leg weakness	*Anterior circulation*—anterior cerebral artery (ACA)
	Includes stem of circle of Willis connecting internal carotid artery to ACA, and the segment distal to ACA and its anterior choroidal branch

(table continues on page 336)

Table 17-1 Types of Stroke (*continued*)

Clinical Features and Vascular Territories of Stroke (*continued*)

Major Clinical Features	Vascular Territory
Contralateral face, arm > leg weakness, sensory loss, field cut, aphasia (left MCA) or neglect, apraxia (right MCA)	*Anterior circulation*—middle cerebral artery (MCA) Largest vascular bed for stroke
Contralateral motor or sensory deficit without cortical signs	*Subcortical circulation*—lenticulostriate deep penetrating branches of MCA Small vessel subcortical *lacunar infarcts* in internal capsule, thalamus, or brainstem. Four common syndromes: pure motor hemiparesis; pure sensory hemianesthesia; ataxic hemiparesis; clumsy hand—dysarthria syndrome
Contralateral field cut	*Posterior circulation*—posterior cerebral artery (PCA) Includes paired vertebral arteries, the basilar artery, paired posterior cerebral arteries. Bilateral PCA infarction causes cortical blindness but preserved pupillary light reaction.
Dysphagia, dysarthria, tongue/palate deviation and/or ataxia with crossed sensory/motor deficits (= ipsilateral face with contralateral body)	*Posterior circulation*—brainstem, vertebral, or basilar artery branches
Oculomotor deficits and/or ataxia with crossed sensory/motor deficits	*Posterior circulation*—basilar artery Complete basilar artery occlusion—"locked-in syndrome" with intact consciousness but inability to speak and quadriplegia

Source: Adapted from American College of Physicians. *Stroke, in Neurology. Medical Knowledge Self-Assessment Program (MKSAP) 14*. Philadelphia, PA: American College of Physicians; 2006:52.

Table 17-2   Disorders of Speech

Disorders of speech fall into three groups affecting: (1) phonation of the voice, (2) the articulation of words, and (3) the production and comprehension of language.

- *Aphonia* refers to a loss of voice that accompanies disease affecting the larynx or its nerve supply. *Dysphonia* refers to less severe impairment in the volume, quality, or pitch of the voice. For example, a person may be hoarse or only able to speak in a whisper. Causes include laryngitis, laryngeal tumors, and unilateral vocal cord paralysis (CN X).

- *Dysarthria* refers to a defect in the muscular control of the speech apparatus (lips, tongue, palate, or pharynx). Words may be nasal, slurred, or indistinct, but the central symbolic aspect of language remains intact. Causes include motor lesions of the central or peripheral nervous system, parkinsonism, and cerebellar disease.

- *Aphasia* refers to a disorder in producing or understanding language. It is often caused by lesions in the dominant cerebral hemisphere, usually the left.

(table continues on page 338)

Table 17-2 Disorders of Speech (*continued*)

Compared below are two common types of aphasia: (1) Wernicke, a fluent (receptive) aphasia, and (2) Broca, a nonfluent (or expressive) aphasia. There are other less common kinds of aphasia, which are distinguished by differing responses on the specific tests listed. Neurologic consultation is usually indicated.

	Wernicke Aphasia	Broca Aphasia
Qualities of Spontaneous Speech	Fluent; often rapid, voluble, and effortless. Inflection and articulation are good, but sentences lack meaning and words are malformed (*paraphasias*) or invented (*neologisms*). Speech may be totally incomprehensible.	Nonfluent; slow, with few words and laborious effort. Inflection and articulation are impaired but words are meaningful, with nouns, transitive verbs, and important adjectives. Small grammatical words are often dropped.
Word Comprehension	Impaired	Fair to good
Repetition	Impaired	Impaired
Naming	Impaired	Impaired, though the patient recognizes objects
Reading Comprehension	Impaired	Fair to good
Writing	Impaired	Impaired
Location of Lesion	Posterior superior temporal lobe	Posterior inferior frontal lobe

Although it is important to recognize aphasia early in your encounter with a patient, integrate this information with your neurologic examination as you generate your differential diagnosis.

Table 17-3   Types of Facial Paralysis

Distinguish peripheral from central lesions of CN VII by closely observing movements of the *upper face*. Because of innervation from both hemispheres, the upper facial movements are *preserved* in central lesions.

CN VII—Peripheral Lesion	CN VII—Central Lesion

Peripheral nerve damage to CN VII paralyzes the entire right side of the face, including the forehead.

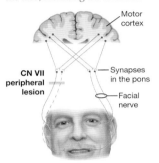

Motor cortex

CN VII peripheral lesion

Synapses in the pons

Facial nerve

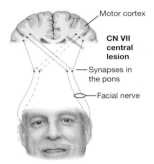

Motor cortex

CN VII central lesion

Synapses in the pons

Facial nerve

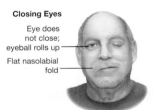

Closing Eyes

Eye does not close; eyeball rolls up

Flat nasolabial fold

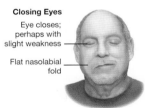

Closing Eyes

Eye closes; perhaps with slight weakness

Flat nasolabial fold

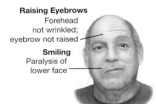

Raising Eyebrows
Forehead not wrinkled; eyebrow not raised

Smiling
Paralysis of lower face

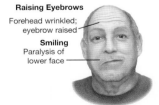

Raising Eyebrows
Forehead wrinkled; eyebrow raised

Smiling
Paralysis of lower face

Table 17-4   Motor Disorders

	Peripheral Nervous System Disorder	Central Nervous System Disorder[a]	Parkinsonism (Basal Ganglia Disorder)	Cerebellar Disorder
Involuntary movements	Often fasciculations	No fasciculations	Resting tremors	Intention tremors
Muscle bulk	Atrophy	Normal or mild atrophy (disuse)	Normal	Normal
Muscle tone	Decreased or absent	Increased, spastic	Increased, rigid	Decreased
Muscle strength	Decreased or lost	Decreased or lost	Normal or slightly decreased	Normal or slightly decreased
Coordination	Unimpaired, though limited by weakness	Slowed and limited by weakness	Good, though slowed and often tremulous	Impaired, ataxic
Reflexes				
Deep tendon	Decreased or absent	Increased	Normal or decreased	Normal or decreased
Plantar	Flexor or absent	Extensor	Flexor	Flexor
Abdominals	Absent	Absent	Normal	Normal

[a]Upper motor neuron.

Table 17-5 Involuntary Movements

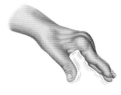

Resting static tremors. Fine, "pill-rolling" tremor seen at rest, usually disappear with movement; seen in basal ganglia disorders like Parkinson disease.

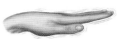

Postural tremor. Seen when maintaining active posture; in anxiety, hyperthyroidism; also familial. From basal ganglia disorder.

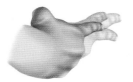

Intention tremor. Seen with intentional movement, absent at rest; in cerebellar disorders, including multiple sclerosis

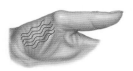

Fasciculations. Fine, rapid flickering of muscle bundles in lower motor neuron disorders.

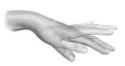

Chorea. Brief, rapid, irregular, jerky; face, head, arms, or hands (e.g., Huntington disease)

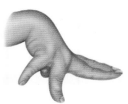

Athetosis. Slow, twisting, writhing; face, distal limbs, often with associated spasticity (e.g., cerebral palsy)

Table 17-6 Disorders of Muscle Tone

Spasticity	**Rigidity**
Location. Upper motor neuron or corticospinal tract systems.	**Location.** Basal ganglia system
Description. Increased muscle tone (*hypertonia*) that is rate-dependent. Tone is greater when passive movement is rapid, and less when passive movement is slow. Tone is also greater at the extremes of the movement arc. During rapid passive movement, initial hypertonia may give way suddenly as the limb relaxes. This spastic "catch" and relaxation is known as "clasp-knife" resistance.	**Description.** Increased resistance that persists throughout the movement arc, independent of rate of movement, is called *lead-pipe rigidity*. With flexion and extension of the wrist or forearm, a superimposed ratchet-like jerkiness is called *cogwheel rigidity*.
Common Cause. Stroke, especially late or chronic stage	**Common Cause.** Parkinsonism
Flaccidity	**Paratonia**
Location. Lower motor neuron at any point from the anterior horn cell to the peripheral nerves	**Location.** Both hemispheres, usually in the frontal lobes
Description. Loss of muscle tone (*hypotonia*), causing the limb to be loose or floppy. The affected limbs may be hyperextensible or even flail-like.	**Description.** Sudden changes in tone with passive range of motion. Sudden loss of tone that increases the ease of motion is called *mitgehen* (moving with). Sudden increase in tone making motion more difficult is called *gegenhalten* (holding against).
Common Cause. Guillain–Barré syndrome; also initial phase of spinal cord injury (spinal shock) or stroke	**Common Cause.** Dementia

Table 17-7 Dermatomes

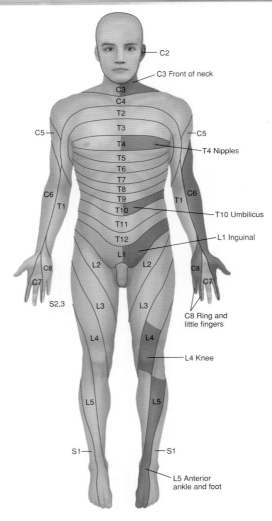

Dermatomes Innervated by Posterior Roots

(table continues on page 344)

Table 17-7 Dermatomes (*continued*)

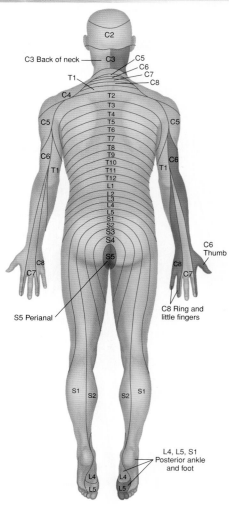

Dermatomes Innervated by Posterior Roots

Table 17-8   Metabolic and Structural Coma

Toxic–Metabolic	Structural
Pathophysiology	
Arousal centers poisoned or critical substrates depleted	Lesion destroys or compresses brainstem arousal areas, either directly or secondary to more distant expanding mass lesions.
Clinical Features	
■ ***Respiratory pattern.*** If regular, may be normal or hyperventilation. If irregular, usually Cheyne–Stokes	***Respiratory pattern.*** Irregular, especially Cheyne–Stokes or ataxic breathing. Also with selected stereotypical patterns like "apneustic" respiration (peak inspiratory arrest) or central hyperventilation.
■ ***Pupillary size and reaction.*** Equal, reactive to light. If *pinpoint* from opiates or cholinergics, you may need a magnifying glass to see the reaction. May be unreactive if *fixed and dilated* from anticholinergics or hypothermia	***Pupillary size and reaction.*** Unequal or unreactive to light (fixed) *Midposition, fixed*—suggests midbrain compression *Dilated, fixed*—suggests compression of CN III from herniation
■ ***Level of consciousness.*** Changes *after* pupils change	***Level of consciousness.*** Changes *before* pupils change
Examples of Cause	
Uremia, hyperglycemia	Epidural, subdural, or intracerebral hemorrhage
Alcohol, drugs, liver failure	
Hypothyroidism, hypoglycemia	Cerebral infarct or embolus
Anoxia, ischemia	Tumor, abscess
Meningitis, encephalitis	Brainstem infarct, tumor, or hemorrhage
Hyperthermia, hypothermia	Cerebellar infarct, hemorrhage, tumor, or abscess

Table 17-9 Glasgow Coma Scale

Activity		Score
Eye Opening		
None	1 = Even to supraorbital pressure	
To pain	2 = Pain from sternum/limb/supraorbital pressure	
To speech	3 = Nonspecific response, not necessarily to command	
Spontaneous	4 = Eyes open, not necessarily aware	_____
Motor Response		
None	1 = To any pain; limbs remain flaccid	
Extension	2 = Shoulder adducted and shoulder and forearm internally rotated	
Flexor response	3 = Withdrawal response or assumption of hemiplegic posture	
Withdrawal	4 = Arm withdraws to pain, shoulder abducts	
Localizes pain	5 = Arm attempts to remove supraorbital/chest pressure	
Obeys commands	6 = Follows simple commands	_____
Verbal Response		
None	1 = No verbalization of any type	
Incomprehensible	2 = Moans/groans, no speech	
Inappropriate	3 = Intelligible, no sustained sentences	
Confused	4 = Converses but confused, disoriented	
Oriented	5 = Converses and is oriented	_____

TOTAL (3–15)[a]

[a]Interpretation: Patients with scores of 3–8 usually are considered to be in a coma.
Source: Teasdale G, Jennett B. Assessment of coma and impaired consciousness. A practical scale. *Lancet.* 1974;304(7872):81.

Table 17-10 Pupils in Comatose Patients

Small or Pinpoint Pupils

Bilaterally small pupils (1–2.5 mm) suggest (1) damage to the sympathetic pathways in the hypothalamus or (2) metabolic encephalopathy (a diffuse failure of cerebral function from drugs and other causes). Light reactions are usually normal.

Pinpoint pupils (<1 mm) suggest (1) a hemorrhage in the pons or (2) the effects of morphine, heroin, or other narcotics. Use a magnifying glass to see the light reactions.

Midposition Fixed Pupils

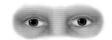

Midposition or *slightly dilated pupils* (4–6 mm) and *fixed to light* suggest damage in the midbrain.

Large Pupils

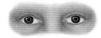

Bilaterally fixed and dilated pupils in severe anoxia with sympathomimetic effects, may be seen with cardiac arrest. They also result from atropine-like agents, phenothiazines, or tricyclic antidepressants.

One Large Pupil

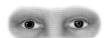

One fixed and dilated pupil warns of herniation of the temporal lobe, causing compression of the oculomotor nerve and midbrain. Also seen in diabetes with CN III infarction.

Assessing Children: Infancy through Adolescence

Child Development

Children display tremendous variations in physical, cognitive, and social development compared with adults.

Key Principles of Child Development

- Child development proceeds along a predictable pathway.
- The range of normal development is wide.
- Various physical, psychological, social, and environmental factors, as well as diseases, can affect child development and health.
- The child's developmental level affects how you conduct the history and physical examination.

The Health History

The child's history follows the same outline as the adult's history, with certain *additions* presented here.

Identifying Data

Record date and place of birth, nickname, and first and last names of parents.

Chief Complaints

Determine if they are the concerns of the child, the parent(s), a school-teacher, or some other person.

Present Illness

Determine how each family member responds to the child's symptoms, why he or she is concerned, and impact on the child's functioning.

History

Birth History. This is especially important when neurologic or developmental problems are present. Get hospital records if necessary.

- Prenatal—maternal health: medications; tobacco, drug, and alcohol use; weight gain; duration of pregnancy

- Natal—nature of labor and delivery, birth weight, Apgar scores at 1 and 5 minutes

- Neonatal—resuscitation efforts, cyanosis, jaundice, infections, bonding

Feeding History. This is particularly important with either undernutrition or obesity.

- Breast-feeding—frequency and duration of feeds, difficulties, timing and method of weaning

- Bottle-feeding—type; amount; frequency; vomiting; colic; diarrhea

- Vitamins, iron, and fluoride supplements; introduction of solid foods

- Eating habits—types and amounts of food eaten, parental attitudes and responses to feeding problems

Growth and Developmental History. This is particularly important with delayed growth or development and behavioral disturbances.

- Physical growth—weight and height at all ages; head circumference at birth and younger than 2 years; periods of slow or rapid growth; BMI after age 2 years

- Developmental milestones, speech development, performance in preschool and school

- Social development—day and night sleeping patterns; toilet training; habitual behaviors; discipline problems; school behavior; relationships with family and peers; social risks such as poverty, food insecurity and adverse experiences

Current Health Status

Allergies. Pay particular attention to history of eczema, urticaria, perennial allergic rhinitis, asthma, food intolerance, insect hypersensitivity, and recurrent wheezing.

Immunizations. Include dates given and any untoward reactions.

Screening Tests. These vary according to the child's medical and social conditions. Include newborn screening results, anemia screening, blood lead, sickle cell disease, vision, hearing, developmental screening, and others (e.g., tuberculosis).

Health Promotion and Counseling: Evidence and Recommendations

For the most up-to-date Bright Futures recommendations for preventive health care, see https://www.aap.org/en-us/Documents/periodicity_schedule.pdf. Each child and family is unique; therefore, such recommendations are designed for the care of children who are receiving competent parenting, have no manifestation of any important health problems, and are growing and developing in satisfactory fashion.

1. Age-appropriate developmental achievement of the child
   - Physical (maturation, growth, puberty)
   - Motor (gross and fine motor skills)
   - Cognitive (milestones, language, school performance)
   - Emotional (self-regulation, self-efficacy, self-esteem, independence)
   - Social (social competence, self-responsibility, integration with family and community)

2. Health supervision visits (per health supervision schedule)
   - Periodic assessment of medical and oral health
   - Adjustment of frequency for children or families with special needs

3. Integration of physical examination findings

4. Immunizations

5. Screening procedures

6. Anticipatory guidance
   - Healthy habits
   - Nutrition and healthy eating
   - Emotional and mental health
   - Oral health
   - Safety and prevention of injury
   - Sexual development and sexuality
   - Self-responsibility and efficacy and self-esteem
   - Family relationships (interactions, strengths, supports)
   - Prevention or recognition of illness

- Prevention of risky behaviors and addictions

- School and vocation

- Peer relationships

- Community interactions

7. Partnership between health provider, child, and family

Techniques of Examination

Sequence of Examination

The sequence of examination varies according to the child's age and comfort level.

- For infants and young children, *perform nondisturbing maneuvers early and potentially distressing maneuvers toward the end.* For example, palpate the head and neck and auscultate the heart and lungs early; examine the ears and mouth and palpate the abdomen near the end. If the child reports pain in an area, examine that part last.

- For older children and adolescents, use the same sequence as with adults, except examine the most painful areas last.

Assessing Newborns

EXAMINATION TECHNIQUES | POSSIBLE FINDINGS

Immediate Assessment at Birth

Listen to the anterior thorax with your stethoscope. Palpate the abdomen. Inspect the head, face, oral cavity, extremities, genitalia, and perineum.

Apgar Score. Score each newborn according to the following table, at 1 and 5 minutes after birth, according to the 3-point scale (0, 1, or 2) for each component.

If the 5-minute score is 8 or more, proceed to a more complete examination.

The Apgar Scoring System

Clinical Sign	Assigned Score		
	0	1	2
Heart rate	Absent	<100	>100
Respiratory effort	Absent	Slow and irregular	Good; strong
Muscle tone	Flaccid	Some flexion of the arms and legs	Active movement
Reflex irritability[a]	No responses	Grimace	Crying vigorously, sneeze, or cough
Color	Blue, pale	Pink body, blue extremities	Pink all over

1-Minute Apgar Score		5-Minute Apgar Score	
8–10	Normal	8–10	Normal
5–7	Some nervous system depression	0–7	High risk for subsequent central nervous system and other organ system dysfunction
0–4	Severe depression, requiring immediate resuscitation		

[a]Reaction to suction of nares with bulb syringe.

Gestational Age and Birth Weight. Classify newborns according to their gestational age and birth weight (see Table 18-1, Classification of Newborn's Level of Maturity, p. 373).

Classification by Gestational Age and Birth Weight

Gestational Age

Classification	Gestational Age
Preterm	<34 wks
Late preterm	34–36 wks
Term	37–42 wks
Postterm	>42 wks

Birth Weight

Classification	Weight
Extremely low birth weight	<1,000 g
Very low birth weight	<1,500 g
Low birth weight	<2,500 g
Normal birth weight	≥2,500 g

EXAMINATION TECHNIQUES	POSSIBLE FINDINGS

Newborn Classifications

Category	Abbreviation	Percentile
Small for gestational age	SGA	<10th
Appropriate for gestational age	AGA	10–90th
Large for gestational age	LGA	>90th

Assessment Several Hours After Birth

During the first day of life, newborns should have a comprehensive examination following the technique outlined under "Infants." Wait until 1 or 2 hours after a feeding, when the newborn is more responsive. Ask parents to remain.

Observe the baby's color, size, body proportions, nutritional status, posture, respirations, and movements of the head and extremities.

Most newborns are *bowlegged,* reflecting their curled up intrauterine position.

Inspect the newborn's *umbilical cord* to detect abnormalities. Normally, there are two thick-walled umbilical arteries and one larger but thin-walled umbilical vein, which is usually located at the 12-o'clock position.

A *single umbilical artery* may be associated with congenital anomalies. *Umbilical hernias* in infants are from a defect in the abdominal wall.

The neurologic screening examination of all newborns should include assessment of mental status, gross and fine motor function, tone, cry, deep tendon reflexes, and primitive reflexes.

Signs of *severe neurologic disease* include extreme irritability; persistent asymmetry of posture or extension of extremities; constant turning of head to one side; marked extension of head, neck, and extremities (opisthotonus); severe flaccidity; and limited pain response.

EXAMINATION TECHNIQUES | POSSIBLE FINDINGS

Assessing Infants

Mental and Physical Status

Observe the parents' affect when talking about the baby and their manner of holding, moving, and dressing the baby. Observe a breast or bottle-feeding. Determine attainment of developmental milestones, optimally using a standardized developmental screening test.

Common causes of *developmental delay* include abnormalities in embryonic development, hereditary and genetic disorders, environmental and social problems, other pregnancy or perinatal problems, childhood diseases such as infection (e.g., meningitis), trauma, and severe chronic disease.

General Survey

Growth, reflected in increases in height and weight within expected limits, is an excellent indicator of health during infancy and childhood. Deviations from normal may be early indications of an underlying problem. To assess growth, compare a child's parameters with respect to:

Failure to thrive is a condition reflecting significantly low weight gain (e.g., below 2nd percentile) for gestational-age corrected age and sex. Causes can be environmental or psychosocial, or various gastrointestinal, neurologic, cardiac, endocrine, renal, and other diseases.

- Normal values according to age and sex

- Prior readings to assess trends

Measures above the 97th or below the 3rd percentile, or recent rises or falls from prior levels, require investigation.

Height and Weight. Plot each child's height and weight on standard growth charts to determine progress.

Reduced growth in height may indicate *endocrine disease,* other *causes of short stature,* or, if weight is also low, other *chronic diseases.*

Head Circumference. Determine head circumference at every physical examination during the first 2 years (Fig. 18-1).

Premature closure of the sutures or microcephaly may cause small head size. Hydrocephalus, subdural hematoma, or, rarely, brain tumor or inherited syndromes may cause an abnormally large head size.

EXAMINATION TECHNIQUES

POSSIBLE FINDINGS

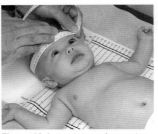

Figure 18-1 Head circumference is a vital metric during early childhood.

Vital Signs

Blood Pressure. Measure blood pressure at least once during infancy. Although the hand-held method is shown in Figure 18-2, the most easily used measure of systolic blood pressure in infants and young children is obtained with the *Doppler method*.

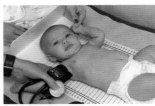

Figure 18-2 Practice is required to accurately measure blood pressure in early childhood.

Causes of Sustained Hypertension in Children	
Newborn	**Middle Childhood**
Renal artery disease (stenosis, thrombosis)	Primary hypertension
Congenital renal malformations	Renal parenchymal or arterial disease
Coarctation of the aorta	Coarctation of the aorta
Infancy and Early Childhood	**Adolescence**
Renal parenchymal or artery disease	Primary hypertension
Coarctation of the aorta	Renal parenchymal disease
	Drug induced

Pulse. The heart rate is quite variable and will increase markedly with excitement, crying, or anxiety. Therefore, measure the pulse when the infant or child is quiet.

Tachycardia (>180–200 beats per minute) usually indicates *paroxysmal supraventricular tachycardia.* Bradycardia may result from serious underlying disease.

EXAMINATION TECHNIQUES

POSSIBLE FINDINGS

Respiratory Rate. The respiratory rate has a very wide range and is more responsive to illness, exercise, and emotion than in adults.

Respiratory diseases such as *bronchiolitis* or *pneumonia* may cause rapid respirations (up to 80 to 90 breaths per minute), *and* increased work of breathing. Peaceful tachypnea (without increased work of breathing) may be a sign of *cardiac failure*.

The Skin

Assess:

- Texture and appearance

  Cutis marmorata

- Vasomotor changes

  Acrocyanosis; cyanotic congenital heart disease

- Pigmentation (e.g., Mongolian spots)

  Café-au-lait spots

- Hair (e.g., lanugo)

  Midline hair tuft on back

- Common skin conditions (e.g., milia, erythema toxicum)

  Herpes simplex

- Color

  Jaundice can be from hemolytic disease.

- Turgor

  Dehydration

The Head

Examine *sutures* and *fontanelles* carefully (Fig. 18-3).

Head small with *microcephaly*, enlarged with *hydrocephaly*; fontanelles full and tense with *meningitis*, closed with *microcephaly*, separated with *increased intracranial pressure* (hydrocephaly, subdural hematoma, and brain tumor)

Swelling from subperiosteal hemorrhage (cephalohematoma) does not cross suture lines; swelling from bleeding associated with a fracture does.

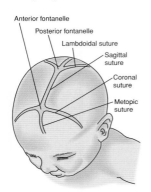

Anterior fontanelle
Posterior fontanelle
Lambdoidal suture
Sagittal suture
Coronal suture
Metopic suture

Figure 18-3 Sutures and fontanelles.

EXAMINATION TECHNIQUES	POSSIBLE FINDINGS

Check the *face* for symmetry. Examine for an overall impression of the *facies*; comparing with the faces of the parents is helpful.

Abnormal facies occurs in a child with a constellation of facial features that appear abnormal. A variety of syndromes can cause abnormal facies (see box below for evaluation). Examples include *Down syndrome* and *fetal alcohol syndrome*.

Pearls to Evaluate Potentially Abnormal Facies

Carefully review the history, especially the *family history*, *pregnancy*, and *perinatal history*.

Note abnormalities of growth/development or dysmorphic somatic features.

Measure and plot percentiles, especially of *head circumference*, *height*, and *weight*.

Consider the three mechanisms of facial dysmorphogenesis:

- Deformations from intrauterine constraint
- Disruptions from amniotic bands or fetal tissue
- Malformations from intrinsic abnormality (either face/head or brain)

Examine parents and siblings (similarity may be reassuring but might also point to a familial disorder).

Determine whether facial features fit a recognizable syndrome. Compare against references, pictures, tables, and databases.

The Eyes

Newborns and young infants may look at your face and follow a bright light if you catch them while alert. Examine the red reflex.

Nystagmus, strabismus

Leukocoria is a white papillary reflex (instead of the normal red papillary reflex). It can be a sign of a rare tumor called *retinoblastoma*.

Normal visual milestones are as follows:

Visual Milestones of Infancy

Birth	Blinks, may regard face
1 month	Fixes on objects
1½–2 months	Coordinated eye movements
3 months	Eyes converge, baby reaches
12 months	Acuity around 20/60–20/80

EXAMINATION TECHNIQUES

POSSIBLE FINDINGS

The Ears

Check *position*, *shape*, and *features*.

Small, deformed or low-set auricles may indicate associated *congenital defects*, especially renal disease.

Signs That an Infant Can Hear

Age	Signs
0–2 months	Startle response and blink to a sudden noise
	Calming down with soothing voice or music
2–3 months	Change in body movements in response to sound
	Change in facial expression to familiar sounds
	Turning eyes and head to sound
3–4 months	Turning to listen to voices and conversation
6–7 months	Appropriate language development

The Nose

Test patency of the nasal passages by occluding alternately each nostril while holding the infant's mouth closed.

With *choanal atresia,* the baby cannot breathe if one nostril is occluded.

The Mouth and Pharynx

Inspect (with a tongue blade and flashlight) and palpate.

Supernumerary teeth, Epstein pearls

You may see a whitish covering on the tongue. If this coating is from milk, you can easily remove it by scraping or wiping it away.

Oral candidiasis (thrush)

Vesicles in the mouth can be caused by *enteroviral infections* and *herpes simplex virus infections.*

The Neck

Palpate the *lymph nodes,* and assess for any additional masses (e.g., *congenital cysts*), as shown in Figure 18-4.

Lymphadenopathy is usually from viral or bacterial infections.

Other neck masses include *malignancy, branchial cleft* or *thyroglossal duct cysts, and periauricular cysts and sinuses.*

EXAMINATION TECHNIQUES

POSSIBLE FINDINGS

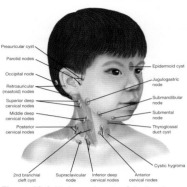

Figure 18-4 Nodes and cysts of the head and neck.

The Thorax and Lungs

Carefully assess respirations and breathing pattern.

Apnea

Do not rush to the stethoscope, but observe the patient carefully first.

Upper respiratory infections may cause nasal flaring.

Examination of the Lungs in Infants—Before You Touch the Child!

Assessment	Possible Findings	Explanation
General appearance	Inability to feed or smile Lack of consolability	*Lower respiratory infections* (e.g., *bronchiolitis, pneumonia*) are common in infants.
Respiratory rate	Tachypnea	Cardiac or respiratory disease (e.g., pneumonia)
Color	Pallor or cyanosis	Cardiac or pulmonary disease
Nasal component of breathing	Nasal flaring (enlargement of both nasal openings during inspiration)	Upper or lower respiratory infection

(*continued*)

EXAMINATION TECHNIQUES

POSSIBLE FINDINGS

Examination of the Lungs in Infants—Before You Touch the Child! (Continued)

Assessment	Possible Findings	Explanation
Audible breath sounds	Grunting (repetitive, short expiratory sound)	Lower respiratory disease
	Wheezing (musical expiratory sound)	Asthma or bronchiolitis
	Stridor (high-pitched, inspiratory noise)	Croup, epiglottitis, bacterial tracheitis
	Obstruction (lack of breath sounds)	Foreign body
Work of breathing	Nasal flaring	In infants, abnormal work of breathing combined with abnormal findings on auscultation is the best finding for ruling in *pneumonia*.
	Grunting	
	Retractions (chest indrawing):	
	Supraclavicular (motion of soft tissue above clavicles)	
	Intercostal (indrawing of the skin between ribs)	
	Substernal (at xiphoid process)	
	Subcostal (just below the costal margin)	

Auscultate the chest, and try to distinguish upper airway from lower airway sounds.

Distinguishing Upper Airway from Lower Airway Sounds

Technique	Upper Airway	Lower Airway
Compare sounds from nose/stethoscope	Same sounds	Often different sounds
Listen to harshness of sounds	Harsh and loud	Variable
Note symmetry (left/right)	Symmetric	Often asymmetric
Compare sounds at different locations (higher or lower)	Sounds louder as stethoscope is moved up chest	Sounds louder lower in chest
Inspiratory vs. expiratory	Almost always inspiratory	Often has expiratory phase

The Heart

Inspection. Observe carefully for any cyanosis. The best body part to assess cyanosis is the tongue or inside of the mouth.

At birth: *Transposition of the great arteries; pulmonary valve atresia or stenosis*

Within a few days of birth: The above; also *total anomalous pulmonary venous return, hypoplastic left heart*

Palpation. Palpate the *peripheral pulses.* The *point of maximal impulse* (*PMI*) is not always palpable in infants. *Thrills* are palpable when enough turbulence is within the heart or great vessels.

No or diminished femoral pulses suggest *coarctation of the aorta.* Weak or thready, difficult-to-feel pulses may reflect *myocardial dysfunction* and *heart failure.*

Auscultation. *Heart rhythm* is evaluated more easily in infants by listening to the heart than by feeling the peripheral pulses.

The most common dysrhythmia in children is *paroxysmal supraventricular tachycardia.*

Evaluate S_1 and S_2 carefully. They are normally crisp with intermittent splitting of S_1 and S_2 (fused in expiration).

A louder-than-normal pulmonic component suggests *pulmonary hypertension.* Persistent splitting of S_2 may indicate *atrial septal defect.*

Listen for heart murmurs. Two common benign systolic murmurs are from a closing ductus or peripheral pulmonary flow murmur.

Most infants with cardiac pathology have signs beyond heart murmurs.

The Breasts

The breasts of males and females may be enlarged for months after birth as a result of maternal estrogen.

The Abdomen

You will find it easy to palpate an infant's abdomen, because infants like being touched. Palpate the liver and spleen and assess for hepatosplenomegaly.

Abnormal abdominal masses can be associated with kidney, bladder, or bowel tumors. In *pyloric stenosis,* deep palpation in the right upper quadrant or midline can reveal an "olive," or a 2-cm firm pyloric mass.

EXAMINATION TECHNIQUES	POSSIBLE FINDINGS

Male Genitalia

Inspect with the infant supine. The foreskin of a newborn is nonretractable at birth or just enough to visualize the urethral meatus.

Common scrotal masses are *hydroceles* and *inguinal hernias.*

In 3% of infants, one or both testes cannot be felt in the scrotum or inguinal canal. Try to milk the testes into the scrotum.

Inability to palpate testes, even with maneuvers, indicates *undescended testicles.*

Female Genitalia

In females, genitalia may be prominent for several months after birth from the effects of maternal estrogen.

Ambiguous genitalia involves masculinization of the female external genitalia.

The Musculoskeletal System

Examine the extremities by inspection and palpation to detect congenital abnormalities, particularly in the hands, spine, hips, legs, and feet.

Skin tags, remnants of digits, polydactyly (extra fingers), or syndactyly (webbed fingers) are congenital defects. Fracture of the clavicle can occur during a difficult delivery.

Examine the *hips* carefully at each visit for signs of dislocation. There are two major techniques: one to test for a posteriorly dislocated hip (*Ortolani test*), as shown in Figure 18-5, and the other to test for the ability to sublux or dislocate an intact but unstable hip (*Barlow test*), as shown in Figure 18-6.

Congenital hip dysplasia may have a positive Ortolani or Barlow test, particularly during the first 3 months of age. With a *hip dysplasia,* you feel a "clunk."

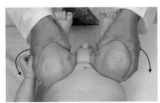

Figure 18-5 Ortolani test, overhead view.

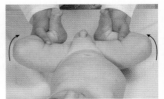

Figure 18-6 Barlow test, overhead view.

EXAMINATION TECHNIQUES	POSSIBLE FINDINGS

Some normal infants exhibit twisting or *torsion of the tibia* inwardly or outwardly on its longitudinal axis.

Pathologic tibial torsion occurs only in association with *deformities of the feet or hips.*

The Nervous System

Evaluate the developing central nervous system by assessing *infantile automatisms,* called *primitive reflexes.*

Suspect a *neurologic* or *developmental abnormality* if primitive reflexes are absent at appropriate age, present longer than normal, asymmetric, or associated with posturing or twitching.

Neurologic abnormalities in infants often present as developmental abnormalities such as failure to do age-appropriate tasks.

Hypotonia can be a sign of a variety of neurologic abnormalities.

Assessing Children (1 to 10 Years)

Tips for Interviewing Children

- **Establish rapport.** Refer to children by name and meet them on their own level. Maintain eye contact at their level (e.g., sit on the floor if needed). Participate in play and talk about their interests.
- **Work with families.** Ask simple, open-ended questions such as "Are you sick? Tell me about it," followed by more specific questions. Once the parent has started the conversation, direct questions back to the child. Also observe how parents interact with the child.
- **Identify multiple agendas.** Your job is to discover as many perspectives and agendas as possible.
- **Use the family as the key resource.** View parents as experts in the care of their child and you as their consultant.
- **Note hidden agendas.** As with adults, the chief complaint may not relate to the real reason the parent has brought the child to see you.

The following discussion focuses on those areas of the comprehensive physical examination that are different for children than for infants and for adults.

| POSSIBLE FINDINGS

Mental and Physical Status

In *children age 1 to 5 years,* observe the degree of sickness or wellness, mood, nutritional state, speech, cry, facial expression, and developmental skills. Note parent–child interaction, including separation tolerance, affection, and response to discipline.

This overall examination can uncover evidence of *chronic disease, developmental delay, social* or *environmental disorders,* and *family problems.*

In *children 6 to 10 years,* determine orientation to time and place, factual knowledge, and language and number skills. Observe motor skills used in writing, tying laces, buttoning, cutting, and drawing.

Observing children performing tasks can reveal signs of inattentiveness or impulsivity, which may indicate *attention deficit disorder.*

Body Mass Index for Age.
Age- and sex-specific charts are now available to assess body mass index (BMI) in children.

Underweight is <5th percentile, *at risk of overweight* is ≥85th percentile, and *overweight* is ≥95th percentile.

Blood Pressure. Hypertension during childhood is more common than previously thought. Recognizing, confirming, and appropriately managing it is important. Blood pressure readings should be part of the physical examination of every child older than 2 years (see Table 18-2, Hypertension in Childhood, p. 374). *Proper cuff size is essential for accurate determination of blood pressure in children.*

The most frequent "cause" of elevated blood pressure in children is probably an *improperly performed examination,* often from an incorrect cuff size.

Causes of *sustained hypertension* in childhood include renal disease, coarctation of the aorta, and primary hypertension. Hypertension is often related to *childhood obesity.*

The Eyes

Test visual acuity in each eye and determine whether the gaze is conjugate or symmetric.

Any difference in visual acuity between eyes is abnormal.

Myopia or hyperopia often present in school-aged children.

EXAMINATION TECHNIQUES	POSSIBLE FINDINGS

Special Technique

The corneal light reflex test (Fig. 18-7) and the cover–uncover test (Fig. 18-8) are particularly useful in young children.

Strabismus can lead to *amblyopia*.

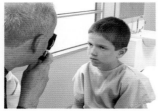

Figure 18-7 Corneal light reflex test.

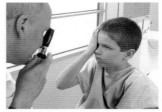

Figure 18-8 Cover–uncover test.

Visual Acuity	
Age	**Visual Acuity**
3 months	Eyes converge, baby reaches
12 months	20/60–20/80
Younger than 4 years	20/40
4 years and older	20/30

The Ears

Examine the ear canal and drum. There are two positions for the child (lying down or sitting), and also two ways to hold the otoscope, as shown in Figures 18-9 and 18-10.

Pain on movement of the pinna occurs with *otitis externa*.

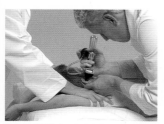

Figure 18-9 Gently holding the child's arms reduces reactions to the otoscope.

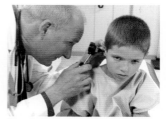

Figure 18-10 Gently pulling up on the auricle gives a better otoscope view with many children.

EXAMINATION TECHNIQUES	POSSIBLE FINDINGS

■ Insert the speculum, obtaining a proper seal.

Acute otitis media involves a red and bulging tympanic membrane.

Pneumatic Otoscope. Learn to use a *pneumatic otoscope* to improve accuracy of diagnosis of otitis media. When air is introduced into the normal ear canal, the tympanic membrane and its light reflex move inward. When air is removed, the tympanic membrane moves outward toward you.

Diminished movement of tympanic membrane with *acute otitis media;* no movement with *otitis media with effusion.*

The Mouth and Pharynx

For anxious or young children, leave this examination toward the end. The best technique for a tongue blade is to push down and pull slightly forward toward you while the child says "ah." Do not place the blade too far posteriorly, eliciting a gag reflex.

A common cause of a strawberry tongue, red uvula, and pharyngeal exudate is *streptococcal pharyngitis.*

Examine the *teeth* for the timing and sequence of eruption, number, character, condition, and position.

Abnormalities of the enamel may reflect local or general disease.

Carefully inspect the inside of the upper teeth, as shown in Figure 18-11.

Nursing bottle caries; dental caries; staining of the teeth, which may be intrinsic or extrinsic

Dental caries are the most common health problem of children and are particularly prevalent in impoverished children.

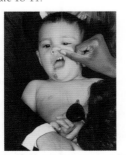

Figure 18-11 Lift the lip to check for dental caries.

EXAMINATION TECHNIQUES	POSSIBLE FINDINGS

Look for abnormalities of tooth position.

Malocclusion

Note the size, position, symmetry, and appearance of the *tonsils*.

Peritonsillar abscess

The Heart

A challenging aspect to cardiac evaluation of children is evaluation of *heart murmurs,* particularly distinguishing common benign murmurs from unusual or pathologic ones. Most children have one or more *functional,* or *benign, heart murmurs* at some point in time (Fig. 18-12).

See Table 18-3, Characteristics of Pathologic Heart Murmurs, pp. 375–376.

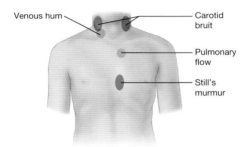

Venous hum

Carotid bruit

Pulmonary flow

Still's murmur

Figure 18-12 Location of benign heart murmurs in children.

The Abdomen

Most children are ticklish when you first place your hand on their abdomens for palpation. This reaction tends to disappear, particularly if you distract the child.

A pathologically enlarged liver in children usually is palpable more than 2 cm below the costal margin, has a round, firm edge, and often is tender.

A common condition of childhood that can occasionally cause a protuberant abdomen is *constipation*.

EXAMINATION TECHNIQUES

POSSIBLE FINDINGS

Male Genitalia

There is an art to palpation of the young boy's scrotum and testes, because many have an active cremasteric reflex causing the testes to retract upward into the inguinal canal and appear undescended. A useful technique is to have the boy sit cross-legged on the examining table.

In *precocious puberty,* the penis and testes are enlarged, with signs of pubertal changes.

A painful testicle requires rapid treatment and may indicate *torsion.*

Inguinal hernias in older boys present as they do in adult men.

Female Genitalia

Use a calm, gentle approach, including a developmentally appropriate explanation.

Examine the genitalia in an efficient and systematic manner. The normal hymen can have various configurations (Fig. 18-13).

Vaginal discharge in early childhood can result from *perineal irritation* (e.g., from bubble baths, soaps), *foreign body, vaginitis,* or *sexually transmitted infections* from sexual abuse. *Vaginal bleeding, abrasions,* or signs of trauma to the external genitalia can result from *sexual abuse* (see Table 18-7, Physical Signs of Sexual Abuse, p. 381).

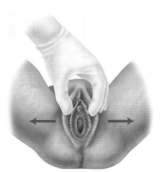

Figure 18-13 Separate labia to assess genital structures.

|

The Musculoskeletal System

Abnormalities of the upper extremities are rare in the absence of injury. To assess the lower extremities, observe the child standing and walking barefoot, and ask the child to touch the toes, rise from sitting, run a short distance, and pick up objects. You will detect most abnormalities by watching carefully.

A screening musculoskeletal examination for children participating in sports can detect injuries or abnormalities that may result in problems during athletics.

Extreme bowing or unilateral bowing may be from pathologic causes such as rickets or tibia vara (*Blount disease*).

The Nervous System

Beyond infancy, the neurologic examination includes the components evaluated in adults. Again, combine the neurologic and developmental assessments. You can turn this into a game with the child to assess optimal development and neurologic performance.

Delayed language or cognitive skills can be due to neurologic disease as well as developmental disorders.

Soft neurologic signs can suggest *minor developmental abnormalities*.

Assessing Adolescents

The key to successfully examining teens is a comfortable, confidential environment that makes the examination relaxed and informative. Adolescents are more likely to open up when the interview focuses on them rather than on their problems.

Consider the patient's cognitive and social development when deciding issues of privacy, parental involvement, and confidentiality. Explain to both teens and parents that the purpose of confidentiality is to improve health care, not keep secrets. Your goal is to help adolescents bring their concerns or questions to their parents. Never make confidentiality unlimited, however. Always state to teens explicitly that you may need to act on information that makes you concerned about safety.

The physical examination of the adolescent is similar to that of the adult. Keep in mind issues particularly relevant to teens, such as puberty, growth, development, family and peer relationships, sexuality, decision making, and risk behaviors. For more details on specific techniques of examination, the reader should refer to the corresponding chapter for the regional examination of interest or concern. Following are special areas to highlight when examining adolescents.

EXAMINATION TECHNIQUES

The Breasts

Assess normal maturational development.

See Table 18-4, Sex Maturity Ratings in Girls: Breasts, p. 377.

Special Technique

Testing for Scoliosis. Inspect any child who can stand for *scoliosis*. Make sure the child bends forward with the knees straight (*Adams bend test*). Evaluate any asymmetry in positioning or gait. If you detect scoliosis, use a *scoliometer* to test for the degree of scoliosis (Fig. 18-14).

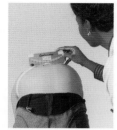

Figure 18-14 Measure and record scoliosis with a scoliometer.

Male and Female Genitalia

An important goal when examining adolescent males and females is to assign a sexual maturity rating, regardless of chronologic age.

See Table 18-5, Sex Maturity Ratings in Boys, pp. 378–379, and Table 18-6, Sex Maturity Ratings in Girls: Pubic Hair, p. 380.

Recording Your Findings

The format of the pediatric medical record is the same as that of the adult. Thus, although the sequence of the physical examination may vary, convert your written findings back to the traditional format.

Recording the Physical Examination— The Pediatric Patient

Brian is a chubby, active, and energetic toddler. He plays with the reflex hammer, pretending it is a truck. He appears closely bonded with his mother, looking at her occasionally for comfort. She seems concerned that Brian will break something. His clothes are clean.

(continued)

Recording the Physical Examination—
The Pediatric Patient (Continued)

Vital Signs. Ht 90 cm (90th percentile). Wt 16 kg (>95th percentile). BMI 19.8 (>95th percentile). Head circumference 50 cm (75th percentile). BP 108/58. Heart rate 90 and regular. Respiratory rate 30; varies with activity. Temperature (ear) 37.5°C. Obviously no pain.

Skin. Normal except for bruises on legs, and patchy, dry skin over external surface of elbows.

HEENT. *Head:* Normocephalic; no lesions. *Eyes:* Difficult to examine because he won't sit still. Symmetric with normal extraocular movements. Pupils 4 to 5 mm constricting. Discs difficult to visualize; no hemorrhages noted. *Ears:* Normal pinna; no external abnormalities. Normal external canals and tympanic membranes (TMs). *Nose:* Normal nares; septum midline. *Mouth:* Several darkened teeth on inside surface of upper incisors. One clear cavity on upper right incisor. Tongue normal. Cobblestoning of posterior pharynx; no exudates. Tonsils large but adequate gap (1.5 cm) between them.

Neck. Supple, midline trachea, no thyroid palpable.

Lymph Nodes. Easily palpable (1.5 to 2 cm) tonsillar lymph nodes bilaterally. Small (0.5 cm) nodes in inguinal canal bilaterally. All lymph nodes mobile and nontender.

Lungs. Good expansion. No tachypnea or dyspnea. Congestion audible, but seems to be upper airway (louder near mouth, symmetric). No rhonchi, rales, or wheezes. Clear to auscultation.

Cardiovascular. PMI in 4th or 5th interspace and midsternal line. Normal S_1 and S_2. No murmurs or abnormal heart sounds. Normal femoral pulses; dorsalis pedis pulses palpable bilaterally.

Breasts. Normal, with some fat under both.

Abdomen. Protuberant but soft; no masses or tenderness. Liver span 2 cm below right costal margin (RCM) and not tender. Spleen and kidneys not palpable.

Genitalia. Tanner I circumcised penis; no pubic hair, lesions, or discharge. Testes descended, difficult to palpate because of active cremasteric reflex. Normal scrotum both sides.

Musculoskeletal. Normal range of motion of upper and lower extremities and all joints. Spine straight. Gait normal.

Neurologic. *Mental Status:* Happy, cooperative child. *Developmental:* Gross motor—Jumps and throws objects. Fine motor—Imitates vertical line. Language—Does not combine words; single words only, three to four noted during examination. Personal–social—Washes face, brushes teeth, and puts on shirt. Overall—Normal, except for language, which appears delayed. *Cranial Nerves:* Intact, although several difficult to elicit. *Cerebellar:* Normal gait; good balance. *Deep tendon reflexes (DTRs):* Normal and symmetric throughout with downgoing toes. *Sensory:* Deferred.

Aids to Interpretation

Table 18-1   Classification of Newborn's Level of Maturity

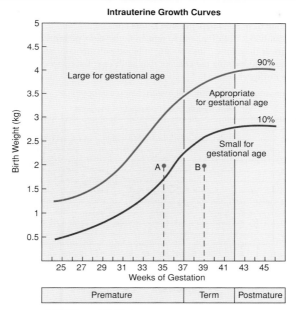

Intrauterine Growth Curves

Weight Small for Gestational Age (SGA) = Birth weight <10th percentile on the intrauterine growth curve

Weight Appropriate for Gestational Age (AGA) = Birth weight within the 10th and 90th percentiles on the intrauterine growth curve

Weight Large for Gestational Age (LGA) = Birth weight >90th percentile on the intrauterine growth curve

Level of intrauterine growth based on birth weight and gestational age of liveborn, single, white infants. Point A represents a premature infant, while point B indicates an infant of similar birth weight who is mature but small for gestational age; the growth curves are representative of the 10th and 90th percentiles for all of the newborns in the sampling.

Adapted from Sweet YA. Classification of the low-birth-weight infant. In: Klaus MH, Fanaroff AA. *Care of the High-Risk Neonate,* 3rd ed. Philadelphia, PA: WB Saunders; 1986. Reproduced with permission.

Table 18-2 Hypertension in Childhood

Hypertension can start in childhood. Although young children with elevated blood pressure are more likely to have a renal, cardiac, or endocrine cause older children and adolescents with hypertension are most likely to have primary or essential hypertension. Hypertension is often related to obesity.

This child developed hypertension before adolescence, and it "tracked" into adulthood. Children tend to remain in the same percentile for blood pressure as they grow. This tracking of blood pressure continues into adulthood, supporting the concept that adult essential hypertension begins during childhood.

The consequences of untreated hypertension can be severe.

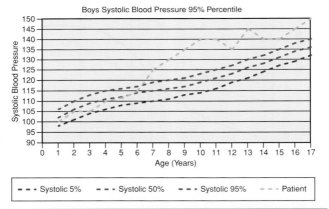

Boys Systolic Blood Pressure 95% Percentile

Legend: Systolic 5%, Systolic 50%, Systolic 95%, Patient

Table 18-3	Characteristics of Pathologic Heart Murmurs

Congenital Defect	Characteristics of Murmur
Pulmonary Valve Stenosis	*Location.* Upper left sternal border
Mild 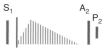	*Radiation.* In mild degrees of stenosis, the murmur may be heard over the course of the pulmonary arteries in the lung fields.
	Intensity. Increases in intensity and duration as the degree of obstruction increases
Severe 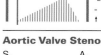	*Quality.* Ejection, peaking later in systole as the obstruction increases
Aortic Valve Stenosis 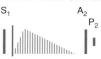	*Location.* Midsternum, upper right sternal border
	Radiation. To the carotid arteries and suprasternal notch; may also be a thrill
	Intensity. Varies, louder with increasingly severe obstruction
	Quality. An ejection, often harsh, systolic murmur
Tetralogy of Fallot	*General.* Variable cyanosis, increasing with activity
With Pulmonic Stenosis 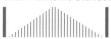	*Location.* Mid to upper left sternal border. If pulmonary atresia, there is no systolic murmur but the continuous murmur of ductus arteriosus flow at upper left sternal border or in the back.
With Pulmonic Atresia 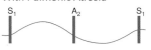	*Radiation.* Little, to upper left sternal border, occasionally to lung fields
	Intensity. Usually grade III–IV
	Quality. Midpeaking, systolic ejection murmur

(table continues on page 376)

Table 18-3	Characteristics of Pathologic Heart Murmurs (*continued*)
Congenital Defect	**Characteristics of Murmur**
Transposition of the Great Arteries	*General.* Intense generalized cyanosis
	Location. No characteristic murmur. If present, it may reflect an associated defect such as VSD.
	Radiation and quality. Depends on associated abnormalities
Ventricular Septal Defect	*Location.* Lower left sternal border
Small to Moderate	*Radiation.* Little
S_1 A_2 P_2	*Intensity.* Variable, only partially determined by the size of the shunt. Small shunts with a high-pressure gradient may have very loud murmurs. Large defects with elevated pulmonary vascular resistance may have no murmur. Grade II–IV/VI, with a thrill if grade IV/VI or higher.

Table 18-4   Sex Maturity Ratings in Girls: Breasts

Stage 1

Preadolescent—elevation of nipple only

Stage 2   ### Stage 3

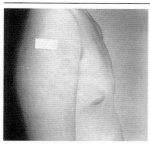   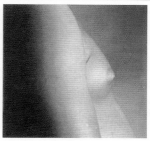

Breast bud stage. Elevation of   Further enlargement and
breast and nipple as a small   elevation of breast and areola,
mound; enlargement of areolar   with no separation of the
diameter   contours

Stage 4   ### Stage 5

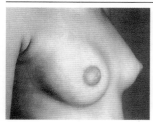   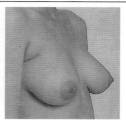

Projection of areola and nipple to   Mature stage; projection of nipple
form a secondary mound above the   only. Areola has receded to
level of the breast   general contour of the breast
                                      (although may continue to form
                                      a secondary mound).

Photos reprinted, with permission from the American Academy of Pediatrics, *Assessment of
Sexual Maturity Stages in Girls*, 1995.

Table 18-5   Sex Maturity Ratings in Boys

In assigning SMRs in boys, observe each of the three characteristics separately. Record two separate ratings: pubic hair and genital. If the penis and testes differ in their stages, average the two into a single figure for the genital rating.

Stage 1	**Pubic Hair:** Preadolescent—no pubic hair except for the fine body hair (vellus hair) similar to that on the abdomen
	Genitalia
	■ **Penis, Testes, and Scrotum:** Preadolescent—same size and proportions as in childhood

Stage 2 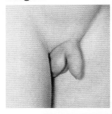	**Pubic Hair:** Sparse growth of long, slightly pigmented, downy hair, straight or only slightly curled, chiefly at the base of the penis
	Genitalia
	■ **Penis:** Slight to no enlargement
	■ **Testes and Scrotum:** Testes larger; scrotum larger, somewhat reddened, and altered in texture

Stage 3 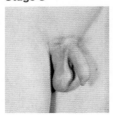	**Pubic Hair:** Darker, coarser, curlier hair spreading sparsely over the pubic symphysis
	Genitalia
	■ **Penis:** Larger, especially in length
	■ **Testes and Scrotum:** Further enlarged

Table 18-5   Sex Maturity Ratings in Boys (*continued*)

Stage 4

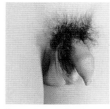

Pubic Hair: Coarse and curly hair, as in the adult; area covered greater than in stage 3 but less than adult and not yet on thighs

Genitalia

- **Penis:** Further enlarged in length and breadth, with development of the glans
- **Testes and Scrotum:** Further enlarged; scrotal skin darkened

Stage 5

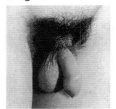

Pubic Hair: Hair adult quantity and quality, spread to the medial surfaces of the thighs but not up over the abdomen

Genitalia

- **Penis:** Adult in size and shape
- **Testes and Scrotum:** Adult in size and shape

Photos reprinted from *Pediatric Endocrinology and Growth,* 2nd ed., Wales & Wit, 2003, with permission from Elsevier.

Table 18-6 Sex Maturity Ratings in Girls: Pubic Hair

Stage 1	Preadolescent—no pubic hair except for the fine body hair (vellus hair) similar to that on the abdomen
Stage 2 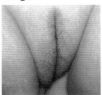	Sparse growth of long, slightly pigmented, downy hair, straight or only slightly curled, chiefly along the labia
Stage 3 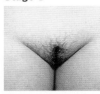	Darker, coarser, curlier hair, spreading sparsely over the pubic symphysis
Stage 4 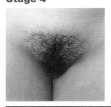	Coarse and curly hair as in adults; area covered greater than in stage 3 but not as great as in the adult and not yet including the thighs
Stage 5 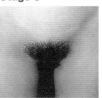	Hair adult in quantity and quality, spread on the medial surfaces of the thighs but not up over the abdomen

Photos reprinted, with permission from the American Academy of Pediatrics, *Assessment of Sexual Maturity Stages in Girls,* 1995.

Table 18-7   Physical Signs of Sexual Abuse

Physical Signs That May Indicate Sexual Abuse in Children[a]

1. Marked and immediate dilatation of the anus in knee–chest position, with no constipation, stool in the vault, or neurologic disorders
2. Hymenal notch or cleft that extends >50% of the inferior hymenal rim (confirmed in knee–chest position)
3. Condyloma acuminata in a child older than 3 years
4. Bruising, abrasions, lacerations, or bite marks of labia or perihymenal tissue
5. Herpes of the anogenital area beyond the neonatal period
6. Purulent or malodorous vaginal discharge in a young girl (all discharges should be cultured and viewed under a microscope for evidence of a sexually transmitted infection)

Physical Signs That Strongly Suggest Sexual Abuse in Children[a]

1. Lacerations, ecchymoses, and newly healed scars of the hymen or the posterior fourchette
2. No hymenal tissue from 3 to 9 o'clock (confirmed in various positions)
3. Healed hymenal transections, especially between 3 and 9 o'clock (complete cleft)
4. Perianal lacerations extending to external sphincter

A sexual abuse expert must evaluate a child with concerning physical signs for a complete history and sexual abuse examination.

[a]Any physical sign must be evaluated in light of the entire history, other parts of the physical examination, and laboratory data.

The Pregnant Woman

Common Concerns

- Initial prenatal history
  - Confirmation of pregnancy
  - Symptoms of pregnancy
  - Concerns about and attitudes toward the pregnancy
  - Current health and past medical history
  - Past obstetric history
  - Risk factors for maternal and fetal health
  - Family history of patient and father of the newborn
  - Plans for breastfeeding
  - Plans for postpartum contraception
- Gestational age and expected date of delivery
- Subsequent prenatal visits

Initial Prenatal Visit. Focus the *initial prenatal visit* on the health status of the mother and fetus. Confirm the pregnancy and estimate gestational age, develop a plan for continuing care, and counsel the mother about her expectations and concerns. At the end of the visit, reaffirm your commitment to the patient's health and any ongoing concerns, review your findings, and discuss any questions or tests or screenings that are needed. Ask about the following topics:

▩ *Confirmation of pregnancy.* Has the patient had a confirmatory urine pregnancy test, and when? When was her last menstrual period (LMP)? Has an ultrasound been done to establish dates? Explain that serum pregnancy tests are rarely required to confirm pregnancy.

▩ *Symptoms of pregnancy.* Has the patient had absence of menses, breast fullness or tenderness, nausea or vomiting, fatigue, and urinary frequency? Explain that serum or urine testing for beta human chorionic gonadotropin (HCG) offers the best confirmation of pregnancy.

■ *Maternal concerns and attitudes.* Review the mother's feelings about the pregnancy and whether she plans to continue to term. Ask about any fears and about support from the father. Respect diverse family structures, such as extended family support, single motherhood, or pregnancy conceived by sperm donation with or without a partner of either gender.

■ *Current health and past medical history.* Does the patient have any acute or chronic medical concerns, past or present? Pay particular attention to issues that affect pregnancy, such as abdominal surgeries, hypertension, diabetes, cardiac conditions including any that were surgically corrected in childhood, asthma, hypercoagulability states involving lupus or anticardiolipin antibodies, mental health disorders including postpartum depression, HIV, sexually transmitted infections, abnormal Pap smears, and exposure to diethylstilbestrol (DES) in utero.

■ *Past obstetric history.* Ask about prior pregnancies and outcomes. Has she had any complications during past pregnancies? Were there any complications during labor and delivery such as large babies (*fetal macrosomia*), fetal distress, or emergency interventions? Were deliveries by vaginal delivery, assisted delivery (vacuum or forceps), or cesarean section?

■ *Risk factors for maternal and fetal health.* Does the patient use tobacco, alcohol, or illicit drugs? Does she take any medications, over-the-counter drugs, or herbal prescriptions? Does she have any toxic exposures at work, home, or otherwise? Is her nutritional intake adequate, or is she at risk from obesity? Does she have an adequate social support network and income? Is there unusual stress at home or work? Is there any history of physical abuse or domestic violence?

■ *Family history* of chronic illnesses or genetically transmitted diseases: sickle cell anemia, cystic fibrosis, muscular dystrophy, and others.

■ *Plans for breastfeeding.* Education and encouragement during pregnancy increase adoption and duration of breastfeeding.

■ *Plans for postpartum contraception.* Initiate this discussion early, as postpartum contraception reduces the risk of unintended pregnancy and shortened interpregnancy intervals, which are linked to adverse pregnancy outcomes.

Gestational Age and Expected Date of Delivery. Accurate dating is best done early and contributes to appropriate management of the pregnancy. Dating establishes the timeframe for reassuring the patient about normal progress, establishing paternity, timing screening tests, tracking fetal growth, and effectively triaging preterm and postdated labor.

Determining Gestational Age and the Expected Date of Delivery

- *Gestational age.* Count the number of weeks and days from the first day of the LMP. Counting this *menstrual age* from the LMP–although biologically distinct from the date of conception, is the standard means of calculating fetal age, yielding an average pregnancy length of 40 weeks. If the actual date of conception is known (as with in vitro fertilization), a conception age which is 2 weeks less than the menstrual age can be used to calculate menstrual age (i.e., a corrected or adjusted LMP dating) to establish dating.
- *Expected date of delivery (EDD).* The expected date of delivery is 40 weeks from the first date of the LMP. Using the *Naegele rule,* the EDD can be estimated by taking the LMP, adding 7 days, subtracting 3 months, and adding 1 year.
- *Tools for calculations.* Pregnancy wheels and online calculators are commonly used to calculate the EDD, but they should be checked for accuracy.
- *Limitations on pregnancy dating.* Patient recall of the LMP is highly variable. The LMP can also be biased by hormonal contraceptives, menstrual irregularities, or variations in ovulation that result in atypical cycle lengths. Check LMP dating against physical examination markers such as fundal height, clarifying discrepancies against ultrasound evaluation.

Subsequent Prenatal Visits. During subsequent visits, assess interim changes in the health status of the mother and fetus, review specific physical examination findings related to the pregnancy, and provide counseling and timely preventive screenings. Obstetric visits traditionally follow a set schedule: monthly until 28 gestational weeks, then biweekly until 36 weeks, then weekly until delivery. Update and document the history at every visit, especially fetal movement, contractions, leakage of fluids and vaginal bleeding. At every visit, assess: vital signs (especially blood pressure and weight), fundal height, verification of FHR, and fetal position and activity. At each visit, test the urine for infection and protein.

Health Promotion and Counseling: Evidence and Recommendations

Important Topics for Health Promotion and Counseling

- Nutrition
- Weight gain
- Immunizations
- Exercise
- Substance abuse
- Intimate partner violence
- Prenatal laboratory screenings

Nutrition and Weight Gain. Evaluate nutritional status, especially inadequate nutrition and obesity.

■ Assess diet history; measurement of height, weight, and body mass index (BMI); and a hematocrit. Prescribe needed vitamin and mineral supplements.

■ To help prevent listeriosis, encourage pregnant patients to avoid: unpasteurized milk and foods made with unpasteurized milk; raw and undercooked seafood, eggs, and meat; refrigerated paté, meat spreads, and smoked salmon; and hot dogs, luncheon meats, and cold cuts unless served steaming hot.

■ Recommend two servings a week of selected fish low in mercury and shellfish.

■ Make a nutritional plan tailored to the patient's BMI. Use the Pregnancy Weight Gain Calculator and Super Tracker at the user-friendly Choose-MyPlate.gov website (http://www.choosemyplate.gov/pregnancy-weight-gain-calculator). This calculator displays the daily recommended intake of each of the five food groups for each trimester, based on height, prepregnancy weight, due date, and levels of weekly exercise.

Monitor weight gain at each visit, with the results plotted on a graph, using the updated recommendations below.

Recommendations for Total and Rate of Weight Gain During Pregnancy, by Prepregnancy BMI, 2009

Prepregnancy BMI[a]	Total Weight Gain (Range in lbs)	Rates of Weight Gain[b] 2nd and 3rd Trimesters	
		(lbs/wk)	Mean Range
Underweight, or <18.5	28–40	1	1.0–1.3
Normal weight, or 18.5–24.9	25–35	1	0.8–1.0
Overweight, or 25.0–29.9	15–25	0.6	0.5–0.7
Obese, or ≥30.0	11–20	0.5	0.4–0.6

[a]To calculate BMI, go to Calculate Your Body Mass Index, National Heart, Lung, and Blood Institute at http://www.nhlbi.nih.gov/health/educational/lose_wt/BMI/bmicalc.htm.
[b]Calculations assume a 1.1–4.4 lbs-weight gain in the first trimester.
Source: Rasmussen KM, Yaktine AL (eds.) and Institute of Medicine. *Committee to Re-examine IOM Pregnancy Weight Guidelines. Weight gain during pregnancy: re-examining the guidelines.* Washington, DC: National Academies Press, 2009. Available at http://www.ncbi.nlm.nih.gov/books/NBK32799/table/summary.t1/?report = objectonly. Accessed September 4, 2015.

Immunizations. Administer Tdap during each pregnancy, ideally at 27 to 36 weeks of gestation, regardless of the prior immunization history, and to caretakers in direct contact with the infant. Give inactivated influenza vaccination in any trimester during the influenza season.

Safe and Unsafe Vaccines during Pregnancy

Safe during Pregnancy	Not Safe during Pregnancy
• Pneumococcal polysaccharide • Meningococcal polysaccharide and conjugate • Hepatitis A • Hepatitis B	• Measles/mumps/rubella • Polio • Varicella

All women should have rubella titers drawn during pregnancy and be immunized after birth if found to be nonimmune. Check Rh(D) and antibody typing at the first prenatal visit, at 28 weeks, and at delivery. Anti-D immunoglobulin should be given to all Rh-negative women at 28 weeks' gestation and again within 3 days of delivery to prevent sensitization if the infant is Rh-D positive.

Exercise. Recommend ≥30 minutes of moderate exercise on most days of the week unless there are contraindications. Women initiating exercise during pregnancy should be cautious and consider programs developed specifically for pregnant women. Water-based exercises can temporarily help alleviate musculoskeletal aches, but immersion in hot water should be avoided. After the first trimester, women should avoid exercise in the supine position, which compresses the inferior vena cava and can cause dizziness and decreased placental blood flow. Because the center of gravity shifts in the third trimester, advise against exercises that cause loss of balance. Contact sports or activities that risk abdominal trauma are contraindicated throughout pregnancy. Pregnant women also should avoid overheating, dehydration, and any exertion that causes notable fatigue or discomfort.

Substance Abuse. Promote abstinence as the immediate goal during pregnancy. Pursue universal screening in a neutral manner for:

■ *Tobacco.* Tobacco use accounts for up to 20% of all low-birth-weight babies. It doubles the risk of placenta previa, placental abruption, and preterm labor and increases risk of spontaneous abortion, fetal death, and fetal digit anomalies. Cessation is the goal, but any decrease in use is favorable.

■ *Alcohol.* Fetal alcohol syndrome is the leading cause of preventable mental retardation in the United States. The American Congress of Obstetricians and Gynecologists (ACOG) strongly recommends that women abstain throughout pregnancy.

■ *Illicit drugs including narcotics.* Women with addictions should be referred for treatment immediately and counseled and screened for hepatitis C and HIV.

■ *Abuse of prescription drugs.* Ask about commonly abused prescription drugs, including narcotics, stimulants, benzodiazepines.

Intimate Partner Violence. Pregnancy is a time of increased risk from intimate partner violence ranging from verbal to physical abuse or from mild to severe physical abuse. Up to one in five women experiences some form of abuse during pregnancy, contributing to delayed prenatal care, low infant birth weight, or even murder of the mother and fetus. ACOG recommends universal screening of all women for domestic violence at the first prenatal visit and at least once each trimester. For a direct nonjudgmental approach, ACOG recommends the statement and simple questions listed below.

ACOG Screening Approach for Intimate Partner Violence

Initial Statement: "Because violence is so common in many women's lives and because there is help available for women being abused, I now ask every patient about domestic violence."

Screening Questions:
1. "Within the past year—or since you have been pregnant—have you been hit, slapped, kicked or otherwise physically hurt by someone?"
2. "Are you in a relationship with a person who threatens or physically hurts you?"
3. "Has anyone forced you to have sexual activities that made you feel uncomfortable?"

Source: American Congress of Obstetricians and Gynecologists. Screening tools–domestic violence. Available at http://www.acog.org/About-ACOG/ACOG-Departments/Violence-Against-Women/Screening-Tools–Domestic-Violence. Accessed September 2, 2015.

Watch for nonverbal clues of abuse such as frequent last-minute appointment changes, unusual behavior during visits, partners who refuse to leave the patient alone during the visit, and bruises or other injuries. Once the patient acknowledges abuse, ask about the best way for you to help her. Respect limits she places on sharing information, with the caveat that if children are involved, you may be required to report harmful behaviors to the authorities. Maintain an updated list of shelters, counseling centers, hotline numbers, and other trusted local referrals. Plan future appointments at more frequent intervals. Perform as thorough a physical examination as the patient permits, and document all injuries on a body diagram.

National Domestic Violence Hotline

- Website: www.thehotline.org
- 1–800–799-SAFE (7233)
- TTY for hearing impaired: 1–800–787–3224

Prenatal Laboratory Screenings. Initially include blood type and Rh, antibody screen, complete blood count—especially hematocrit and platelet count, rubella titer, syphilis test, hepatitis B surface antigen, HIV, STI screen for gonorrhea and chlamydia, and urinalysis with culture. Scheduled screenings include an oral glucose tolerance test for gestational diabetes around 24 weeks; a vaginal swab for group B streptococcus between 35 to 37 weeks' gestation; and for obese pregnant patients, a glucose tolerance in the first trimester. Pursue additional tests related to the mother's risk factors, such as screening for aneuploidy, Tay–Sachs, or other genetic diseases, or amniocentesis.

Techniques of Examination

Preparing for the Examination

Be responsive to the patient's comfort and privacy, as well as her individual and cultural sensitivities. During the initial visit, take the history while she is clothed. Ask her to wear her gown with the opening in front to ease the examination of both breasts and the pregnant abdomen.

Positioning
- The semisitting position with the knees bent (see p. 391) affords the most comfort and protects abdominal organs and vessels from the weight of the gravid uterus.
- Avoid prolonged periods of lying on the back. Make your abdominal palpation efficient and accurate.
- The pelvic examination also should be relatively quick.

Equipment
- *Gynecologic speculum and lubrication:* Because of vaginal wall relaxation during pregnancy, a larger-than-usual speculum may be needed.
- *Sampling materials:* The cervical brush may cause bleeding, so the "broom" sampling device is preferred during pregnancy. Use additional swabs if needed to screen for sexually transmitted infections, group B strep, and wet mount preparations.
- *Tape measure:* Use a plastic or paper tape measure to assess the size of the uterus after 20 gestational weeks.
- *Doppler fetal heart rate monitor and gel:* Apply a "Doppler" or "Doptone" to the gravid abdomen to assess fetal heart rate after 10 weeks of gestation.

Height, Weight, and Vital Signs

Observe the general health, emotional state, nutritional status, and coordination as the pregnant woman comes into the room.

Measure height and weight. Calculate the BMI with standard tables, using 19 to 25 as normal for the prepregnant state.

Weight loss of more than 5% in excessive vomiting, or *hyperemesis*

Measure blood pressure at every visit. In midpregnancy, it may be lower than in the nonpregnant state.

Hypertension in Pregnancy

- *Gestational hypertension:* Systolic blood pressure (SBP) >140 or diastolic blood pressure (DBP) >90 first documented after 20 weeks, without proteinuria or preeclampsia, that resolves by 12 weeks' postpartum.
- *Chronic hypertension:* SBP >140 or DBP >90 that predates pregnancy.
- *Preeclampsia:* SBP ≥140 or DBP ≥90 after 20 weeks on two occasions at least 4 hours apart in a woman with previously normal BP or BP ≥160/110 confirmed within minutes *and* proteinuria ≥300 mg/24 hours, protein:creatinine ≥0.3, or dipstick 1+; or new onset hypertension without proteinuria and any of the following: thrombocytopenia (platelets <100,000/μL), impaired liver function (liver transaminase levels more than twice normal), new renal insufficiency (creatinine >1.1 mg/dL or doubles in the absence of renal disease), pulmonary edema, or new onset cerebral or visual symptoms.

Head and Neck

◼ *Face.* Inspect for the mask of pregnancy, *chloasma,* or irregular brownish patches around the forehead and cheeks, across the bridge of the nose, or along the jaw.

Facial edema after 20 weeks in possible preeclampsia

◼ *Hair*

Hair loss should not be attributed to pregnancy.

◼ *Eyes.* Note the conjunctival color.

Anemia of pregnancy may cause conjunctival pallor.

◼ *Nose,* including nasal congestion

Nosebleeds are more common during pregnancy. Erosion of nasal septum if use of intranasal cocaine.

◼ *Mouth*

Gingival enlargement common

◼ *Thyroid gland.* Inspect and palpate. Modest symmetric enlargement is common.

Thyroid enlargement, goiters, and nodules are abnormal and should be investigated.

EXAMINATION TECHNIQUES

Thorax and Lungs

Inspect the thorax for contours. Observe the pattern of breathing. Auscultate the lungs.

Respiratory alkalosis in later trimesters. Increased respiratory rate, cough, rales, or respiratory distress in infection, asthma, pulmonary embolus, peripartum cardiomyopathy.

Heart

Palpate the apical impulse.

Impulse may be rotated upward and to the left toward the 4th intercostal space by the enlarging uterus.

Auscultate the heart. A venous hum and systolic or continuous mammary souffle (see p. 185) are common.

Murmurs may signal anemia; new diastolic murmurs should be investigated. If signs of heart failure, consider *peripartum cardiomyopathy*.

Breasts

Inspect the breasts and nipples for symmetry and color. Venous pattern, darkened nipples and areolae, and prominent Montgomery glands are normal.

Inverted nipples at the time of birth may hamper breastfeeding.

Palpate for masses. Tender nodular breasts are normal.

Focal tenderness in *mastitis*. Investigate any new discrete masses.

Compress each nipple between your index finger and thumb.

This may express colostrum from the nipples; investigate if abnormal bloody or purulent discharge.

Abdomen

Place the pregnant woman in a semisitting position with her knees flexed (Fig. 19-1).

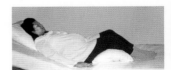

Figure 19-1 The semisitting position.

■ Inspect any scars or striae, the shape and contour of the abdomen, and the fundal height.

Purplish striae and linea nigra are normal.

EXAMINATION TECHNIQUES	POSSIBLE FINDINGS

- Assess the shape and contour to estimate pregnancy size (Fig. 19-2).

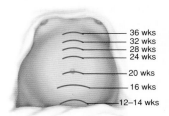

```
                    36 wks
                    32 wks
                    28 wks
                    24 wks
                    20 wks
                    16 wks
                    12–14 wks
```

Figure 19-2 Growth patterns of the uterine fundus by weeks of pregnancy.

- Palpate for:

  - *Organs and masses*

  - *Fetal movements,* usually detected after 24 weeks

  Ultrasound confirmation of fetal health and movement may be needed.

  - *Uterine contractility*

  - Irregular contractions after 12 weeks or after palpation during the third trimester

  Prior to 37 weeks, regular uterine contractions or bleeding are abnormal, suggesting *preterm labor.*

  - If woman is >20 weeks pregnant, *measure fundal height* with a tape measure from the top of the symphysis pubis to the top of the uterine fundus. After 20 weeks, measurement in centimeters should roughly equal the weeks of gestation.

  If fundal height is more than 4 cm higher than expected, consider multiple gestation, a large fetus, extra amniotic fluid, or uterine leiomyoma. If more than 4 cm lower, consider low level of amniotic fluid, missed abortion, transverse lie, growth retardation, or fetal anomaly.

- *Auscultate the fetal heart tones,* noting rate (FHR), location, and rhythm. A Doptone detects the FHR after 10 weeks. The FHR is audible with a fetoscope after 18 weeks.

  Lack of an audible FHR may indicate pregnancy of fewer weeks than expected, fetal demise, or false pregnancy. If unable to locate the FHR, investigate with formal ultrasound.

  - *Location.* From 10 to 18 weeks, the FHR is in the midline of the lower abdomen; later depends on fetal position. Use modified Leopold's maneuvers to palpate the fetal head and back and identify where to listen.

EXAMINATION TECHNIQUES	POSSIBLE FINDINGS

▨ *Rate.* The *rate* usually is 120 to 160 beats per minute. After 32 to 34 weeks, the FHR should increase with fetal movement.

Sustained dips in FHR, or "decelerations," always warrant investigation, at least by formal FHR monitoring.

▨ *Rhythm.* In the third trimester, expect a variance of 10 to 15 beats per minute (BPM) over 1 to 2 minutes.

Lack of beat-to-beat variability late in pregnancy warrants investigation with an FHR monitor.

Genitalia, Anus, and Rectum

Inspect the *external genitalia.*

Parous relaxation of the introitus, labial varicosities, enlargement of the labia and clitoris, scars from an *episiotomy* or perineal lacerations

Palpate *Bartholin* and *Skene glands.* Check for a *cystocele* or *rectocele.*

Bartholin cyst

Examine the internal genitalia.

Speculum Examination

▨ Inspect the *cervix* for color, shape, and healed lacerations.

Purplish color of pregnancy; lacerations from prior deliveries, cervical erosion, erythema, discharge, or irritation in cervicitis and STIs

▨ Perform a *Pap smear,* if indicated.

Specimens may be needed for diagnosis of vaginal or cervical infection

▨ Inspect the *vaginal walls.*

Bluish or violet color, deep rugae, leukorrhea in normal pregnancy; vaginal discharge in candidiasis and bacterial vaginosis (can affect pregnancy outcome)

Bimanual Examination. Insert two lubricated fingers into introitus, palmar side down, with slight pressure downward on the perineum. Slide the fingers into the posterior vaginal vault. Maintaining downward pressure, gently turn the fingers palmar side up.

EXAMINATION TECHNIQUES	POSSIBLE FINDINGS

■ Assess the cervical os and degree of effacement. Place your finger gently in the os, and then sweep it around the *surface of the cervix.*

Closed external os if nulliparous; os open to size of fingertip if multiparous

■ Estimate the *length of the cervix.* Palpate the lateral surface from the cervical tip to the lateral fornix.

Prior to 34 to 36 weeks, cervix should retain normal length of ≥3 cm. Effacement prior to 37 weeks in preterm labor.

■ Palpate the *uterus* for size, shape, consistency, and position.

Hegar sign, or early softening of the isthmus; pear-shaped uterus up to 8 weeks, then globular

■ Estimate *uterine size.* With your internal fingers placed at either side of cervix, palmar surfaces upward, gently lift the uterus toward the abdominal hand. Capture the fundal portion of the uterus between your two hands and gently estimate size.

An irregularly shaped uterus suggests uterine myomata or a *bicornuate uterus,* two distinct uterine cavities separated by a septum.

■ Palpate the *left and right adnexa.*

Early in pregnancy, it is important to rule out tubal (*ectopic*) pregnancy.

■ Evaluate pelvic floor strength as you withdraw the examining fingers.

■ Inspect the anus. Rectal and rectovaginal examinations are usually not indicated.

Hemorrhoids may engorge later in pregnancy.

Extremities

Inspect the legs for *varicose veins.*

Varicose veins may worsen during pregnancy.

Palpate the hands and legs for *edema.*

Watch for swelling of *preeclampsia* or deep venous thrombosis.

Check knee and ankle deep tendon reflexes.

Hyperreflexia may signal *preeclampsia.*

EXAMINATION TECHNIQUES

Special Techniques
Leopold Maneuvers

Identify:

■ The upper and lower fetal poles, namely, the proximal and distal fetal parts

■ The maternal side where the fetal back is located

■ The descent of the presenting part into the maternal pelvis

■ The extent of flexion of the fetal head

■ Estimated fetal weight and size

Common deviations include *breech presentation* (fetal buttocks present at the outlet of the maternal pelvis) and absence of the presenting part well down into the maternal pelvis at term.

First Maneuver (Upper Fetal Pole). Stand at the woman's side, facing her head. Keep the fingers of both examining hands together. Palpate gently with the fingertips to determine what part of the fetus is in the upper pole of the uterine fundus (Fig. 19-3).

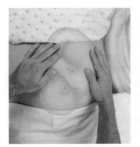

Figure 19-3 Palpate upper fetal pole.

Second Maneuver (Sides of the Maternal Abdomen). Place one hand on each side of the woman's abdomen, capturing the fetal body between them (Fig. 19-4). Steady the uterus with one hand and palpate the fetus with the other, looking for the back on one side and extremities on the other.

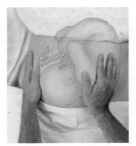

Figure 19-4 Palpate fetal back and extremities.

| EXAMINATION TECHNIQUES | POSSIBLE FINDINGS |

Third Maneuver (Lower Fetal Pole and Descent into Pelvis). Face the woman's feet. Palpate the area just above the symphysis pubis (Fig. 19-5). Note whether the hands diverge with downward pressure or stay together to learn if the presenting part of the fetus, head or buttocks, is descending into the pelvic inlet.

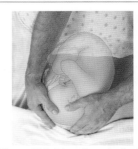

Figure 19-5 Palpate lower fetal pole.

Fourth Maneuver (Flexion of the Fetal Head). This maneuver assesses the flexion or extension of the fetal head, presuming that the fetal head is the presenting part in the pelvis. Still facing the woman's feet, with your hands positioned on either side of the gravid uterus as in the third maneuver, identify the fetal front and back sides (Fig. 19-6). Using one hand at a time, slide your fingers down each side of the fetal body until you reach the "cephalic prominence," that is, where the fetal brow or occiput juts out.

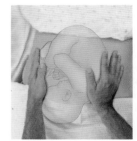

Figure 19-6 Palpate for the cephalic prominence.

Recording Your Findings

Pregnant women are described in terms of number of pregnancies (Gravida, or "G") and labors (Para, or "P") they have experienced. Parity is further broken down into term deliveries, preterm deliveries, abortions (spontaneous abortions and terminated pregnancies), and living children, (which yields the mnemonic "TPAL").

■ For example, a woman who has had two prior children and is pregnant with her third pregnancy would be referred to simply as "G3P2."

■ A woman with two spontaneous losses prior to 20 weeks' gestation, three living children who delivered at term, and a current pregnancy, would be referred to as "G6P3023."

■ One common error is to assign a multiple pregnancy, for example, twins, as a count of two for either gravity or parity. In practice, each pregnancy receives only one count in any of the categories regardless of the number of fetuses, except for living children, when all are counted. So, designate a first pregnancy with twins delivered at term as G1P1002.

Typically, the write-up follows a standard order: age, Gs and Ps, weeks of gestation, means of determining gestational age (ultrasound vs. LMP), followed by chief complaint, chief pregnancy complications, then important history and examination findings, as below.

Recording the Physical Examination—The Pregnant Woman

"32-year-old G3,P1102 at 18 weeks' gestation as determined by LMP presents to establish prenatal care. Patient endorses fetal movement; denies contractions, vaginal bleeding, and leakage of fluids. On external examination, low transverse cesarean scar is evident; fundus is palpable just below umbilicus. On internal examination, cervix is open to fingertip at the external os but closed at the internal os; cervix is 3 cm long; uterus enlarged to size consistent with 18-week gestation. Speculum examination shows leukorrhea with positive Chadwick sign. FHT by Doppler are between 140 and 145 BPM." *(This describes a healthy woman at 18 weeks' gestation.)*

The Older Adult

Older Americans now number more than 43 million people and are expected to reach 80 million by 2040, over 20% of the population. Life span at birth is currently 81 years for women and 76 years for men. The "demographic imperative" is to maximize not only life span but also "health span" so that older adults maintain full function for as long as possible, enjoying rich and active lives in their homes and communities. This entails a focus on healthy or "successful" aging; understanding and mobilizing family, social, and community supports; skills directed to functional assessment, "the sixth vital sign"; and promoting long-term health and safety.

The aging population displays marked heterogeneity. Investigators distinguish "usual" aging, with its complex of diseases and impairments, from optimal aging. Optimal aging occurs in those people who escape debilitating disease entirely and maintain healthy lives late into their 80s and 90s. Studies of centenarians show that genes account for approximately 20% of the probability of living to 100, with healthy lifestyles accounting for approximately 20% to 30%.

The Geriatric Approach for Primary Care

1. Learn to quickly identify frail elderly patients; they are most vulnerable to adverse outcomes and most benefit from a holistic geriatric approach.
2. Look for common geriatric syndromes, including falls, delirium/cognitive impairment, functional dependence, and urinary incontinence in every patient.
3. Learn about efficient assessment tools for geriatrics and geriatric syndromes and teach clinical staff to administer them when possible.
4. Be familiar with community resources, such as fall prevention programs, PACE programs, and senior centers.
5. Take into account a patient's goals, life expectancy, and functional status before considering any test or procedure.
6. Review advanced directives and goals of care periodically.
7. Be knowledgeable about the Beers Criteria (*J Am Geriatr Soc.* 2012;60:616); use them to identify potentially inappropriate medications in the elderly and inform periodic comprehensive medication review.
8. Adopt an evidence-based approach to health screening, especially in the frail elderly.

(*continued*)

The Geriatric Approach for Primary Care *(Continued)*

9. Watch carefully for mood disorders in the frail elderly and consider using geriatric-specific screening tools, such as the five-item Geriatric Depression Scale.

10. Provide caregiver support when possible.

Source: Carlson C, Merel SE, Yukawa M. Geriatric syndromes and geriatric assessment for the generalist. *Med Clin N Am.* 2015;99:263; Adapted from American Geriatrics Society 2012 Beers Criteria Update Expert Panel. American Geriatrics Society updated Beers criteria for potentially inappropriate medication use in older adults. *J Am Geriatr Soc.* 2012;60:616; and Hoyl MT, Alessi CA, Harker JO, et al. Development and testing of a five-item version of the geriatric depression scale. *J Am Geriatr Soc.* 1999;47:873.

The Health History

Approach to the Older Adult

As you talk with older adults, convey respect, patience, and cultural awareness. Be sure to address patients by their last name.

Adjusting the Office Environment. Make sure the office is neither too cool nor too warm. Face the patient directly, sitting at eye level. A well-lit room allows the older adult to see your facial expressions and gestures.

More than 50% of older adults have hearing deficits. Free the room of distractions or noise. Consider using a "pocket talker," a microphone that amplifies your voice and connects to an earpiece inserted by the patient. Chairs with higher seating and a wide stool with a handrail leading up to the examining table help patients with quadriceps weakness.

Shaping the Content and Pace of the Visit. Older people often reminisce. Listen to this process of life review to gain important insights and help patients as they work through painful feelings or recapture joys and accomplishments. Balance the need to assess complex problems with the patient's endurance and possible fatigue. Consider dividing the initial assessment into two visits.

Eliciting Symptoms in the Older Adult. Older patients may overestimate their health even when increasing disease and disability are apparent. To reduce the risk of late recognition and delayed intervention, adopt more directed questions or *health screening tools.* Consult with family members and caretakers.

Acute illnesses present differently in older adults. Be sensitive to unusual presentations of myocardial infarction and thyroid disease. Older patients with infections are less likely to have fever.

Recognize the symptom clusters of different *geriatric syndromes,* characterized by interacting clusters of symptoms that lead to functional decline, for example, falls, dizziness, depression, urinary incontinence, and functional impairment. Searching for the usual "unifying diagnosis" may pertain to fewer than 50% of older adults.

Although cognitive impairment may alter the patient's history, most older adults even with mild cognitive impairment can provide sufficient history to reveal current disorders. Use simple sentences with prompts to trigger necessary information. If impairments are more severe, confirm symptoms with family members or caregivers.

Addressing Cultural Dimensions of Aging

Geriatric Diversity—Now and in 2050

- *Hispanic Americans* over age 65 will increase from 2.7 million in 2010, or 6.9% of older adults, to 17.5 million in 2050, or 19.8% of the older population.
- *African American* older adults will increase from 3.4 million (8.5%), to 10.5 million in 2050 (11.9%).
- *Asian Americans* and other ethnic groups, although smaller in number currently, will increase from 1.4 million to 7.5 million, or from 3.4% to 8.5%.
- *Non-Hispanic whites* will increase from 32.2 million to 58.5 million in 2050, but will drop as a percentage of the older population from 80% to 58.5%.

Source: Federal Interagency Forum on Aging Related Statistics. Older Americans 2012, Key Indicators of Well Being. Indicator 2, Racial and Ethnic Composition, p. 86. Federal Interagency Forum on Aging-Related Statistics. Washington, DC: U.S. Government Printing Office. June 2012. Available at http://agingstats.gov/agingstatsdotnet/Main_Site/ Data/2012_Documents/Docs/EntireChartbook.pdf. Accessed August 11, 2015.

Cultural differences affect the epidemiology of illness and mental health, acculturation, the specific concerns of the elderly, the potential for misdiagnosis, and disparities in health outcomes. Review the components of self-awareness needed for cultural responsiveness, discussed in Chapter 3 (pp. 49–50). Ask about spiritual advisors and native healers. Cultural values particularly affect decisions about the end of life. Elders, family, and even an extended community group may make these decisions with or for the older patient.

Common Concerns

- Activities of daily living
- Instrumental activities of daily living
- Medications
- Acute and persistent pain
- Smoking and alcohol
- Nutrition
- Frailty
- Advance directives and palliative care

Place symptoms in the context of your overall *functional assessment,* always focusing on helping the older adult to maintain optimal well-being and level of function.

Activities of Daily Living. Daily activities provide an important baseline for future evaluations. Ask, "Tell me about your typical day" or "Tell me about your day yesterday." Then move to a greater level of detail: "You got up at 8 AM? How is it getting out of bed?"

Activities of Daily Living and Instrumental Activities of Daily Living	
Physical Activities of Daily Living (ADLs)	**Instrumental Activities of Daily Living (IADLs)**
Bathing	Using the telephone
Dressing	Shopping
Toileting	Preparing food
Transferring	Housekeeping
Continence	Laundry
Feeding	Transportation
	Taking medicine
	Managing money

Medications. Adults older than 65 take approximately 30% of all prescriptions. Almost 40% take five or more prescription drugs daily. Older adults have more than 50% of all reported adverse drug reactions. Take a thorough medication history, including name, dose, frequency, and indication for each drug. Explore all components of polypharmacy, including concurrent use of multiple drugs, underuse, inappropriate use, and nonadherence. Ask about use of over-the-counter medications, vitamin and nutrition supplements, and mood-altering drugs. Medications are the most common modifiable risk factor associated with falls. "Start low, go slow" when prescribing doses.

Acute and Persistent Pain. Pain and associated complaints account for 80% of clinician visits, usually for musculoskeletal complaints like back and joint pain. Older patients are less likely to report pain, leading to undue suffering, depression, social isolation, physical disability, and loss of function.

Inquire about pain each time you meet with the older patient. Ask specifically, "Are you having any pain right now? How about over the past week?" Unidimensional scales such as the Visual Analog Scale, graphic pictures, and the Verbal 0–10 Scale have all been validated and are easiest to use.

Characteristics of Acute and Persistent Pain

Acute Pain	Persistent Pain
Distinct onset	Lasts more than 3 months
Obvious pathology	Often associated with psychological or functional impairment
Short duration	Can fluctuate in character and intensity over time
Common causes: postsurgical, trauma, headache	Common causes: arthritis, cancer, claudication, leg cramps, neuropathy, radiculopathy

Source: Reuben DB, Herr KA, Pacala JT, et al. *Geriatrics at Your Fingertips: 2004.* 6th ed. Malden, MA: Blackwell Publishing, for the American Geriatrics Society; 2004:149.

Smoking and Alcohol. At each visit, advise elderly smokers to quit. From 10% to 15% of older patients in primary care practices have problem drinking. Rates of detection and treatment are low. Screen all older adults for excess alcohol use, which contributes to drug interactions and worsens comorbid illnesses. Use the CAGE questions to uncover problem drinking (see p. 56), and watch for clues of excess consumption such as memory loss, depression, and self-neglect.

Nutrition. Taking a diet history and using rapid screening tools (p. 73) are especially important in older adults.

Frailty. The prevalence of this multifactorial syndrome is 4% to 59%. Screen for three key features and pursue related interventions: weight loss of more than 5% over 3 years, inability to do five chair stands, and self-reported exhaustion.

Advance Directives and Palliative Care. Initiate these discussions *before* serious illness develops. Advance care planning involves providing information, invoking the patient's preferences, identifying surrogate decision makers, and conveying empathy and support. Use clear, simple language. Clarify preferences related to "Do Not Resuscitate" orders specifying life support measures "if the heart or lungs were to stop or give out." Seek a written health care proxy or durable power of attorney for health care, "someone who can make decisions reflecting your wishes in case of confusion or emergency." Discuss these decisions in the office rather than in the pressured environments of the emergency room or hospital.

When needed, provide *palliative care* "to relieve suffering and improve the quality of life for patients with advanced illnesses and their families through specific knowledge and skills, including communication with patients and family members; management of pain and other symptoms; psychosocial, spiritual, and bereavement support; and coordination of an array of clinical and social services."

Health Promotion and Counseling: Evidence and Recommendations

Important Topics for Health Promotion and Counseling

- When to screen
- Cancer screening
- Depression, dementia, and cognitive impairment
- Elder mistreatment and abuse

When to Screen. As the life span for older adults extends into the 80s, base screening decisions on the older adult's individual health and functional status, including presence of comorbidity, rather than age alone. The American Geriatrics Society recommends a five-step approach: assess patient preferences, interpret the available evidence, estimate prognosis, consider treatment feasibility, and optimize therapies and care plans. If life expectancy is short, adopt treatments that benefit the patient in the time that remains. Defer screening if it overburdens the older adults who have multiple clinical problems, shortened life expectancy, or dementia.

- Screen for age-related changes in *vision* and *hearing*. These are included in the 10-Minute Geriatric Screener (p. 407).

- Recommend aerobic *exercise,* such as brisk walking for 150 minutes every week and graded resistance training in major muscle groups to increase strength.

- Promote *household safety.* Correct poor lighting, chairs at awkward heights, slippery or irregular surfaces, and environmental hazards.

- *Immunizations.* Recommend vaccination for influenza; pneumonia, both PPSV23 and PCV13; herpes zoster (shingles); and tetanus/diphtheria and pertussis (Tdap and Td). Consult the updated annual guidelines and contraindications provided by the CDC at http://www.cdc.gov/vaccines.

Cancer Screening. Cancer screening can be controversial because of limited evidence about adults older than age 70 to 80. The U.S. Preventive Services Task Force (USPSTF) guidelines are summarized below.

Screening Recommendations for Older Adults: U.S. Preventive Services Task Force

- **Breast cancer (2016):** Recommends mammography every 2 years for women ages 50 to 74 and cites insufficient evidence for screening women ages ≥75 years.

(continued)

Screening Recommendations for Older Adults:
U.S. Preventive Services Task Force *(Continued)*

- **Cervical cancer (2012):** Recommends against routine screening for women over age 65 if they have had adequate recent screening with normal Pap smears and are not otherwise at high risk for cervical cancer, based on fair evidence.
- **Colorectal cancer (2008):** Recommends screening with colonoscopy every 10 years, sigmoidoscopy every 5 years with high-sensitivity fecal occult blood tests (FOBTs) every 3 years, or FOBTs every year beginning age 50 years through age 75 years. Recommends against routine screening for adults ages 76 to 85 years, due to moderate certainty that the net benefit is small.
- **Prostate cancer (2012):** Recommends against prostate-specific antigen-based screening for prostate cancer in men of all ages due to evidence that expected harms are greater than expected benefits.
- **Lung cancer (2013):** For adults ages 55 to 80 years with a 30-pack/year smoking history, and those who currently smoke or have quit within the past 15 years, recommends annual screening with low-dose computed tomography. Screening should be discontinued once a person has not smoked for 15 years or develops a health problem that substantially limits life expectancy or the ability or willingness to have curative lung surgery.
- **Skin cancer (2009; updated in 2015):** States that evidence is insufficient to balance the benefits and harms of whole-body skin examination.

Depression, Dementia, and Cognitive Impairment. *Depression* affects 5% to 7% of community-dwelling older adults and approximately 10% of older men and 18% of older women, but is often undiagnosed. Use the two validated screening questions in Chapter 5 on pp. 85–86.

Dementia is "an acquired condition that is characterized by a decline in at least two cognitive domains (e.g., loss of memory, attention, language, or visuospatial or executive functioning) that is severe enough to affect social or occupational functioning." Alzheimer disease (AD), the predominant form, affects 11% of Americans over age 65 years; over two thirds are women.

Probable AD, based on DSM-5 criteria, consists of evidence of a causative genetic mutation from family history or genetic testing, or the presence of cognitive decline in two or more cognitive domains, with all three of the following features:

- Clear evidence of a decline in memory and learning and at least one other cognitive domain (as described for dementia above);

- Steady progressive decline in cognition without extended plateaus; and

- No evidence of mixed etiology from other neurodegenerative, cerebro-vascular, mental, or systemic disease.

Most dementias represent AD (50% to 85%) or vascular multi-infarct dementia (10% to 20%). Other dementias include frontotemporal dementia, dementia with Lewy bodies, Parkinson disease with dementia, and dementia of mixed etiology.

The spectrum of cognitive decline includes:

■ *Age-related cognitive decline:* with occasional mild forgetfulness, difficulty remembering names, and mildly reduced concentration but preservation of daily function.

■ *Mild cognitive impairment (MCI):* Daily function is preserved, but there is evidence of modest cognitive decline in one or more cognitive domains (complex attention, executive function, learning and memory, language, perceptual-motor, or social cognition) based on objective tasks, as reported by the patient, an informant, or the clinician or on clinical testing. Alertness and attention is preserved (unlike delirium).

Use recommended screening tests for dementia such as the Mini-Cog and the Montreal Cognitive Assessment (MoCA). See Table 20-3, p. 420, and Table 20-4, p. 421.

Elder Mistreatment and Abuse. Screen older patients for possible *elder mistreatment,* which includes abuse, neglect, exploitation, and abandonment. Prevalence ranges from 5% to 10% of older adults; however, many cases remain undetected.

Techniques of Examination

Assessment of the older adult departs from the traditional history and physical examination. Enhanced interviewing, emphasis on daily function and the key topics described above, and functional assessment are especially important.

Assessing Functional Status: The "Sixth Vital Sign"
Assessing Functional Ability. Functional status is the ability to perform tasks and fulfill social roles associated with daily living across a wide range of complexity. The 10-Minute Geriatric Screener is brief, has high interrater agreement, and can be used easily by office staff. It covers the three important domains: physical, cognitive, and psychosocial function and addresses key sensory modalities and urinary incontinence, an often unreported problem. Mnemonics that help students assess incontinence are: DIAPERS (**D**elirium, **I**nfection, **A**trophic urethritis/vaginitis, **P**harmaceuticals, **E**xcess urine output from conditions like hyperglycemia or heart

failure, **R**estricted mobility, and **S**tool impaction) and **DDRRIIPP** (**D**elirium, **D**rug side effects, **R**etention of feces, **R**estricted mobility, **I**nfection of urine, **I**nflammation, **P**olyuria, and **P**sychogenic).

10-Minute Geriatric Screener

Problem and Screening Measure	Positive Screen
Vision: Two Parts: Ask: "Do you have difficulty driving, or watching television, or reading, or doing any of your daily activities because of your eyesight?" If yes, then: Test each eye with Snellen chart while patient wears corrective lenses (if applicable).	Yes to question and inability to read >20/40 on Snellen chart
Hearing: Use audioscope set at 40 dB. Test hearing using 1,000 and 2,000 Hz.	Inability to hear 1,000 or 2,000 Hz in both ears or either of these frequencies in one ear
Leg mobility: Time the patient after instructing: "Rise from the chair. Walk 20 feet briskly, turn, walk back to the chair, and sit down."	Unable to complete task in 15 seconds
Urinary incontinence: Two Parts: Ask: "In the last year, have you ever lost your urine and gotten wet?" If yes, then ask: "Have you lost urine on at least 6 separate dates?"	Yes to both questions
Nutrition/weight loss: Two parts: Ask: "Have you lost 10 lb over the past 6 months without trying to do so?" Weigh the patient.	Yes to the question or weight <100 lb
Memory: Three-item recall	Unable to remember all three items after 1 minute
Depression: Ask: "Do you often feel sad or depressed?"	Yes to the question
Physical disability: Six questions: "Are you able to . . . : • "Do strenuous activities like fast walking or bicycling?" • "Do heavy work around the house like washing windows, walls, or floors?" • "Go shopping for groceries or clothes?" • "Get to places out of walking distance?" • "Bathe, either a sponge bath, tub bath, or shower?" • "Dress, like putting on a shirt, buttoning and zipping, or putting on shoes?"	No to any of the questions

Source: More AA, Siu AL. Screening for common problems in ambulatory elderly: clinical confirmation of a screening instrument. *Am J Med.* 1996;100:438.

Further Assessment for Preventing Falls. Compelling evidence links falls, a multifactorial geriatric syndrome, to fatal and nonfatal injuries, mortality, and burgeoning clinical costs that exceed $34 billion annually. One in three older adults falls each year. Falls are the most common cause of traumatic brain injury in older adults and cause 95% of hip fractures.

The American Geriatrics Society, the British Geriatrics Society, and the CDC's Injury Center has launched the *STEADI (Stopping Elderly Accidents, Deaths, and Injuries) falls prevention toolkit* to help primary care providers better assess, treat, and refer patients at risk. Also see Figure 20-1.

STEADI Falls Prevention Algorithm: Key Features for Clinical Practice

- Screen *all* community-dwelling older adults about risk for falls.
- Encourage *all* older patients to pursue gait and balance exercise.
- Do a gait, strength, and balance assessment with the Timed Get Up and Go test in patients who screen positive.
- Stratify patients according to low, moderate, and high risk.
- *Identify high-risk older adults,* namely, those with a gait, strength, or balance problem and at least one fall with an injury.
- In *high-risk older adults,* conduct a multifactorial risk assessment, including:
  - review of the Stay Independent brochure;
  - a falls history and medication review;
  - physical examination including assessment of visual acuity, postural hypotension, a cognitive screen, inspection of the feet and use of footwear, and use of mobility aids;
  - functional assessment; and
  - environmental or home safety assessment.
- Implement individualized interventions, including physical therapy and follow-up in 30 days.

EXAMINATION TECHNIQUES	POSSIBLE FINDINGS

Physical Examination of the Older Adult

Vital Signs. Measure blood pressure, checking for increased systolic blood pressure (SBP) and widened pulse pressure (PP), defined as SBP minus diastolic blood pressure (DBP).

Isolated systolic hypertension (SBP ≥140) after age 50 years and PP ≥60 increase risk of stroke, renal failure, and heart disease.

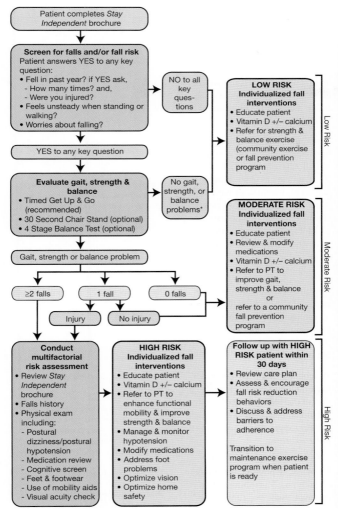

*For these patients, consider additional risk assessment (e.g. medication review, cognitive screen, syncope)

Figure 20-1 STEADI algorithm. Source: Centers for Disease Control and Prevention. National Center for Injury Prevention and Control. STEADI—Stopping Elderly Accidents, Deaths and Injuries. Available at http://www.cdc.gov/steadi/pdf/algorithm_2015–04-a.pdf. Accessed August 23, 2015.

EXAMINATION TECHNIQUES

POSSIBLE FINDINGS

For adults ages ≥60 years, the JNC8 recommends blood pressure targets of ≤150/90 but notes that if treatment results in SBP <140 and is "well tolerated and without adverse effects to health or quality of life, treatment does not need to be adjusted."

Assess the patient for *orthostatic hypotension*, defined as a drop in SBP of ≥20 mm Hg or DBP of ≥10 mm Hg or HR increase of ≥20 BPM, within 3 minutes of standing. Measure in two positions: supine after the patient rests for up to 10 minutes, then within 2 to 3 minutes after standing up.

Orthostatic hypotension occurs in 10% to 20% of older adults and in up to 30% of frail nursing home residents, especially when they first arise in the morning. Watch for lightheadedness, weakness, unsteadiness, visual blurring, and, in 20% to 30% of patients, syncope.

Assess medications and causes such as autonomic disorders, diabetes, prolonged bed rest, volume depletion, amyloidosis, postprandial state, and cardiovascular disorders.

Measure heart rate, respiratory rate, and temperature. Check the apical heart rate to help detect arrhythmias in older adults. Use thermometers accurate for lower temperatures.

Respiratory rate ≥25 breaths per minute indicates lower respiratory infection or possible CHF or COPD.

Hypothermia is more common in elderly patients.

Weight and height are especially important and needed for calculation of the BMI (p. 63). Weight should be measured at every visit. Obtain oxygen saturation using a pulse oximeter.

Low weight is a key indicator of poor nutrition.

Undernutrition in depression, alcoholism, cognitive impairment, malignancy, chronic organ failure (cardiac, renal, pulmonary), medication use, poor dentition, social isolation, and poverty

Skin. Note physiologic changes of aging, such as thinning, loss of elastic tissue and turgor, and wrinkling.

Dry, flaky, rough, and often itchy

Benign comedones, or blackheads, on the cheeks or around the eyes; cherry angiomas (p. 113); and seborrheic keratoses (p. 112)

Inspect the extensor surface of the hands and forearms.

White depigmented patches (*pseudoscars*); well-demarcated, vividly purple macules or patches that may fade after several weeks (*actinic purpura*)

EXAMINATION TECHNIQUES

Look for changes from sun exposure: *actinic lentigines,* or "liver spots," and *actinic keratoses,* superficial flattened papules covered by a dry scale (p. 108).

Distinguish such lesions from a *basal cell carcinoma* and *squamous cell carcinoma* (p. 108). Dark, raised, asymmetric lesions with irregular borders are suspicious for *melanoma*

Inspect for painful vesicular lesions in a dermatomal distribution.

Herpes zoster from reactivation of latent varicella-zoster virus in the dorsal root ganglia

In older bedbound patients, especially when emaciated or neurologically impaired, inspect for damage or ulceration.

Pressure sores if obliteration of arteriolar and capillary blood flow to the skin or shear forces with movement across sheets or lifting upright incorrectly

HEENT. Inspect the eyelids, the bony orbit, and the eye.

Senile ptosis arising from weakening of the levator palpebrae, relaxation of the skin, and increased weight of the upper eyelid

Ectropion or *entropion* of lower lids (p. 133)

Yellowing of the sclera and *arcus senilis,* a benign whitish ring around the limbus

Test visual acuity, using a pocket Snellen chart or wall-mounted chart.

More than 40 million Americans have refractive errors—*presbyopia.*

Examine the lenses and fundi.

Cataracts, glaucoma, and macular degeneration all increase with aging.

Inspect each lens for opacities.

Cataracts are the world's leading cause of blindness.

Assess the cup-to-disc ratio, usually ≤1:2.

Increased cup-to-disc ratio suggests open-angle *glaucoma* and possible loss of peripheral and central vision, and blindness. Prevalence is three to four times higher in African Americans.

Inspect the fundi for colloid bodies causing alterations in pigmentation called *drusen.* These may be hard and sharply defined, or soft and confluent with altered pigmentation.

Macular degeneration causes poor central vision and blindness: types include *dry atrophic* (more common but less severe) and *wet exudative* (or neovascular).

EXAMINATION TECHNIQUES	POSSIBLE FINDINGS

Test hearing by the whispered voice test (see p. 124) or audioscope. Inspect ear canals for cerumen.

Removing cerumen often quickly improves hearing.

Examine the oral cavity for odor, appearance of the gingival mucosa, any caries, mobility of the teeth, and quantity of saliva.

Malodor in poor oral hygiene, periodontitis, or caries

Gingivitis if periodontal disease

Inspect for lesions on mucosal surfaces. Ask patient to remove dentures so you can check gums for denture sores.

Dental plaque and cavitation if caries. Increased tooth mobility; risk of tooth aspiration

Decreased salivation from medications, radiation, Sjögren syndrome, or dehydration

Oral tumors, usually on lateral borders of tongue and floor of mouth

Thorax and Lungs. Percuss and auscultate the lungs. Note subtle signs of changes in pulmonary function.

Increased anteroposterior diameter, purse-lipped breathing, and dyspnea with talking or minimal exertion in *chronic obstructive pulmonary disease*

Cardiovascular System. Review blood pressure and heart rate.

Isolated systolic hypertension and a widened pulse pressure are cardiac risk factors. Search for *left ventricular hypertrophy (LVH).*

Inspect the jugular venous pulsation (JVP), palpate the carotid upstrokes, and listen for any overlying carotid bruits.

A *tortuous atherosclerotic aorta* can raise pressure in the left jugular veins by impairing drainage into right atrium.

Carotid bruits in possible *carotid stenosis.*

Assess the point of maximal impulse (PMI), and then heart sounds.

Sustained PMI is found in LVH, hypertension, and aortic stenosis; diffuse PMI in heart failure (see p. 180).

In older adults, S_3 in dilatation of the left ventricle from heart failure or cardiomyopathy; S_4 in hypertension

EXAMINATION TECHNIQUES

POSSIBLE FINDINGS

Listen for cardiac murmurs in all six listening areas (see p. 185). Describe timing, shape, location of maximal intensity, radiation, intensity, pitch, and quality of each murmur.

A systolic crescendo–decrescendo murmur in the second right interspace in *aortic sclerosis* or *aortic stenosis*. Both carry increased risk of cardiovascular disease and death.

A harsh holosystolic murmur at the apex suggests *mitral regurgitation,* common in older adults.

Breasts and Axillae. Palpate the breasts carefully for lumps or masses.

Possible breast cancer

Abdomen. Listen for bruits over the aorta, renal arteries, and femoral arteries.

Bruits in atherosclerotic vascular disease

Inspect the upper abdomen; palpate to the left of the midline for aortic pulsations.

Widened aorta of ≥3 cm and pulsatile mass in *abdominal aortic aneurysm.*

Peripheral Vascular System. Auscultate the abdomen for aortic, renal, femoral artery bruits.

Bruits over these vessels in *atherosclerotic disease.*

Palpate pulses.

Diminished or absent pulses in *arterial occlusion.* Confirm with an office ankle–brachial index (see pp. 230–231).

Female Genitalia and Pelvic Examination. Take special care to explain the steps of examination and allow time for careful positioning. For the woman with arthritis or spinal deformities who cannot flex her hips or knees, an assistant can gently raise and support the legs, or help the woman into the left lateral position.

Inspect the vulva for changes related to menopause; identify any labial masses. Bluish swellings may be varicosities.

Benign masses include condylomata, fibromas, leiomyomas, and sebaceous cysts. Bulging of the anterior vaginal wall below the urethra in urethrocele

Erythema with satellite lesions in *Candida* infection; erythema with ulceration or a necrotic center in vulvar carcinoma.

EXAMINATION TECHNIQUES	POSSIBLE FINDINGS
Inspect the urethra for *caruncles,* or prolapse of fleshy erythematous mucosal tissue at the urethral meatus.	Clitoral enlargement in *androgen-producing tumors* or use of androgen creams
Speculum Examination. Inspect vaginal walls, which may be atrophic, and cervix.	Estrogen-stimulated cervical mucus with ferning in use of hormone replacement therapy, *endometrial hyperplasia,* and *estrogen-producing tumors;* lichen sclerosus
If indicated, obtain endocervical cells for the Pap smear. Use a blind swab if the atrophic vagina is too small.	
Removing speculum, ask patient to bear down.	Uterine prolapse, cystocele, urethrocele, or rectocele.
Perform the bimanual examination.	Note any uterine retroversion, retroflex-ion, porolapse, or myomas (fibroids)
	Mobility of cervix restricted if inflamma-tion, malignancy, or surgical adhesion
	Palpable ovaries in *ovarian cancer.*
Perform the rectovaginal examina-tion if indicated.	Enlarged, fixed, or irregular uterus if adhesions or malignancy. Rectal masses in *colon cancer.*

Male Genitalia and Prostate.
Examine the penis; retract foreskin if present. Examine the scrotum, testes, and epididymis.

Smegma, penile cancer, and scrotal hydroceles

Do a rectal examination.

Rectal masses in *colon cancer.* Prostate hyperplasia if enlargement; *prostate cancer* if nodules or masses.

Musculoskeletal System.
Screen general range of motion and gait. Conduct *timed "get up and go"* test.

Review examination techniques for individual joints in Chapter 16, Musculoskeletal System.

See Table 20-1, Timed Get Up and Go Test, p. 417.

If joint deformity, deficits in mobil-ity, or pain with movement, conduct a more thorough examination.

Degenerative joint changes in *osteoar-thritis;* joint inflammation in *rheumatoid* or *gouty arthritis.* See Tables 16-1 to 16-4, pp. 304–308.

EXAMINATION TECHNIQUES

POSSIBLE FINDINGS

Nervous System. Review results of 10-Minute Geriatric Screener, p. 407. Pursue further examination if any deficits. Focus especially on memory and affect.

Distinguish delirium from depression and dementia. See Table 20-2, Delirium and Dementia, pp. 418–419 and Table 20-3, Screening for Dementia: The Mini-Cog, p. 420. Table 20-4, Montreal Cognitive Assessment, p. 421.

Assess gait and balance, particularly standing balance; timed 8-foot walk; stride characteristics like width, pace, and length of stride; and careful turning.

Abnormalities of gait and balance, especially widening of base, slowing and lengthening of stride, and difficulty turning, are correlated with risk of falls.

Although neurologic abnormalities are common in older adults, their prevalence without identifiable disease increases with age, ranging from 30% to 50%.

Physiologic changes of aging: unequal pupil size, decreased arm swing and spontaneous movements, increased leg rigidity and abnormal gait, presence of the snout and grasp reflexes, and decreased toe vibratory sense.

Assess any tremor, rigidity, bradykinesia, micrographia, shuffling gait, and difficulty turning in bed, opening jars, and rising from a chair.

In Parkinson disease, tremor is slow frequency and at rest, with a "pill-rolling" quality, aggravated by stress and inhibited during sleep or movement.

Essential tremor is often bilateral, symmetric, with positive family history, and diminished by alcohol.

Recording Your Findings

As you read through this physical examination, you will notice some atypical findings. Test yourself to see if you can interpret these findings in the context of all you have learned about the examination of the older adult.

Recording the Physical Examination—The Older Adult

Mr. J is an older adult who appears healthy but underweight, with good muscle bulk. He is alert and interactive, with good recall of his life history. He is accompanied by his son.

Vital Signs: Ht (without shoes) 160 cm (5′). Wt (dressed) 65 kg (143 lb). BMI 28. BP 145/88 right arm, supine; 154/94 left arm, supine. Heart rate (HR) 98 and regular. Respiratory rate (RR) 18. Temperature (oral) 98.6°F.

(continued)

Recording the Physical Examination— The Older Adult (Continued)

10-Minute Geriatric Screener: (see p. 407)

Vision: Patient reports difficulty reading. Visual acuity 20/60 on Snellen chart.

Needs further evaluation for glasses and possibly hearing aid.

Hearing: Cannot hear whispered voice in either ear. Cannot hear 1,000 or 2,000 Hz with audioscope in either ear.

Leg Mobility: Can walk 20 feet briskly, turn, walk back to chair, and sit down in 14 seconds.

Urinary Incontinence: Has lost urine and gotten wet on 20 separate days.

Needs further evaluation for incontinence, including "DIAPER" assessment (see p. 406), prostate examination, and postvoid residual, which is normally ≤50 mL (requires bladder catheterization).

Nutrition: Has lost 15 lb over the past 6 months without trying.

Needs nutritional screen (see p. 73).

Memory: Can remember three items after 1 minute.

Depression: Does not often feel sad or depressed.

Physical Disability: Can walk fast but cannot ride a bicycle. Can do moderate but not heavy work around the house. Can go shopping for groceries or clothes. Can get to places out of walking distance. Can bathe each day without difficulty. Can dress, including buttoning and zipping, and can put on shoes.

Consider exercise regimen with strength training.

Physical Examination: Carefully describe your findings for each relevant segment of the peripheral examination, using terminology found in the "Recording Your Findings" sections of the prior chapters.

Aids to Interpretation

Table 20-1 Timed Get Up and Go Test

Performed with patient wearing regular footwear, using usual walking aid if needed, and sitting back in a chair with armrest.

On the word, "Go," the patient is asked to do the following:

1. Stand up from the arm chair
2. Walk 3 m (in a line)
3. Turn
4. Walk back to chair
5. Sit down

Time the second effort.

Observe patient for postural stability, steppage, stride length, and sway.

Scoring:
1. **Normal:** completes task in <10 seconds
2. **Abnormal:** completes task in >20 seconds

Low scores correlate with good functional independence; high scores correlate with poor functional independence and higher risk of falls.

Reproduced from: Get-up and Go Test. In: Mathias S, Nayak USL, Isaacs B. "Balance in elderly patient" The "Get Up and Go" Test. *Arch Phys Med Rehabil.* 1986;67:387; Podsiadlo D, Richardson S. The Timed "Up and Go": A test of basic functional mobility for frail elderly persons. *J Am Geriatr Soc.* 1991;39:142.

Table 20-2 Delirium and Dementia

	Delirium	**Dementia**
Clinical Features		
Onset	Acute	Insidious
Course	Fluctuating, with lucid intervals; worse at night	Slowly progressive
Duration	Hours to weeks	Months to years
Sleep/Wake Cycle	Always disrupted	Sleep fragmented
General Clinical Illness or Drug Toxicity	Either or both present	Often absent, especially in Alzheimer disease
Mental Status		
Level of Consciousness	Disturbed. Person less clearly aware of the environment and less able to focus, sustain, or shift attention	Usually normal until late in the course of the illness
Behavior	Activity often abnormally decreased (somnolence) or increased (agitation, hypervigilance)	Normal to slow; may become inappropriate
Speech	May be hesitant, slow or rapid, incoherent	Difficulty in finding words, aphasia
Mood	Fluctuating, labile, from fearful or irritable to normal or depressed	Often flat, depressed
Thought Processes	Disorganized, may be incoherent	Impoverished. Speech gives little information
Thought Content	Delusions common, often transient	Delusions may occur
Perceptions	Illusions, hallucinations, most often visual	Hallucinations may occur.

Table 20-2 Delirium and Dementia (*continued*)

	Delirium	**Dementia**
Judgment	Impaired, often to a varying degree	Increasingly impaired over the course of the illness
Orientation	Usually disoriented, especially for time. A known place may seem unfamiliar.	Fairly well maintained, but becomes impaired in the later stages of illness
Attention	Fluctuates. Person easily distracted, unable to concentrate on selected tasks	Usually unaffected until late in the illness
Memory	Immediate and recent memory impaired	Recent memory and new learning especially impaired
Examples of Cause	Delirium tremens (due to withdrawal from alcohol)	*Reversible:* Vitamin B_{12} deficiency, thyroid disorders
	Uremia	
	Acute hepatic failure	*Irreversible:* Alzheimer disease, vascular dementia (from multiple infarcts), dementia due to head trauma
	Acute cerebral vasculitis	
	Atropine poisoning	

Table 20-3   Screening for Dementia: The Mini-Cog

Administration

The test is administered as follows:

1. Instruct the patient to listen carefully to and remember three unrelated words and then to repeat the words.
2. Instruct the patient to draw the face of a clock, either on a blank sheet of paper or on a sheet with the clock circle already drawn on the page. After the patient puts the numbers on the clock face, ask him or her to draw the hands of the clock to read a specific time.
3. Ask the patient to repeat the three previously stated words.

Scoring

Word Recall: Give 1 point for each recalled word without cueing after doing the clock drawing test (CDT).

Patients recalling none of the three words are classified as demented (Score = 0). Patients recalling all three words are classified as nondemented (Score = 3). Patients with intermediate word recall of one to two words are classified based on the CDT (Abnormal = demented; Normal = nondemented).

Clock Draw: The CDT is considered normal if all numbers are present in the correct sequence and position, and the hands readably display the requested time. Scoring is 2 (normal) or 0 (abnormal).

Total Score (0–5 points): Score <3 has been validated for dementia.

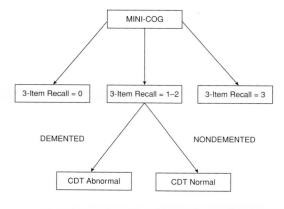

From Borson S, Scanlan J, Brush M, et al. The Mini-Cog: a cognitive "vital signs" measure for dementia screening in multi-lingual elderly. *Int J Geriatr Psychiatry*. 2000;15(11):1021. Copyright John Wiley & Sons Limited. Reproduced with permission.

Table 20-4 Screening for Dementia: The Montreal Cognitive Assessment (MoCA)

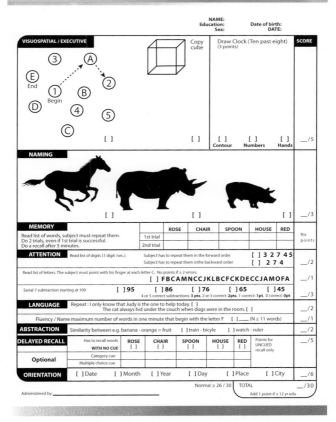

Source: © Z. Nasreddine MD. Reproduced with permission. Copies are available at www.mocatest.org.

Index

Note: Page numbers followed by "b," "f," and "t" indicate boxed material, figure, and end-of-chapter tables, respectively.